Springhouse Certification Review

EMERGENCY NURSING

Springhouse Certification Review

EMERGENCY NURSING

Springhouse Corporation
Springhouse, Pennsylvania

Staff

Executive Director
Matthew Cahill

Editorial Director
June Norris

Art Director
John Hubbard

Managing Editor
David Moreau

Acquisitions Editors
Patricia Kardish Fischer, RN, BSN; Louise Quinn

Clinical Consultant
Collette Bishop Hendler, RN, CCRN

Editors
Carol Munson, Michael Shaw

Copy Editors
Cynthia C. Breuninger (manager), Christine Cunniffe, Barbara Hodgson, Janet Hodgson, Brenna Mayer

Designers
Arlene Putterman (associate art director), Mary Stangl, Lesley Weissman-Cook

Production Coordinator
Margaret Rastiello

Editorial Assistants
Beverly Lane, Mary Madden, Jeanne Napier

Manufacturing
Debbie Meiris (director), Pat Dorshaw (manager), Anna Brindisi, T.A. Landis

---

The clinical procedures described and recommended in this publication are based on research and consultation with nursing, medical, and legal authorities. To the best of our knowledge, these procedures reflect currently accepted practice; nevertheless, they can't be considered absolute or universal recommendations. For individual application, all recommendations must be considered in light of the patient's clinical condition and, before administration of new or infrequently used drugs, in light of the latest package-insert information. The authors and the publisher disclaim responsibility for any adverse effects resulting directly or indirectly from any suggested procedures herein, from any undetected errors, or from the reader's misunderstanding of the text.

Printed in the United States of America.
CREN-021097

℞ A member of the Reed Elsevier plc group

Library of Congress Cataloging-in-Publication Data
Springhouse certification review: emergency nursing.
  p. cm.
  Includes bibliographical references and index.
  1. Emergency nursing—Outlines, syllabi, etc.
  2. Emergency nursing—Examinations, questions, etc.
  I. Springhouse Corporation.
  [DNLM: 1. Emergency Nursing — examination questions. WY 18.2 S7693 1997]
RT120.E4S67 1997
610.73'61—dc20
DNLM/DLC   96-31612
ISBN 0-87434-846-3 (alk. paper)   CIP

Contents

Section I: Clinical Practice

Section II: Professional Issues

Section III: Sample Test

Appendices

Contributors and Reviewers

CONTRIBUTORS

Margaret M. Anderson, RN,C, EdD, CNAA
Assistant Professor of Nursing–
Director of the BSN Program
Northern Kentucky University
Highland Heights

Ruthie Bach, RN, MSN, CCRN, CEN
Cardiovascular Clinical Nurse Specialist
Beaumont (Tex.) Regional Medical Center

Cathleen M. Cassidy, RN, MS, CEN
Base Hospital Coordinator
San Francisco General Hospital

Patricia L. Clutter, RN, MEd, CEN
Staff Nurse, Emergency Trauma Center
St. John's Regional Health Center
Springfield, Mo.

Sheila D. DeVaugh, RN, MSN, CEN, CNS
Assistant Director, Emergency Services
St. Elizabeth Hospital
Beaumont, Tex.

Emmy L. Hunt, RN, MSN, CEN
Head Nurse
Maine Medical Center
Portland

Martha Kowalik, RN, CEN
Assistant Nurse Manager
Albany (N.Y.) Medical Center

Carrie A. McCoy, RN, MSN, CEN
Associate Professor of Nursing
Northern Kentucky University
Highland Heights

Leanna R. Miller, RN, MN, CCRN, CEN
Clinical Nurse Specialist
Medical Center of Central Georgia
Macon

Glen Allen Sinks, RN, BSN, EMT-P, CEN
Outreach Educator, Trauma Division
Cardinal Glennon Children's Hospital
St. Louis, Mo.

David W. Unkle, RN, MSN, CCRN, CEN, FCCM
Nurse Manager
Emergency Department, Intensive Care Unit
West Jersey Hospital
Camden, N.J.

Steven A. Weinman, RN, CEN
Emergency Nurse
Emergency Department
St. Luke's Northland Hospital
Kansas City, Mo.

REVIEWERS

Patti A. Ellison, RN, MSN, CEN
Assistant Professor of Nursing
Raymond Walters College
University of Cincinnati

Reet Henze, RN, BSN, MSN, DSN
Associate Professor
College of Nursing
University of Alabama in Huntsville

Kathleen M. Kearney, RN, MSN, CEN
Clinical Nurse Specialist
Emergency Department
Beth Israel Medical Center
New York

Leanna R. Miller, RN, MN, CCRN, CEN
Clinical Nurse Specialist
Medical Center of Central Georgia
Macon

Catherine A. Parvensky-Barwell, RN, PHRN, MEd
Deputy Director of Training
Chester County Department of Emergency
Services
West Chester, Pa.

Deborah Jane Schwytzer, RN, MSN, CEN
Instructor of Clinical Nursing
College of Nursing and Health
University of Cincinnati

Diane M. Stauffer, RN, MSN, CEN
Clinical Faculty, Department of Nursing
Northern Kentucky University
Highland Heights
Staff Nurse
Good Samaritan Hospital
Cincinnati

Sheryl L. Veurink, RN, BSN, CEN
Clinical Nurse Specialist
Trauma Nurse Coordinator
Saint Mary's Health Services
Grand Rapids, Mich.

Foreword

The commitment to pursue certification reflects professionalism and a desire to demonstrate that you have the knowledge required to be a competent emergency nurse. Passing a rigorous test is one example of your commitment to promote high-quality nursing care for emergency patients.

Without adequate preparation, however, you will find it very difficult to pass the Certified Emergency Nurse (CEN) exam, which is international in scope and comprehensive in content. Relying on your clinical experience as your sole preparation is dangerous because it is a rare emergency nurse who has encountered all situations covered on the exam. *Springhouse Certification Review: Emergency Nursing* can be a valuable preparation tool for several reasons:

• It follows the most recent CEN content outline, addressing clinical practice areas in Section I and professional issues in Section II. Naturally, the questions in this book approximate the weights assigned to content areas and nursing process steps in the actual exam.

• Each question in the clinical practice component of the CEN exam addresses a step in the nursing process. Because questions in *Springhouse Certification Review: Emergency Nursing* are classified according to the same nursing process, you can determine which steps of the process you need to review in greater detail.

• This text reviews all options for each question, so you can better understand not only why one option is correct but also why the other three options are incorrect. Understanding nursing priorities and principles is easier when such thorough rationales are given for all options.

• The book's design simulates the actual test-taking situation (questions on the left, options on the right). Being comfortable with the test format can help improve your performance. Furthermore, this design has an added benefit: Use the enclosed card to cover the right-hand column while you read each question on the left; then lower the card to reveal the answers and rationales. Unlike many other CEN review books that inconveniently bury the answers near the back of the book, *Springhouse Certification Review: Emergency Nursing* gives you instant feedback on your progress.

• The text provides 1,000 review questions in all—more than any other book of its kind—including a comprehensive 250-question sample test (to match the actual exam, which also contains 250 questions). You'll also find an answer sheet to aid your study and, of course, detailed rationales for correct and incorrect options on the sample test.

• *Springhouse Certification Review: Emergency Nursing* also provides helpful appendices on critical laboratory values, common life-support drugs, NANDA taxonomy, triage assessment principles, coma scales, laboratory values in toxicology, and emergency antidotes; a generous list of selected references for further review; and a detailed index to help you find important topics quickly.

• Finally, when you have passed the CEN exam, you can still use this book for continuing education review and designing in-service exams. It becomes a permanent resource.

Many emergency nursing experts have contributed to the development of *Springhouse Certification Review: Emergency Nursing*. Your experience, along with theirs, should provide a firm foundation for review and a positive performance on test day.

Pamela Kidd, RN, PhD, CEN
Associate Professor, College of Nursing
Manager, Motor Vehicle Injury Prevention
Program
University of Kentucky
Lexington

Understanding the CEN Exam

According to the National Specialty Nursing Certifying Organization (NSNCO), certification is the process by which a nongovernmental agency or association validates, based on predetermined standards, a registered nurse's qualifications and knowledge for practice in a defined functional or clinical area of nursing. To enhance your performance on the Certified Emergency Nurse (CEN) examination, review the answers to these commonly asked questions.

Who sponsors the CEN exam?

The Board for Certification of Emergency Nurses (BCEN) sponsors the CEN exam. The BCEN evaluates and recognizes nurses who have attained and applied a defined body of emergency nursing knowledge needed to function at a competent level.

Is the CEN exam as difficult as the NCLEX?

Health care professionals who take a certification examination for a specialty area of practice already have the knowledge required by the basic licensure examination. Because the knowledge measured by the CEN exam is specialized for emergency nursing, the exam is more challenging than the NCLEX.

If I've been an emergency nurse for years, do I need to study?

As an emergency nurse, you have probably mastered complex technical skills related to the care of emergency patients as well as the theoretical knowledge that underlies these skills. You have also probably developed the ability to make sound nursing judgments in crises that often determine whether a patient lives or dies. Despite such advanced education, skill mastery, and decision-making ability, however, many emergency nurses experience high levels of test-taking anxiety that may prevent them from seeking certification. This book can help alleviate test-taking anxiety by providing a thorough review of the material contained in the CEN exam.

What are the eligibility requirements?

The BCEN establishes criteria for eligibility to take the CEN exam. Current criteria are listed below.

• You must possess a current unrestricted license or nursing certificate as a registered nurse in the United States, Canada, Australia, or New Zealand (or their territories or provinces).

• Any restriction, suspension, or probation, or any order arising from a Nursing License Authority that limits your ability to function in an emergency nurse setting and perform those tasks normally associated with emergency nursing practice, will disqualify you to sit for the exam unless you're a qualified individual with a disability who can perform the essential functions of emergency nursing with or without reasonable accommodation.

• Although not a requirement, the BCEN recommends that you have 2 years of experience in emergency nursing practice and membership in the Emergency Nurses Association or the professional emergency nursing society of your country.

How many questions are on the exam?

The CEN exam is a written test, with a maximum of 250 multiple-choice questions and a maximum testing time of 4 hours.

What topics does the exam cover?

The content of the CEN exam, based on recognized standards and practices for emergency nursing, is divided into two major areas: clinical practice and professional issues.

Clinical practice

About 96% of the questions on the CEN exam focus on clinical practice. The list below specifies the topics covered and the percentage of exam questions devoted to each topic. The questions in Chapters 1 to 19 of this book approximate the percentages shown below; the sample test reflects the percentages exactly.

- Abdominal Emergencies (5%)
- Cardiovascular Emergencies (9%)
- Disaster Management (2%)
- Environmental Emergencies (4%)
- Maxillofacial Emergencies (3%)
- Medical Emergencies and Communicable Diseases (8%)
- Genitourinary and Gynecologic Emergencies (4%)
- Neurologic Emergencies (7%)
- Obstetric Emergencies (2.5%)
- Ocular Emergencies (2.5%)
- Orthopedic Emergencies (6%)
- Mental Health Emergencies (4.5%)
- Patient Care Management (9%)
- Respiratory Emergencies (9%)
- Shock and Multisystem Trauma Emergencies (7%)
- Substance Abuse and Toxicologic Emergencies (6%)
- Wound Management (4%)
- Stabilization and Transfer (2%)
- Patient and Community Education (1.5%)

When studying for the exam, keep in mind that clinical practice questions also are designed to test your knowledge of the four steps of the nursing process: Assessment, Analysis/Nursing diagnosis, Planning/Intervention, and Evaluation. The outline below shows the percentages of test items and examples of specific nursing behaviors associated with each step. The CEN examination uses only the NANDA-approved list of nursing diagnoses in test items. Potential nursing diagnoses are presented as such.

Assessment

About 30.5% of the questions test your ability to collect data. These questions focus on such nursing behaviors as:

- assessing the patient's physiologic, psychosocial, health, and safety needs
- collecting information from the patient, family, friends, hospital records, and health team members
- recognizing symptoms and findings
- communicating findings to other team members
- challenging orders and decisions by health team members, as appropriate.

Analysis/Nursing diagnosis

About 19% of the questions test your ability to identify real or potential health care needs and problems. These questions focus on such nursing behaviors as:

- organizing, interpreting, and validating assessment data
- gathering additional data when necessary
- identifying and communicating nursing diagnoses to the health care team
- determining the patient's needs and the staff's ability to meet them.

Planning/Intervention

About 28.5% of the questions test your ability to initiate and complete actions that accomplish defined goals. These questions focus on such nursing behaviors as:

- including the patient, family, friends, and other health team members in setting goals
- mutually establishing goal priorities
- providing a safe, effective care environment for the patient
- involving the patient, family, friends, and other health team members in developing care strategies
- documenting all information needed to manage the patient's needs

• planning for the patient's comfort and the maintenance of optimum functioning
• selecting the best nursing measures to deliver effective care
• identifying community resources to assist the patient and family
• coordinating the patient's care with other health care providers
• delegating care responsibilities to other health care providers
• supervising and validating the activities of other health team members
• formulating outcomes of nursing interventions
• teaching the patient and family
• recording all appropriate information, orally and in written reports.

Evaluation

About 18% of the questions test your ability to measure goal achievement. These questions focus on such nursing behaviors as:
• comparing actual outcomes with expected outcomes
• evaluating the patient's compliance with the prescribed plan of care
• documenting the patient's response to care
• revising the plan of care and reordering priorities as needed.

Professional issues

About 4% of the questions on the CEN exam (2% for legal issues and 2% for organizational issues) focus on such topics as informed consent, confidentiality, and quality improvement. The questions in Chapters 20 and 21 of this book approximate these percentages; the sample test reflects the percentages exactly. The professional issues portion of the exam does not include a nursing process dimension.

What's the "best" way to study for the exam?
That depends entirely on you. Some test candidates prefer studying alone, others opt for group study, and still others enjoy a combination of the two.

Individual study

No matter what other study strategies you use, individual preparation for the CEN examination is highly recommended. This preparation can take several forms.
• Read review books such as this one to help you pinpoint areas that need improvement. You can then concentrate on reviewing materials in those areas.
• Consult emergency nursing textbooks and study guides. As you read the material, ask yourself multiple-choice questions about the information. Consider how the CEN exam might test your knowledge of this material.
• Answer practice questions similar to those on the test. Spend about 30 minutes each day answering 10 to 20 questions (don't try to answer 100 questions on your day off). After you answer the questions, compare your answers with the correct answers listed in the review book; also review the rationales provided. If you answer some questions incorrectly and are not sure why, return to the textbook or review book to find the rationale. By doing this, you'll become more familiar and comfortable with the exam's format while reinforcing the information you've studied.

Group study

Studying with others can effectively prepare you for the CEN examination. To get the most from your sessions, follow these guidelines:
• Be choosy about whom to include in your study group. Limit the number of people (the recommended size is four to six people); larger groups can disrupt study.
• Ask each member to prepare one section of the study topic before the group meets. For example,

have one person discuss anatomy and physiology, another review the drugs used for treatments, and a third cover key elements of emergency nursing care.

• Meet regularly (once or twice weekly) to maintain a studious atmosphere.

• Limit each study session to 2 hours. Longer sessions invite participants to wander off the topic and promote a negative attitude toward the examination.

• Avoid turning study sessions into a party. Although snacks and refreshments can help maintain the group's energy, a party atmosphere will render the session ineffective.

How can I master a multiple-choice test?
Multiple-choice questions are one of the most commonly used test formats for such standardized tests as the CEN examination. Once you've mastered the following test-taking strategies, you'll be able to score better on multiple-choice tests.

• Read the question and all options carefully and completely.

• Treat each question individually. Use only the information provided for that question, and avoid reading into a question information that isn't provided.

• Monitor your time. You'll have more than 60 seconds per question; because most test-takers average 45 seconds per question, you may finish well before the time limit.

• Narrow your choices by using the process of elimination. If you can identify even one option as incorrect, you can focus your attention on the more plausible answers (and improve your chances of answering correctly).

• Don't change your answer. Studies show that test-takers who change an answer on a multiple-choice examination usually change it from a correct answer to an incorrect one or from one incorrect answer to another incorrect answer. Rarely do they change to a correct answer.

• For the same reason, don't review questions that you've already answered, even if you have extra time.

• Look for qualifying words in the question (such as *first*, *best*, *most*, *better*, and *highest*) that ask you to judge the priority of the options; then select the answer that has the highest priority.

• Look for negative words in the question (such as *not*, *least*, *unlikely*, *inappropriate*, *unrealistic*, *lowest*, *contraindicated*, *except*, *inconsistent*, *all but*, *atypical*, and *incorrect*). In general, when you're asked a negative question, three of the choices are appropriate actions, and one is inappropriate. You are being asked to select the inappropriate choice as your answer.

• Avoid selecting answers that contain absolute words (including *always*, *every*, *only*, *all*, *never*, and *none*); these options usually are incorrect.

• Never choose an option that refers the patient to a doctor. Because the CEN exam is for nurses and includes conditions and problems that nurses should be able to solve independently, an answer that refers a patient to the doctor usually is incorrect and can be eliminated from consideration.

• Don't look for a pattern (such as C, C, A, B, C, C, A, B) when selecting answers. The questions and answers on the exam are randomly arranged.

• Don't panic if you read a question that you don't understand. Some questions may refer to diseases, drugs, or laboratory tests that you're unfamiliar with. In such cases, remember that nursing care is similar in many situations, even when disease processes differ markedly. Just select the answer that seems logical and involves general nursing care.

• Think positively about the examination. People who have a positive attitude score higher than those who don't.

Are there any other tips I should know about?
Proper planning can go a long way toward ensuring your success on the CEN exam. Try these suggestions.

Before exam day

• A week or so before the exam, drive to the test site to familiarize yourself with parking facilities and to locate the test room. Knowing where to go will greatly reduce your anxiety on the day of the exam.

• Follow as normal a schedule as possible on the day before the examination. If you need to travel to the exam site and stay away from home overnight, try to follow your usual nightly routine; avoid the urge to do something different.

• The night before the exam, avoid drinking alcoholic beverages. Alcohol, a central nervous system (CNS) depressant, interferes with your ability to concentrate. Also avoid eating foods you've never eaten before; they may cause adverse gastrointestinal effects the next day.

• Avoid taking sleep medications you've never taken before. Like alcohol, most sleep aids are CNS depressants; some have a hangover effect, while others produce drowsiness for an extended period.

• Don't stay up late to study; this will make you tired during the test, which will decrease your ability to concentrate. Besides, you're probably as prepared as you can be. Review formulas, charts, and lists for no more than 1 hour. Then relax, perhaps by watching television or reading a magazine or book. These activities will help decrease your anxiety. Go to bed at your usual time.

Exam day

• On the morning of the exam, don't attempt a major review of the material. The likelihood of learning something new is slim, and intensive study may only increase your anxiety.

• Don't drink excessive amounts of coffee, tea, or caffeine-containing beverages. Caffeine will increase your nervousness and stimulate your renal system. (Restroom visits are permitted, but the allotted test time is not extended if you leave the room during the exam.)

• Eat breakfast, even if you usually do not, and include foods high in glucose and protein to maintain your energy level. Shun greasy, heavy foods. They tend to form an uncomfortable knot in your stomach and may decrease your ability to concentrate.

• Bring mints or hard candy to the test room to relieve dry mouth.

• Dress in comfortable, layered clothing. Jogging suits are popular. Many rooms are air-conditioned in the summer and may be cool even if it's hot outside. Be prepared by taking a sweater or sweatshirt.

• Arrive at the test site 30 to 45 minutes early, and make sure you have the required papers and documents for admittance to the test room. Latecomers are not admitted to the examination.

• Take several sharpened lead pencils. Calipers may be taken into the examination room. Calculators are permitted in the testing room provided they are silent, do not require electrical outlets, do not print tape, and do not have a key for each letter of the alphabet. Calculators with a memory key are permissible. You may not bring a cellular phone into the testing room.

• Think positively about how you'll do. Taking the CEN examination shows confidence in your knowledge of emergency nursing. When you receive your passing results, plan to celebrate your success, a significant achievement in your professional life that deserves to be rewarded.

Who can I contact for more information?

Contact the Board of Certification of Emergency Nursing (BCEN), 216 Higgins Road, Park Ridge, IL 60068-5736 USA, or phone (708) 698-9400. All correspondence and requests for information concerning applications for or administration of the CEN exam should be directed to: Applied Measurement Professionals, Inc. (AMP), Candidate Services – CEN Examination, 8310 Nieman Road, Lenexa, KS 66214 USA, or phone (913) 541-0400.

ABDOMINAL EMERGENCIES

CHAPTER 1

Abdominal Emergencies

1. A patient is complaining of right lower quadrant abdominal pain, nausea, and vomiting. Which of the following interventions is not appropriate?
A. Offering clear liquids
B. Obtaining a urine specimen
C. Obtaining a blood specimen for a complete blood count
D. Assisting patient to a position of comfort

CORRECT ANSWER—A. *Rationales:* A patient with undiagnosed abdominal pain should receive nothing by mouth in case surgery is required. Obtaining a urine specimen and a complete blood count can help diagnose the cause of abdominal pain. Repositioning can sometimes diminish the patient's pain.
Nursing process step: Intervention

2. A patient complains of abdominal pain and distention, fever, tachycardia, and diaphoresis. An abdominal X-ray shows free air under the diaphragm. The emergency nurse should suspect which of these conditions?
A. Intestinal obstruction
B. Acute appendicitis
C. Intestinal perforation
D. Acute cholelithiasis

CORRECT ANSWER—C. *Rationales:* Intestinal perforation is associated with free air under the diaphragm. Intestinal obstruction, acute appendicitis, and acute cholelithiasis are not associated with free air.
Nursing process step: Assessment

3. A patient has an intestinal perforation. Which of the following interventions is considered inappropriate?
A. Inserting a nasogastric (NG) tube
B. Offering clear liquids
C. Administering I.V. antibiotics
D. Preparing the patient for surgery

CORRECT ANSWER—B. *Rationales:* The patient with intestinal perforation will require surgery and should receive nothing by mouth. An NG tube should be inserted to decompress the GI tract. Antibiotics should be administered I.V. to prevent sepsis, which can be caused by leakage from the perforation.
Nursing process step: Intervention

4. Serum amylase levels may be elevated 3 to 5 times above normal during the first 24 to 48 hours after onset of acute pancreatitis symptoms. What is the normal serum amylase level?
A. 8.4 to 10.2 U/L
B. 850 to 975 U/L
C. 150 to 250 U/L
D. 25 to 125 U/L

CORRECT ANSWER—D. *Rationales:* The normal serum amylase level is 25 to 125 U/L.
Nursing process step: Assessment

5. What is the most appropriate nursing diagnosis for a patient with acute pancreatitis?
  A. Fluid volume deficit
  B. Fluid volume excess
  C. Increased cardiac output
  D. Altered tissue perfusion

CORRECT ANSWER—A. *Rationales:* Patients with acute pancreatitis commonly experience fluid volume deficit, sometimes resulting in hypovolemic shock. Causes include vomiting, bleeding that results in hemorrhagic pancreatitis, and plasma leakage into the peritoneal cavity. Hypovolemic shock decreases cardiac output. It also causes altered tissue perfusion, but this is not the primary nursing diagnosis for this patient.
Nursing process step: Analysis

6. Peritoneal lavage is a diagnostic tool used in detecting abdominal injuries. Which of the following is a contraindication for peritoneal lavage?
  A. An unconscious patient
  B. A history of abdominal surgery
  C. A distended bladder
  D. An allergy to radiopaque dye

CORRECT ANSWER—C. *Rationales:* A distended bladder is an absolute contraindication for peritoneal lavage. An indwelling urinary catheter should be inserted before the procedure. Peritoneal lavage is especially useful for diagnosing abdominal injuries in unconscious patients because they are unable to report pain. A history of abdominal surgery is not a contraindication for this procedure. Peritoneal lavage involves the instillation and withdrawal of fluid from the abdominal cavity; radiopaque dye is not required.
Nursing process step: Intervention

7. Which organ is most frequently injured in blunt abdominal trauma?
  A. Large bowel
  B. Spleen
  C. Liver
  D. Stomach

CORRECT ANSWER—B. *Rationales:* A highly vascular and encapsulated organ, the spleen is compressed against the vertebral column during blunt abdominal trauma. Injuries to the spleen are commonly seen in patients with left lower rib injuries. Injuries to the liver are common in patients with right lower rib fractures. The large bowel and stomach are seldom injured in blunt abdominal trauma.
Nursing process step: Assessment

8. A 4-year-old child is brought to the emergency department after being hit in the abdomen with a baseball bat. Which of the following is not a normal finding for this child?
  A. High-pitched tympanic sound over the stomach
  B. Cylindrical contour of the abdomen
  C. Failure of the abdomen to move with respirations
  D. Crying during exam

CORRECT ANSWER—C. *Rationales:* Children under age 9 are abdominal breathers, so chest movements are normally synchronized with abdominal movements. Failure of the abdomen to move with respirations could indicate serious abdominal injury. The high-pitched tympanic sounds indicate air in the stomach, a condition common in mouth breathers. Young children have a spinal lordosis that gives the abdomen a cylindrical, prominent contour. They may express their fear by crying during the exam; speaking softly and allowing a caregiver to stay nearby may help ease their fear.
Nursing process step: Assessment

9. What is the primary nursing diagnosis for a patient with a bowel obstruction?
   A. Fluid volume deficit
   B. Knowledge deficit
   C. Pain
   D. Alteration in tissue perfusion

CORRECT ANSWER—**A.** *Rationales:* Feces, fluid, and gas accumulate above a bowel obstruction. Then the absorption of fluids decreases, and gastric secretions increase. This process leads to a loss of fluids and electrolytes in circulation. Options B, C, and D are applicable but are not the primary nursing diagnosis.
Nursing process step: Analysis

10. Which of the following is not a priority nursing diagnosis for a patient with acute GI bleeding?
   A. Coagulation defect
   B. Fluid volume deficit
   C. High risk for systemic infection
   D. Decreased tissue perfusion

CORRECT ANSWER—**C.** *Rationales:* A patient with GI bleeding is not necessarily at risk for systemic infection. However, this patient may experience coagulation defects from multiple transfusions or underlying liver disease. Blood loss causes fluid volume deficit and decreased tissue perfusion.
Nursing process step: Analysis

11. The patient with liver failure will have which of these laboratory values?
   A. Increased albumin, increased prothrombin time
   B. Increased albumin, decreased prothrombin time
   C. Decreased albumin, decreased prothrombin time
   D. Decreased albumin, increased prothrombin time

CORRECT ANSWER—**D.** *Rationales:* Albumin decreases because the liver cannot synthesize blood proteins. Prothrombin time increases because the diseased liver cannot make clotting factors in sufficient amounts. These patients are prone to bleeding.
Nursing process step: Assessment

12. A 2-month-old infant is brought to the emergency department by his mother. His abdomen is distended, and he has been vomiting forcefully and with increasing frequency over the past 2 weeks. On examination, the emergency nurse notes signs of dehydration and a palpable mass to the right of the umbilicus. Peristaltic waves are visible, moving from left to right. The nurse should suspect which of the following conditions?
   A. Colic
   B. Failure to thrive
   C. Intussusception
   D. Pyloric stenosis

CORRECT ANSWER—**D.** *Rationales:* These are classic symptoms of pyloric stenosis caused by hypertrophy of the circular pylorus muscle. Surgery is the standard treatment for this disorder. Abdominal masses and abnormal peristalsis are not necessarily related to colic or failure to thrive. Intussusception is usually characterized by acute onset and severe abdominal pain.
Nursing process step: Assessment

13. Pneumatic antishock garments are appropriate for which of the following conditions?
   A. Tension pneumothorax
   B. Intrathoracic hemorrhage
   C. Abdominal evisceration
   D. Intra-abdominal hemorrhage

CORRECT ANSWER—**D.** *Rationales:* Pneumatic antishock garments (PASG) are used to slow blood loss in patients with suspected intra-abdominal hemorrhage while they wait for surgical intervention. PASG are contraindicated in tension pneumothorax because they may increase tension pressures. They may also increase bleeding in intrathoracic hemorrhage. Because PASG decrease tissue perfusion to eviscerated organs, the emergency nurse should consider inflating the leg sections only.
Nursing process step: Intervention

14. A Sengstaken-Blakemore tube, which controls bleeding, is inserted in a patient with esophageal varices. Shortly after the procedure, the patient develops severe respiratory distress. What should the emergency nurse do first?
   A. Verify placement by taking a chest X-ray
   B. Place the patient in high Fowler's position and administer oxygen by way of a face mask
   C. Cut the tube
   D. Suction the oropharynx

CORRECT ANSWER—**C.** *Rationales:* The Sengstaken-Blakemore tube should be cut and removed immediately; the tube may have been improperly placed and is obstructing the airway. Taking a chest X-ray to verify placement would delay treatment and serves no useful purpose. Administering oxygen without a patent airway is ineffective. Suction should be available during removal of the tube.
Nursing process step: Intervention

15. A patient in the emergency department has severe nausea and has been vomiting every 30 to 45 minutes for the past 8 hours. This patient is at risk for developing which of these conditions?
   A. Metabolic acidosis and hyperkalemia
   B. Metabolic acidosis and hypokalemia
   C. Metabolic alkalosis and hyperkalemia
   D. Metabolic alkalosis and hypokalemia

CORRECT ANSWER—**D.** *Rationales:* Excessive vomiting, which reduces hydrochloric acid in the stomach, causes metabolic alkalosis. It also leads to hypokalemia.
Nursing process step: Assessment

16. A patient with abdominal pain arrives in the emergency department. What should the emergency nurse do first?
   A. Palpate the abdomen
   B. Percuss the abdomen
   C. Ask the patient to press the spot that hurts
   D. Visually inspect the abdomen

CORRECT ANSWER—**D.** *Rationales:* The abdomen should be examined in the following sequence: inspection, auscultation, percussion, and palpation. Palpation may interfere with bowel sounds and increase the patient's pain, which leads to guarding.
Nursing process step: Intervention

17. Which of the following is not indicative of a stomach injury?
A. Blood in the nasogastric aspirate
B. Bowel sounds in the chest
C. Epigastric pain and tenderness
D. Decreased or absent bowel sounds

CORRECT ANSWER—**B.** *Rationales:* The patient with a stomach injury may have blood in the nasogastric aspirate as well as epigastric pain and tenderness. Bowel sounds may be decreased or absent. Signs of peritonitis may be present if acidic gastric contents have been released. Bowel sounds in the chest are indicative of diaphragmatic rupture, not stomach injury.
Nursing process step: Evaluation

18. Which of the following is the most distinguishing factor of a pancreatic injury?
A. Positive Turner's sign
B. Positive Ballance's sign
C. Right upper quadrant tenderness with guarding
D. Rectal bleeding

CORRECT ANSWER—**A.** *Rationales:* Turner's sign is ecchymosis in the flank area. It suggests retroperitoneal bleeding and is often associated with pancreatic injury. Ballance's sign is characterized by two types of dullness: (1) a fixed dullness to percussion in the left flank and (2) a dullness that disappears with a change in position in the right flank. It is usually associated with splenic injuries. Option C is associated with liver injuries; option D is associated with colon injuries. Patients with pancreatic injuries may also demonstrate ileus; epigastric pain radiating to the back or left upper quadrant; pain, nausea, and vomiting; and a positive Kehr's sign (pain in the left shoulder secondary to diaphragmatic irritation by blood).
Nursing process step: Assessment

19. Decreased or absent bowel sounds may result from what condition?
A. Irritants inside the bowel
B. Irritants outside the bowel
C. Hypovolemia
D. Anxiety

CORRECT ANSWER—**B.** *Rationales:* Decreased or absent bowel sounds may be caused by an irritant, such as blood or intestinal contents, outside the bowel. Irritants inside the bowel usually cause hyperactive bowel sounds. Hypovolemia and anxiety do not cause decreased or absent bowel sounds.
Nursing process step: Evaluation

20. Which of the following statements about a penetrating abdominal trauma is true?
A. The outside appearance of the wound reflects the extent of internal injury.
B. The outside appearance of the wound does not reflect the extent of internal injury.
C. Death occurs more frequently after penetrating trauma than after blunt trauma.
D. Objects impaled in the abdomen should be removed soon after the patient arrives in the emergency department.

CORRECT ANSWER—**B.** *Rationales:* The appearance of entrance and exit wounds does not determine the extent of internal injury. For example, a bullet may fragment and change direction once inside the body. Death occurs more frequently after blunt abdominal trauma, in which case external signs of injury are not obvious; therefore, detection and treatment may be delayed. Impaled objects should not be removed but be stabilized with a dressing to prevent further injury to the patient.
Nursing process step: Evaluation

21. A patient with upper GI bleeding and a history of liver disease arrives at the emergency department. The emergency nurse may need to administer which of the following drugs by way of a nasogastric tube?
A. Vasopressin (Pitressin)
B. Heparin
C. Magnesium citrate
D. All of the above

CORRECT ANSWER—C. *Rationales:* Magnesium citrate helps rid the bowel of blood and fecal matter; digested blood releases ammonia and other toxins into the blood stream, increasing the risk of hepatic encephalopathy. Vasopressin is administered I.V. to control bleeding. Heparin is contraindicated because the patient may have coagulation defects from the liver disease.
Nursing process step: Intervention

22. Which of the following patients should be admitted to the hospital?
A. A 10-year-old child with moderate dehydration
B. A 5-year-old child with moderate dehydration
C. A 6-month-old infant with moderate dehydration
D. None of the above

CORRECT ANSWER—C. *Rationales:* Most children with moderate dehydration may be rehydrated safely in the emergency department. However, infants, who risk sudden decompensation, should be admitted.
Nursing process step: Analysis

23. For a patient with upper GI bleeding, gastric lavage is used to achieve the following with which exception?
A. Removing blood from the stomach
B. Reducing acid-peptide activity in the stomach
C. Reducing gastric mucosal blood flow
D. Sclerosing bleeding varices

CORRECT ANSWER—D. *Rationales:* Gastric lavage with room temperature saline solution or water removes blood from the stomach. (The absorption of this blood may increase the patient's ammonia levels.) Lavage also reduces acid-peptide activity in the stomach, reduces gastric mucosal blood flow, and prepares the patient for diagnostic procedures such as endoscopy. Gastric lavage is not effective in sclerosing bleeding varices.
Nursing process step: Intervention

24. Assessment of the abdomen should be performed in which of the following sequences?
A. Percussion, palpation, auscultation, inspection
B. Inspection, percussion, auscultation, palpation
C. Inspection, auscultation, percussion, palpation
D. Auscultation, percussion, palpation, inspection

CORRECT ANSWER—C. *Rationales:* Inspection, followed by auscultation, should be the first part of an abdominal assessment. Percussion and palpation may alter bowel sounds, so they should be done after auscultation. Palpation should be the last step in the exam because it may cause patient discomfort and guarding.
Nursing process step: Assessment

25. Which of the following complications may be caused by inserting a Sengstaken-Blakemore tube?
A. Rupture of the esophagus
B. Aspiration
C. Obstruction of the upper airway
D. All of the above

CORRECT ANSWER—D. *Rationales:* Rupture of the esophagus, aspiration, and upper airway obstruction are all potential complications of inserting a Sengstaken-Blakemore tube. The patient must be closely monitored while the tube is in place, and scissors should be kept at the bedside. If any of the complications above occurs, the lumens should be cut immediately and the tube removed.
Nursing process step: Evaluation

26. Patients with upper GI bleeding may require medications to reduce the acidity of gastric secretions, which can irritate the bleeding site. Which of the following drugs does not reduce gastric secretion acidity?
   A. Cimetidine (Tagamet)
   B. Vasopressin (Pitressin)
   C. Famotidine (Pepcid)
   D. Ranitidine hydrochloride (Zantac)

CORRECT ANSWER—B. *Rationales:* Vasopressin decreases blood flow to the site. The other drugs are histamine antagonists and reduce gastric acidity.
Nursing process step: Intervention

27. What does nursing care for a patient with a Sengstaken-Blakemore tube include?
   A. Assisting the patient to a chair three times daily
   B. Suctioning the patient's mouth frequently
   C. Keeping the patient supine
   D. All of the above

CORRECT ANSWER—B. *Rationales:* A patient with a Sengstaken-Blakemore tube is unable to swallow and requires frequent suctioning of the mouth. This patient should be kept on bed rest, and the head of the bed should be elevated to help prevent airway obstruction.
Nursing process step: Intervention

28. Which of the following interventions is appropriate for a patient with liver failure and elevated ammonia levels?
   A. Administer neomycin
   B. Administer lactulose
   C. Decrease protein intake
   D. All of the above

CORRECT ANSWER—D. *Rationales:* Neomycin decreases bacteria in the colon and, therefore, may increase ammonia levels. Lactulose increases ammonia excretion. Excessive protein intake increases ammonia levels.
Nursing process step: Intervention

29. Peritoneal lavage is appropriate for which of the following?
   A. Rapidly increasing abdominal distention
   B. An impaled object in the abdomen
   C. A blood alcohol level of 0.240 mg/dl and a tender abdomen
   D. Hypotension unresponsive to fluid bolus

CORRECT ANSWER—C. *Rationales:* Peritoneal lavage is commonly used when a patient can't participate in the abdominal examination (because of injuries or intoxication) or when the exam does not rule out the possibility of abdominal injury. A patient with rapidly increasing abdominal distention or with an impaled object in the abdomen has abdominal injuries, and peritoneal lavage would serve no diagnostic purpose. A patient with hypotension that is unresponsive to fluid boluses needs immediate treatment; peritoneal lavage would waste time.
Nursing process step: Intervention

30. A patient with peritonitis is most likely show which of these symptoms?
   A. Guarding
   B. Generalized abdominal pain
   C. Decreased bowel sounds
   D. All of the above

CORRECT ANSWER—D. *Rationales:* Peritoneal irritation causes guarding, generalized abdominal pain, and hypoactive bowel sounds. In addition, this patient may experience nausea, vomiting, low-grade fever, and shallow respirations secondary to the abdominal pain.
Nursing process step: Assessment

31. Which intervention is inappropriate for a patient with acute rectal bleeding?
   A. Insertion of a nasogastric (NG) tube
   B. Administration of enemas until clear
   C. Insertion of an indwelling urinary catheter
   D. Initiation of large-bore I.V. lines

CORRECT ANSWER—B. *Rationales:* Enemas are not appropriate for a patient with lower GI bleeding because they may increase bleeding. Even though rectal bleeding seems to indicate lower GI bleeding, the blood could be coming from a rapid upper GI bleed. Therefore, an NG tube is appropriate. An indwelling urinary catheter is helpful in maintaining accurate intake and output. Because this patient may need fluid resuscitation, large-bore I.V. lines are indicated. **Nursing process step:** Intervention

32. Which is the most appropriate nursing diagnosis for a patient with a small-bowel obstruction?
   A. Altered nutrition, less than body requirements
   B. Pain
   C. Fluid volume deficit
   D. Fluid volume excess

CORRECT ANSWER—C. *Rationales:* Massive fluid volume shifts may occur in a patient with a small-bowel obstruction. The initial symptom is usually pain, then vomiting occurs. This causes the patient to lose sodium and water, a condition that leads to dehydration and altered nutrition. **Nursing process step:** Analysis

33. A child has swallowed a quarter. What is the nurse's primary concern?
   A. Corrosion of the stomach's mucosal lining
   B. Bowel obstruction
   C. Bowel perforation
   D. Airway obstruction

CORRECT ANSWER—D. *Rationales:* First, the child should be assessed to determine if the airway is obstructed by the quarter. Then the child should be observed for signs of mucosal lining corrosion and bowel obstruction or perforation. **Nursing process step:** Evaluation

34. What are the most common causes of acute pancreatitis?
   A. Trauma and postoperative syndrome
   B. Alcohol abuse and biliary tract disease
   C. Hypercalcemia and drug use
   D. Trauma and alcohol abuse

CORRECT ANSWER—B. *Rationales:* Alcoholism and biliary tract disease cause 80% of all cases of pancreatitis. The other options are less common. **Nursing process step:** Evaluation

35. A patient has a bowel obstruction. Which interventions are appropriate?
   A. I.V. fluids and soapsuds enemas
   B. I.V. fluids and nasogastric (NG) tube insertion
   C. NG tube insertion and soapsuds enemas
   D. All of the above

CORRECT ANSWER—B. *Rationales:* Patients with bowel obstructions often have a fluid volume deficit and require I.V. fluids. NG tube insertion is necessary to decompress the GI tract. Soapsuds enemas are contraindicated because they may increase pain. **Nursing process step:** Intervention

36. Which statement about GI bleeding is not true?
A. The color of passed blood is a product of GI transit time.
B. Melena is a chemical interaction of gastric acid with blood over several hours.
C. Bright red rectal bleeding rules out upper GI bleeding.
D. As little as 50 ml of blood can cause clinical melena.

CORRECT ANSWER—**C.** *Rationales:* Brisk upper GI bleeding with a quick passage of blood through the GI tract can result in bright red rectal bleeding. The other statements are accurate.
Nursing process step: Evaluation

37. A patient has corrosive injury to the esophagus from ingesting a liquid alkali substance. What should be included in the treatment?
A. Induce vomiting
B. Insert a nasogastric (NG) tube
C. Manage the airway
D. Administer steroids

CORRECT ANSWER—**C** *Rationales:* Airway management is important in patients with corrosive injury to the esophagus because aspiration of the alkali substance may have occurred. Esophageal perforation may be present. Vomiting should not be induced; this would further expose tissue to the alkali. Insertion of an NG tube should be avoided except with endoscopy or fluoroscopy. The administration of steroids is probably not beneficial to this patient. If the patient is seen within 1 hour of ingestion, water may be given.
Nursing process step: Intervention

38. The nurse would expect to hear which of the following sounds during percussion of the stomach?
A. Resonance
B. Dullness
C. Hyperresonance
D. Tympany

CORRECT ANSWER—**D.** *Rationales:* Tympany is normally heard over air-filled viscera such as the stomach. Hyperresonance and resonance are more often heard over lung tissue. Dullness is heard over solid organs.
Nursing process step: Assessment

39. Which condition is most likely to have a nursing diagnosis of fluid volume deficit?
A. Appendicitis
B. Pancreatitis
C. Cholecystitis
D. Gastric ulcer

CORRECT ANSWER—**B.** *Rationales:* Hypovolemic shock from fluid shifts is a major factor in acute pancreatitis. The other conditions are not as likely to present with fluid volume deficit.
Nursing process step: Analysis

40. Ascites may be caused by which of these conditions?
A. Constrictive pericarditis
B. Liver cirrhosis
C. Peritonitis
D. All of the above

CORRECT ANSWER—**D.** *Rationales:* Ascites is an accumulation of fluid in the peritoneal cavity; it may be caused by various factors, including constrictive pericarditis, cirrhosis, and peritonitis. Other causes include right-sided heart failure, pancreatitis, tumors, and endometriosis.
Nursing process step: Assessment

41. The pain of mesenteric vascular infarction is often associated with which conditions?
A. Abdominal distention and bloody diarrhea
B. Constipation and vomiting
C. Abdominal distention and abdominal free air
D. All of the above

CORRECT ANSWER—**A.** *Rationales:* Mesenteric vascular infarction is often associated with vomiting, bloody diarrhea, abdominal distention and tenderness, and hypotension. Constipation and vomiting are more often associated with intestinal obstruction. Abdominal distention and abdominal free air are associated with perforated viscous.
Nursing process step: Assessment

42. A patient arrives at the emergency department complaining of a burning, gnawing epigastric pain that occurs 1 to 2 hours after meals. Symptoms have been present for 2 weeks. The emergency nurse recognizes these symptoms as indicative of which condition?
A. Pancreatitis
B. Irritable bowel syndrome
C. Peptic ulcer disease
D. Cholecystitis

CORRECT ANSWER—**C.** *Rationales:* These are common symptoms of peptic ulcer disease. Symptoms of pancreatitis include epigastric pain that radiates to the back with nausea and vomiting. Patients with irritable bowel syndrome complain of left lower quadrant pain and constipation or diarrhea. The pain of cholecystitis is epigastric, or, more commonly, in the right upper quadrant.
Nursing process step: Assessment

43. A patient is complaining of dark stools. The nurse should assess for which of the following?
A. Ingestion of beets
B. Ingestion of bismuth-containing compounds
C. Ingestion of red meat
D. None of the above

CORRECT ANSWER—**B.** *Rationales:* Ingestion of bismuth-containing compounds such as Pepto-Bismol may result in black stools. Iron and charcoal may also cause dark stools. Ingestion of beets may cause red stools. Red meat should not alter the color of stools.
Nursing process step: Assessment

44. For a patient with gastroesophageal reflux disease, discharge instructions should include which of the following?
A. "Lie down and rest after each meal."
B. "Avoid fried and fatty foods."
C. "Drink 16 ounces of water with each meal."
D. All of the above

CORRECT ANSWER—**B.** *Rationales:* Foods that irritate the esophagus should be avoided. They include fried and fatty foods, alcoholic beverages, and chocolate. Patients with gastroesophageal reflux disease should be instructed not to lie down for 3 hours after a meal. Overeating and drinking excessively should be avoided; both contribute to lower esophageal sphincter relaxation.
Nursing process step: Evaluation

45. Which of the following is the primary nursing diagnosis for an infant with intussusception?
A. Pain
B. Altered tissue perfusion
C. Fluid volume excess
D. Fluid volume deficit

CORRECT ANSWER—**B.** *Rationales:* Intussusception is a mechanical bowel obstruction in which one part of the intestine slips into a part below it. Blood supply to the bowel and mesentery can be severely compromised and result in gangrene. An infant with intussusception will have sudden severe abdominal pain. Fluid volume deficit may occur from fluid shifts.
Nursing process step: Analysis

46. Which of the following is the priority nursing diagnosis for a patient with peritonitis?
A. Pain
B. Inadequate nutrition
C. Decreased intravascular fluid volume
D. High risk for systemic infection

CORRECT ANSWER—**C.** *Rationales:* A patient with peritonitis may have decreased intravascular fluid volume caused by vomiting as well as a fluid shift in the peritoneal space and decreased oral intake. Pain is another factor that should be addressed. The patient with peritonitis has inadequate nutrition, which is not a priority concern in the emergency department. This patient is also at risk for systemic infection and should receive I.V. antibiotics.
Nursing process step: Analysis

47. A patient with a history of alcohol abuse and cirrhosis is vomiting large amounts of bright red blood. The patient's responses are poor. Vital signs include blood pressure of 80/50 mm Hg, pulse of 140 beats/minute, respirations of 36 breaths/minute, and temperature of 99.8° F (37.7° C). What should the emergency nurse do first?
A. Suction blood from the airway
B. Insert two large-bore I.V. lines
C. Insert a nasogastric tube
D. Administer I.V. vitamin K (AquaMEPHYTON)

CORRECT ANSWER—**A.** *Rationales:* Establishing a clear airway is the first priority. Airway, breathing, and circulation are always included in the primary assessment. The other interventions are important but should not precede the establishment of an airway.
Nursing process step: Intervention

CARDIOVASCULAR EMERGENCIES

CHAPTER 2

Cardiovascular Emergenci

1. Which of the following drugs should not be
given by way of an endotracheal (ET) tube?
A. Atropine sulfate
B. Sodium bicarbonate
C. Epinephrine (Adrenalin)
D. Lidocaine (Xylocaine)

CORRECT ANSWER—B. *Rationales:* Sodium bicarbonate should not be given by way of an ET tube
because of its alkalinity. Also, large amounts of
this drug are required. Atropine, epinephrine,
and lidocaine are absorbed rapidly by the lungs
and may be given safely by way of an ET tube.
Nursing process step: Intervention

2. A patient has these symptoms: dyspnea, depend-
ent edema, hepatomegaly, crackles, and distend-
ed neck veins. The emergency nurse should sus-
pect which of the following conditions?
A. Pulmonary embolism
B. Congestive heart failure
C. Cardiac tamponade
D. Tension pneumothorax

CORRECT ANSWER—B. *Rationales:* A patient with
congestive heart failure has reduced cardiac output because of the heart's decreased pumping
ability. Therefore, fluid builds up and causes
dyspnea, edema, hepatomegaly, crackles, and
distended neck veins. A patient with pulmonary
embolism has acute shortness of breath, pleuritic
chest pain, hemoptysis, and fever. A patient with
cardiac tamponade has muffled heart sounds,
hypotension, and elevated venous pressure. A
patient with tension pneumothorax has a deviat-
ed trachea and no breath sounds on the affected
side. Dyspnea and distended neck veins are present as well.
Nursing process step: Assessment

Questions 3 through 5 refer to the following situation:
A patient arrives in the emergency department complaining of nausea, diaphoresis, shortness of
breath, and squeezing substernal pain that radiates to the left shoulder and teeth. Symptoms began
2 hours ago while the patient was mowing the lawn; they were not relieved by rest.

3. The nurse should perform which of the following interventions?
A. Complete registration information, order an ECG, gain I.V. access, and take vital signs
B. Alert the catheter lab team, administer oxygen, apply a cardiac monitor, notify the doctor
C. Take the patient to the examination room, gain I.V. access, give sublingual nitroglycerin, alert the catheter lab team
D. Administer oxygen, apply a cardiac monitor, take the patient's vital signs, give sublingual nitroglycerin

CORRECT ANSWER—D. *Rationales:* The patient's pain is caused by myocardial ischemia. Oxygen increases the myocardial oxygen supply. Cardiac monitoring reveals life-threatening arrhythmias. The nurse should ensure that the patient is not hypotensive before giving sublingual nitroglycerin for chest pain. Registration may be delayed until the patient is stabilized. Alerting the catheter lab team before completing an initial assessment is premature.
Nursing process step: Intervention

4. The cardiac monitor reveals the following rhythm:

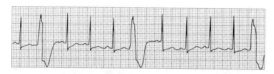

What is the initial pharmacologic treatment for this arrhythmia?
A. Magnesium sulfate 2 g I.V.
B. Bretylium tosylate (Bretylol) 10 mg/kg I.V.
C. Lidocaine (Xylocaine) 1 mg/kg I.V.
D. Atropine sulfate 0.5 mg I.V.

CORRECT ANSWER—C. *Rationales:* Lidocaine is the drug of choice for premature ventricular contractions (PVCs) associated with chest pain and a normal rate. Lidocaine is not used to treat PVCs with severe bradycardia; the heart rate should be treated first. Magnesium sulfate is used in torsades de pointes, suspected hypomagnesemia, or refractory ventricular fibrillation during cardiac arrest. Bretylium is a second-line antiarrhythmic drug. Atropine is used to increase heart rate.
Nursing process step: Intervention

5. The nurse is asked to begin a lidocaine (Xylocaine) infusion. The premixed bag contains 2 g of lidocaine in 500 ml of D5W. What is the drip rate for 2 mg/minute to be delivered?
A. 15 ml/hour
B. 45 ml/hour
C. 30 ml/hour
D. 60 ml/hour

CORRECT ANSWER—C. *Rationales:* First determine the concentration:

$$2 \text{ g} = 2{,}000 \text{ mg}$$
$$\frac{2{,}000 \text{ mg}}{500 \text{ ml}} = 4 \text{ mg/ml}$$

Then determine the drip rate:

$$2 \text{ mg/minute} \times 60 = 120 \text{ mg/hour}$$
$$\frac{120 \text{ mg/hour}}{4 \text{ mg/ml}} = 30 \text{ ml/hour}$$

Nursing process step: Intervention

6. Which of the following is an absolute contraindication for thrombolytic therapy?
A. Active bleeding
B. Current anticoagulant therapy
C. Age over 75 years
D. Severe hepatic disease

CORRECT ANSWER—A. *Rationales:* Active bleeding is an absolute contraindication for thrombolytic therapy. The other options are considered relative risks and should be evaluated before administering thrombolytics.
Nursing process step: Assessment

7. Which are some of the complications of thrombo-lytic therapy?
   A. Puncture site oozing and GI bleeding
   B. Bradycardia and worsening chest pain
   C. Puncture site oozing, GI bleeding, and brady-cardia
   D. All of the above

CORRECT ANSWER—C. *Rationales:* Bleeding is a complication of thrombolytic therapy. Bradycar-dia is a common reperfusion arrhythmia (others are accelerated idioventricular and ventricular ectopy). The patient should have less chest pain.
Nursing process step: Assessment

8. Diuretic therapy is deemed effective in a patient with congestive heart failure if which of the fol-lowing happens?
   A. Dyspnea decreases and jugular venous disten-tion increases
   B. Jugular venous distention increases and urine output increases
   C. Dyspnea decreases, urine output increases, and jugular venous distention decreases
   D. All of the above

CORRECT ANSWER—C. *Rationales:* Diuretics de-crease preload by eliminating sodium and water from the body and decrease dyspnea, increase urine output, and decrease jugular venous dis-tention.
Nursing process step: Evaluation

9. A patient with acute congestive heart failure shows the following hemodynamic parameters: Central venous pressure is 15 mm Hg; blood pressure is 90/50 mm Hg; pulse is 132 beats/minute; and respirations are 36 breaths/minute. What are the therapy goals for this patient?
   A. Decrease myocardial workload, decrease vol-ume, and increase myocardial contractility
   B. Decrease volume, decrease cardiac output, and increase myocardial contractility
   C. All of the above
   D. None of the above

CORRECT ANSWER—A. *Rationales:* Therapy goals for a patient with acute congestive heart failure are to reduce myocardial workload in order to in-crease cardiac output; decrease volume, which causes dyspnea and edema; and increase myo-cardial contractility in order to increase cardiac output. Congestive heart failure is a low cardiac output state.
Nursing process step: Evaluation

10. Pericardiocentesis is performed on a patient with cardiac tamponade caused by blunt chest trauma. This procedure would be deemed effec-tive if which of the following happens?
   A. Aspirated blood clots rapidly
   B. Blood pressure decreases
   C. Blood pressure increases
   D. Heart sounds become muffled

CORRECT ANSWER—C. *Rationales:* Cardiac tam-ponade is associated with decreased cardiac out-put, resulting in decreased blood pressure. Re-moving a small amount of blood may improve blood pressure. Pericardial blood does not clot because it is defibrinated by cardiac motion with-in the pericardial sac. If the blood clots rapidly, the needle may have entered the heart. Patients with cardiac tamponade may have muffled heart sounds. If pericardiocentesis is effective, heart sounds become normal.
Nursing process step: Evaluation

11. A patient comes to the emergency department complaining of severe headache and blurred vision. The symptoms have been present for the past 10 hours. The patient's blood pressure is 230/138 mm Hg. The doctor orders a sodium nitroprusside (Nipride) drip to bring the diastolic pressure to 110 to 120 mm Hg. Which statement is true of Nipride?

A. Nipride reduces afterload and increases cardiac output.

B. Nipride increases myocardial oxygen consumption.

C. Nipride increases heart rate.

D. Nipride is a calcium channel blocker.

CORRECT ANSWER—A. *Rationales:* Nipride reduces afterload and increases cardiac output. It affects both arteriolar and venous dilation. Nipride has an immediate onset and a short half-life. It decreases myocardial oxygen consumption and has no effect on heart rate. Nipride is not a calcium channel blocker.
Nursing process step: Intervention

12. A patient comes to the emergency department complaining of weakness and left-sided chest pain. The symptoms have been present for several weeks after a viral illness. Which of the following is most symptomatic of pericarditis?

A. Pericardial friction rub

B. Bilateral crackles

C. Pain unrelieved by a change in position

D. S₃ heart sound

CORRECT ANSWER—A. *Rationales:* A pericardial friction rub may be present with the pericardial effusion of pericarditis. The lungs are typically clear. Pericarditis pain is often relieved by sitting up and leaning forward. An S₃ heart sound indicates left-sided heart failure and is not usually present with pericarditis.
Nursing process step: Assessment

13. The emergency nurse should prepare a patient with a ruptured aorta for which of the following?

A. Emergency surgery

B. Chest tube insertion

C. Chest computed tomography (CT) scan

D. Immediate intubation

CORRECT ANSWER—A. *Rationales:* A patient with a ruptured aorta requires immediate surgery. Chest tubes should not be inserted. Diagnosis can be made with chest X-ray. A CT scan would delay definitive treatment. Intubation is done at the time of surgery, unless otherwise indicated.
Nursing process step: Intervention

14. A patient with hypotension and dyspnea has the following rhythm:

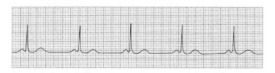

The emergency nurse should immediately do which of the following?

A. Administer lidocaine (Xylocaine) 1 mg/kg I.V. push

B. Prepare for external pacing

C. Administer atropine sulfate 0.5 mg I.V. push

D. Begin a dopamine hydrochloride (Intropin) infusion at 5 g/kg/minute

CORRECT ANSWER—C. *Rationales:* Atropine is the drug of choice for treating symptomatic bradycardia. The 0.5-mg dose may be repeated at 3- to 5-minute intervals until 0.03 to 0.04 mg/kg has been given. Pacing may be indicated if atropine is ineffective. Dopamine is not a first-line drug for treating bradycardia. It is, however, used to treat hypotension. In this case, bradycardia is the cause of hypotension and should be addressed first. Lidocaine should not be given for bradycardia because it may suppress the escape rhythm and lead to further hypotension and, possibly, asystole.
Nursing process step: Intervention

15. The nurse has delivered synchronized cardioversion to a symptomatic patient with supraventricular tachycardia. The patient then develops pulseless ventricular tachycardia. What should the nurse do immediately?
A. Deliver a precordial thump
B. Administer lidocaine (Xylocaine) 1 mg/kg I.V. push
C. Defibrillate at 200 joules
D. Administer adenosine (Adenocard) 6 mg I.V. push

CORRECT ANSWER—C. *Rationales:* Immediately defibrillate at 200 joules per advanced cardiac life support protocol. A precordial thump should be administered only in a witnessed cardiac arrest when a defibrillator is not immediately available. Lidocaine can be administered for persistent pulseless ventricular tachycardia if defibrillation and epinephrine (Adrenalin) are ineffective. Adenosine is not effective for ventricular tachycardias.
Nursing process step: Intervention

16. A patient with atrial fibrillation receives one dose of verapamil hydrochloride (Calan) I.V. push. After 15 minutes, the rate and rhythm are unchanged. Which intervention is inappropriate at this time?
A. Administer a second dose of verapamil 5 to 10 mg I.V. push
B. Administer propranolol (Inderal) I.V. push
C. Perform synchronized cardioversion if the patient becomes unstable
D. Consider diltiazem (Cardizem) I.V. push

CORRECT ANSWER—B. *Rationales:* Beta blockers such as propranolol should not be given within 30 minutes of administering a calcium channel blocker such as verapamil. They potentiate each other and may cause severe bradycardia or asystole. The initial dose of verapamil is usually 2.5 to 5 mg slow I.V. push (over 2 minutes). After 15 to 30 minutes, a second dose of 5 to 10 mg may be given. If the patient becomes unstable (hypotensive), synchronized cardioversion may be necessary. Diltiazem is another calcium channel blocker that may be used to control the rate in atrial fibrillation or flutter.
Nursing process step: Intervention

17. Which of the following best demonstrates the effectiveness of thrombolytic therapy?
A. Greater than 2-mm elevation in the ST segment
B. Oozing from I.V. sites
C. Relief of chest pain
D. Absence of arrhythmias

CORRECT ANSWER—C. *Rationales:* Thrombolytic therapy effectiveness is measured by the relief of chest pain, presence of reperfusion arrhythmias, and normalization of the ST segment. Oozing of blood from I.V. sites may occur because thrombolytic therapy may increase bleeding time, but bleeding does not demonstrate its effectiveness.
Nursing process step: Assessment

18. Which of these interventions is inappropriate for a patient with acute arterial occlusion?
A. Maintain the affected extremity in a dependent position
B. Apply a heating pad to the affected extremity
C. Use a Doppler ultrasound device to auscultate pulses
D. Prepare the patient for possible surgery

CORRECT ANSWER—B. *Rationales:* Increased temperature increases oxygen demands on the extremity. Maintaining the extremity in a dependent position promotes blood flow. Using Doppler ultrasound aids in assessing for worsening of the occlusion. The patient may need surgery.
Nursing process step: Intervention

19. A patient who has been kicked in the chest by a bull arrives in the emergency department. Vital signs are blood pressure 80/50 mm Hg, pulse 144 beats/minute, respirations 36 breaths/minute, and temperature 98.5° F (36.9° C). Heart sounds are muffled, and facial cyanosis is present. A bolus of 1,000 ml of fluid is infused. Blood pressure remains 82/50 mm Hg and pulse 150 beats/minute. The patient is most likely to have which of the following conditions?
A. Myocardial contusion
B. Tension pneumothorax
C. Cardiac tamponade
D. Aortic injury

CORRECT ANSWER—C. *Rationales:* Muffled heart sounds are associated with cardiac tamponade. Volume-depleted patients with cardiac tamponade may not respond to volume infusion. Myocardial contusion presents with chest pain and ECG changes. Tension pneumothorax presents with acute increases in respiratory rate and heart rate, chest pain, tracheal deviation to the unaffected side, and an absence of breath sounds on the affected side. Aortic injury presents with a widened mediastinum by chest X-ray, hypotension, respiratory distress, and chest pain.
Nursing process step: Assessment

20. The aorta is most often injured during which of the following types of trauma?
A. Deceleration trauma that causes shearing
B. Penetrating trauma
C. Blunt chest trauma
D. Chest injuries that cause rib fractures

CORRECT ANSWER—A. *Rationales:* Deceleration may cause laceration to the aorta by shearing forces. The other options may cause aortic injuries but are not the primary mechanisms of injury.
Nursing process step: Assessment

21. A patient is undergoing pericardiocentesis. The rhythm previously showed sinus tachycardia. Premature ventricular contractions are now noted on the monitor. This condition indicates which of the following?
A. It is time for the doctor to begin aspirating the syringe.
B. The pericardial sac has been entered, and it is time to attach a clamp to the needle at the skin level to prevent further insertion.
C. The needle has entered the heart.
D. The needle is touching the myocardium.

CORRECT ANSWER—D. *Rationales:* If the needle touches the myocardium, premature ventricular contractions or ST-segment elevation may be observed. The needle has not necessarily entered the heart. At this time, the needle should be withdrawn slightly. The doctor should aspirate the syringe while advancing the needle and should stop as soon as blood is obtained.
Nursing process step: Intervention

22. Cardiac tamponade may result from which of the following conditions?
A. Chest trauma
B. Pericarditis
C. Systemic lupus erythematosus
D. All of the above

CORRECT ANSWER—D. *Rationales:* All of these conditions may cause an accumulation of fluid in the pericardial sac leading to cardiac tamponade.
Nursing process step: Evaluation

23. A patient with a ruptured descending aorta may exhibit which of the following?
A. Greater pulse amplitude in the arms than in the legs
B. Greater pulse amplitude in the legs than in the arms
C. Blood pressure differences in right and left arms
D. Distended neck veins and muffled heart sounds

CORRECT ANSWER—A. *Rationales:* A patient with a ruptured descending aorta may have a greater pulse amplitude in the arms than in the legs because of decreased perfusion to the legs. Blood pressure differences in arms are indicative of ruptured subclavian arteries. Distended neck veins and muffled heart sounds are not likely to be present in this patient.
Nursing process step: Assessment

24. A patient with ECG changes in leads V_1, V_2, and V_3 may be suffering from which of the following injuries?
A. Inferior wall injury
B. Anterior wall injury
C. Lateral wall injury
D. Posterior wall injury

CORRECT ANSWER—B. *Rationales:* Anterior wall injury is associated with ECG changes in leads V_1, V_2, and V_3. Inferior wall injury is associated with ECG changes in leads II, III, and aVF. Lateral wall injury is associated with ECG changes in leads I, aVL, V_5, and V_6. Posterior wall injury is associated with ECG changes in leads V_1 and V_2.
Nursing process step: Assessment

25. A patient in third-degree block is started on an isoproterenol (Isoprel) infusion while waiting for insertion of a transvenous pacemaker. The patient soon develops the following rhythm:

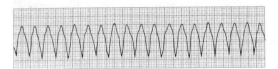

The patient responds poorly with a barely palpable pulse and a blood pressure of 40 mm Hg with a Doppler ultrasound device. The nurse should immediately do which of the following?
A. Administer a precordial thump
B. Defibrillate at 200 joules
C. Stop the isoproterenol infusion
D. Administer lidocaine (Xylocaine) 1 mg/kg I.V. push

CORRECT ANSWER—C. *Rationales:* Isoproterenol possesses beta-adrenergic actions and may cause tachyarrhythmias such as ventricular tachycardia. The infusion should be stopped immediately. Precordial thump and defibrillation are not indicated for ventricular tachycardia with a pulse. Lidocaine is appropriate after the isoproterenol infusion has been discontinued; however, this patient is acutely unstable and requires immediate cardioversion.
Nursing process step: Intervention

26. A patient in ventricular fibrillation has failed to respond to standard treatment — defibrillation, epinephrine (Adrenalin), and lidocaine (Xylocaine). Which of the following is a potentially reversible cause of ventricular fibrillation?
A. Hypothermia
B. Hypovolemia
C. Electrolyte abnormalities
D. All of the above

CORRECT ANSWER—D. *Rationales:* All of the options can potentially cause ventricular fibrillation and may need to be treated before standard measures are effective.
Nursing process step: Evaluation

27. What is the maximum number of times a patient can be defibrillated safely?
A. 10
B. 15
C. 18
D. There is no limit

CORRECT ANSWER—D. *Rationales:* There is no maximum number of times a patient can be defibrillated. However, if the patient remains in ventricular fibrillation for more than 30 minutes, the chances of survival are low. Exceptions would be resuscitation of children, hypothermic individuals, drowning victims, and patients who go in and out of ventricular fibrillation multiple times. These patients may benefit from longer resuscitation.
Nursing process step: Evaluation

28. An elderly patient arrives in the emergency department complaining of diarrhea, weakness, headache, and "yellowish" vision. The patient has a history of hypertension and "heart" problems. Home medications are not available. Vital signs are blood pressure 90/68 mm Hg, pulse 52 beats/minute, respirations 22 breaths/minute, and temperature 98.4° F (36.9° C). The nurse should suspect which of the following conditions?
A. Gastroenteritis
B. Viral syndrome
C. Digoxin (Lanoxin) toxicity
D. Overdose of antihypertensive medication

CORRECT ANSWER—C. *Rationales:* The patient's complaints along with vital signs suggest digoxin toxicity. The nurse should attempt to obtain a list of home medications from the family, the doctor, or medical records. Obtaining a serum digoxin level would be appropriate. The therapeutic digoxin level is 0.8 to 2.0 ng/ml. A patient with gastroenteritis would complain of abdominal cramps, diarrhea, and vomiting. Viral syndrome includes symptoms of malaise and, possibly, fever. A patient with an antihypertensive overdose would exhibit hypotension and weakness but would not have "yellowish" vision.
Nursing process step: Analysis

29. Which of the following is not generally associated with pulseless electrical activity (PEA) or electromechanical dissociation (EMD)?
A. Hypovolemia
B. Alkalosis
C. Massive pulmonary embolism
D. Acidosis

CORRECT ANSWER—B. *Rationales:* These rhythms are not associated with alkalosis. The other options may all be causes of PEA or EMD. Other possible causes include hypoxia, cardiac tamponade, tension pneumothorax, hypothermia, drug overdose, hyperkalemia, and massive myocardial infarction.
Nursing process step: Assessment

30. A patient complaining of severe chest pain is brought to the emergency department and suddenly becomes unresponsive. The monitor shows the following rhythm:

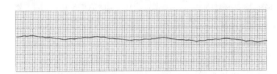

The nurse should immediately do which of the following?
A. Check for pulse and check monitor leads
B. Begin cardiopulmonary resuscitation
C. Administer atropine sulfate 1 mg I.V.
D. Defibrillate at 200 joules

CORRECT ANSWER—A. *Rationales:* Check the patient and monitor before initiating treatment. Cardiopulmonary resuscitation should then be initiated. The patient should be intubated at once and I.V. access obtained. Epinephrine (Adrenalin) 1 mg I.V. is then followed by atropine 1 mg I.V. Defibrillation is not indicated for patients in asystole.
Nursing process step: Intervention

31. Nitrates have which of the following effects?
A. Increase preload, increase afterload
B. Increase preload, decrease afterload
C. Decrease preload, decrease afterload
D. Decrease preload, increase afterload

CORRECT ANSWER—C. *Rationales:* Nitrates decrease preload and afterload and thereby decrease myocardial oxygen demand and increase myocardial oxygen supply.
Nursing process step: Evaluation

32. What is the primary effect of vagal stimulation on the heart?
A. Increases parasympathetic tone
B. Increases sympathetic tone
C. Decreases parasympathetic tone
D. Decreases sympathetic tone

CORRECT ANSWER—A. *Rationales:* Vagal stimulation increases parasympathetic tone, which decreases the heart rate and may slow atrioventricular conduction.
Nursing process step: Analysis

33. How much pressure should be applied to the paddles during defibrillation?
A. 10 pounds
B. 15 pounds
C. 20 pounds
D. 25 pounds

CORRECT ANSWER—D. *Rationales:* Apply 25 pounds of pressure to both paddles. Applying less pressure increases the risk of burns and makes defibrillation less effective. Conductor pads or gel should be used to ensure good contact.
Nursing process step: Intervention

34. A patient in ventricular fibrillation has received initial defibrillation at 200 joules. The monitor continues to show ventricular fibrillation. What is the next action?
A. Charge the defibrillator and deliver 300 joules
B. Check for a pulse
C. Resume cardiopulmonary resuscitation
D. Deliver synchronized cardioversion at 200 joules

CORRECT ANSWER—A. *Rationales:* According to advanced cardiac life support guidelines, the initial three shocks should be delivered one after the other, or "stacked." Cardiopulmonary resuscitation should not be resumed between shocks unless there is an unavoidable delay. Do not pause for a pulse check if the monitor is properly connected and shows persistent ventricular fibrillation.
Nursing process step: Intervention

35. What is the purpose of defibrillation?
A. To produce temporary asystole
B. To "jump start" the heart
C. To produce a sinus rhythm
D. None of the above

CORRECT ANSWER—A. *Rationales:* The purpose of defibrillation is to produce temporary asystole to totally depolarize the myocardium. Depolarizing allows the heart's natural pacemakers to resume normal activity.
Nursing process step: Evaluation

36. Which of the following drugs is inappropriate for a patient with a wide-complex tachycardia?
A. Lidocaine (Xylocaine)
B. Bretylium tosylate (Bretylol)
C. Procainamide hydrochloride (Pronestyl)
D. Verapamil hydrochloride (Calan)

CORRECT ANSWER—D. *Rationales:* Administering verapamil to a patient with ventricular tachycardia can be lethal. Verapamil may accelerate the heart rate and decrease blood pressure, particularly in patients with atrial fibrillation and Wolff-Parkinson-White syndrome. The other options would be appropriate for a patient with wide-complex tachycardia.
Nursing process step: Intervention

37. What is the role of beta blockers in the patient with acute myocardial infarction?
A. To reduce myocardial oxygen consumption
B. To lower blood pressure
C. To decrease catecholamine levels
D. All of the above

CORRECT ANSWER—D. *Rationales:* Beta blockers decrease myocardial oxygen consumption and demands of the ischemic areas of the heart. They are used to reduce infarct size by decreasing sympathetic tone, thereby decreasing afterload. They also lower blood pressure and decrease arrhythmias by decreasing catecholamine levels.
Nursing process step: Analysis

38. A patient with a serum potassium level of 7.8 mEq/L may manifest which of the following ECG changes?
A. Peaked T waves, tachycardia, and widened QRS complex
B. Bradycardia, peaked T waves, and widened QRS complex
C. Tachycardia and widened QRS complex
D. All of the above

CORRECT ANSWER—B. *Rationales:* Patients with hyperkalemia may exhibit peaked T waves, a widened QRS complex with bradycardias, disappearance of P waves and, eventually, idioventricular rhythm and asystole.
Nursing process step: Analysis

39. Which of the following drugs is not considered a positive inotrope?
A. Epinephrine (Adrenalin)
B. Dobutamine (Dobutrex)
C. Propranolol (Inderal)
D. Digoxin (Lanoxin)

CORRECT ANSWER—C. *Rationales:* Options A, B, and D are all positive inotropes; that is, they increase the contractile state of the myocardium. Propranolol is a negative inotrope; it decreases the contractile state of the myocardium.
Nursing process step: Evaluation

40. A patient complaining of severe "tearing" chest pain that radiates to the back is probably experiencing which of the following?

A. Pericarditis
B. Endocarditis
C. Myocardial infarction
D. Dissecting abdominal aneurysm

CORRECT ANSWER—D. *Rationales:* Sudden onset of severe chest pain that radiates to the back with a tearing sensation is the classic presentation of dissecting abdominal aneurysm. A patient with pericarditis may complain of chest pain that is relieved by sitting forward. A patient with endocarditis has a fever, a heart murmur, weight loss, and fatigue but no chest pain. A patient with a myocardial infarction presents with chest pain or pressure radiating to the left arm, neck, or jaw; the pain is unrelieved by rest or change in position.
Nursing process step: Assessment

41. Occlusion of the left coronary artery will probably result in damage to which of the following?

A. Inferior wall of the myocardium
B. Anterior wall of the myocardium
C. Posterior wall of the myocardium
D. Right ventricle

CORRECT ANSWER—B. *Rationales:* The left coronary artery supplies the anterior and lateral walls of the myocardium. The inferior wall is usually supplied by the right coronary artery. The posterior wall is supplied by a branch of the posterior descending artery. The right ventricle is supplied by the right coronary artery.
Nursing process step: Analysis

42. Which of the following is the most appropriate nursing diagnosis for a patient who is receiving thrombolytic therapy?

A. Pain
B. Impaired tissue integrity
C. Knowledge deficit
D. Risk for injury

CORRECT ANSWER—D. *Rationales:* A patient who is receiving thrombolytics is at risk for hemorrhage. The patient may also experience pain, but it is not related to thrombolytic therapy. This patient would not necessarily experience impaired tissue integrity. Although knowledge deficit is always an important nursing diagnosis, it is not the most appropriate one.
Nursing process step: Analysis

43. Which of the following is the primary nursing diagnosis for a patient with acute myocardial infarction?

A. Impaired gas exchange
B. Pain
C. Decreased cardiac output
D. Activity intolerance

CORRECT ANSWER—C. *Rationales:* The injured myocardium contracts poorly, leading to decreased cardiac output. The other options may be appropriate for a patient with acute myocardial infarction but are not priority diagnoses.
Nursing process step: Analysis

44. Which of the following is the term for the force against which a cardiac chamber must eject blood during systole?

A. Systemic vascular resistance
B. Preload
C. Afterload
D. Stroke volume

CORRECT ANSWER—C. *Rationales:* Afterload is the force against which a cardiac chamber must eject blood during systole. Systemic vascular resistance is this force. Preload is the amount of stretch on the myocardium before systole. Stroke volume is the amount of blood ejected by the left ventricle during systole.
Nursing process step: Assessment

45. Which of the following best describes a pericardial friction rub?
  A. Is classified as systolic
  B. Is best heard at the apex with the bell of the stethoscope
  C. Varies in intensity with respiration
  D. May be accentuated by having the patient lean forward and exhale

CORRECT ANSWER—D. *Rationales:* A pericardial friction rub may be heard when the pericardial surfaces are inflamed. The sound can be heard over the entire pericardium by using the diaphragm of the stethoscope. Unlike a pleural friction rub, it does not vary in intensity during respiration. It may be accentuated if the patient leans forward and exhales.
Nursing process step: Assessment

46. Which of the following statements regarding creatine kinase (CK) is true?
  A. A normal CK level in a patient with acute chest pain rules out myocardial infarction (MI).
  B. CK is specific for cardiac muscle.
  C. CK levels after an MI peak between 24 and 28 hours.
  D. CK levels after an MI peak between 6 and 8 hours.

CORRECT ANSWER—C. *Rationales:* CK levels after an MI peak between 24 and 28 hours. They become abnormal between 6 and 8 hours after infarction. A normal CK level does not rule out MI. CK is found in other tissues besides the myocardium.
Nursing process step: Assessment

47. Which of the following is an important sign of left-sided heart failure in adults?
  A. Systolic murmur
  B. S_3, or ventricular gallop
  C. Diastolic murmur
  D. All of the above

CORRECT ANSWER—B. *Rationales:* S_3 is a sign of left-sided heart failure in adults and warrants treatment. It may be heard in early diastole. A systolic murmur is heard with mitral insufficiency; a diastolic murmur is heard with mitral stenosis.
Nursing process step: Assessment

48. Which of the following is the most appropriate nursing diagnosis for a patient with angina?
  A. Altered tissue perfusion
  B. Decreased cardiac output
  C. Impaired gas exchange
  D. Pain

CORRECT ANSWER—A. *Rationales:* The discomfort of angina is caused by ischemia, or altered tissue perfusion to the myocardium. Nursing interventions are aimed at decreasing myocardial oxygen demands. Cardiac output may not be altered in the patient who is experiencing angina. There may not be a problem with gas exchange. Making the patient comfortable is a priority, and the patient should be treated initially with nitroglycerin.
Nursing process step: Analysis

49. Why are diuretics used in the treatment of congestive heart failure?
  A. To increase cardiac output
  B. To decrease myocardial oxygen consumption
  C. To decrease fluid volume
  D. All of the above

CORRECT ANSWER—C. *Rationales:* Diuretics reduce total fluid volume and relieve the symptoms of congestion. They do not affect cardiac output or myocardial oxygen consumption.
Nursing process step: Analysis

50. Which of the following drugs may be used to reduce afterload in a patient with congestive heart failure?
A. Morphine sulfate
B. Digoxin (Lanoxin)
C. Dobutamine hydrochloride (Dobutrex)
D. None of the above

CORRECT ANSWER—A. *Rationales:* Morphine reduces afterload and decreases myocardial oxygen demand. It also decreases anxiety and dyspnea. Digoxin and dobutamine are positive inotropes and increase cardiac contractility.
Nursing process step: Evaluation

51. Which of the following thrombolytic agents is most likely to cause an allergic reaction?
A. Streptokinase
B. Urokinase
C. Tissue plasminogen activator
D. Alteplase (Activase)

CORRECT ANSWER—A. *Rationales:* Allergic reactions, most often manifested by fever and rash, occur in about 5% of patients who are receiving streptokinase. To help prevent allergic reactions, patients are often given steroids and antihistamines before streptokinase is administered.
Nursing process step: Evaluation

52. Which is the most common cause of cardiac arrest in an adult?
A. Electrolyte disturbances
B. Respiratory arrest
C. Ventricular fibrillation
D. Drug toxicity

CORRECT ANSWER—C. *Rationales:* Ventricular fibrillation is the most common cause of cardiopulmonary arrest. Options A, B, and D may result in cardiac arrest but are not the most common causes.
Nursing process step: Evaluation

53. A patient with acute shortness of breath and frothy pink-tinged sputum arrives at the emergency department. Crackles and wheezes are present. Vital signs are blood pressure 90/50 mm Hg, pulse 120 beats/minute, respirations 34 breaths/minute, and temperature 98.6° F (37° C). The patient has a history of diabetes, hypertension, and congestive heart failure. Which of the following should the emergency nurse suspect?
A. Cardiac tamponade
B. Pneumothorax
C. Pulmonary embolus
D. Pulmonary edema

CORRECT ANSWER—D. *Rationales:* These symptoms are typical of acute pulmonary edema related to congestive heart failure. A patient with cardiac tamponade has muffled heart sounds and elevated venous pressure. A patient with a pneumothorax has shortness of breath and chest pain. Breath sounds are decreased on the affected side. Patients with pulmonary embolus often report chest pain.
Nursing process step: Assessment

54. Which of the following drugs are used to treat acute pulmonary edema associated with congestive heart failure?
A. Digoxin (Lanoxin), morphine, and furosemide (Lasix)
B. Furosemide (Lasix), morphine, and nitroglycerin
C. Amrinone (Inocor), digoxin (Lanoxin), and dopamine (Intropin)
D. Norepinephrine (Levophed), amrinone (Inocor), and propranolol (Inderal)

CORRECT ANSWER—B. *Rationales:* Drug therapy in acute pulmonary edema is aimed at reducing preload. Furosemide, morphine, and nitroglycerin are first-line drugs used to reduce preload. Digoxin has little role in the treatment of acute pulmonary edema. Amrinone may be used in cardiogenic shock after other drugs have failed. Norepinephrine has no role in the treatment of acute pulmonary edema.
Nursing process step: Intervention

55. Which is the most common cause of acute cardiac tamponade?
A. Pericarditis
B. Penetrating chest trauma
C. Blunt chest trauma
D. Myocardial infarction (MI)

CORRECT ANSWER—**B.** *Rationales:* Although pericarditis, blunt chest trauma, and MI can cause cardiac tamponade, penetrating chest trauma is the most common cause of acute tamponade.
Nursing process step: Assessment

56. A patient who has had shaking chills and fever for 3 days comes to the emergency department. Assessment reveals splinter hemorrhaging of the nail beds and a systolic murmur. The emergency nurse should suspect which of the following conditions?
A. Pericarditis
B. Endocarditis
C. Myocarditis
D. None of the above

CORRECT ANSWER—**B.** *Rationales:* These are the hallmark symptoms of endocarditis. A patient with pericarditis complains of chest pain that is relieved by leaning forward. A precordial friction rub may be heard on auscultation. A patient with myocarditis may complain of fatigue, dyspnea, palpitations, and mild discomfort. Auscultation may reveal an S_3 and a systolic murmur.
Nursing process step: Assessment

57. Cardiopulmonary resuscitation is being performed on an intubated patient. Gastric distention is present. Which should be the first action?
A. Insert a nasogastric (NG) tube
B. Retract the endotracheal (ET) tube 2 cm
C. Auscultate for bilateral breath sounds
D. Apply direct abdominal pressure

CORRECT ANSWER—**C.** *Rationales:* First, the nurse should be sure that the ET tube is correctly positioned by auscultating for bilateral breath sounds. If the tube is in the correct position, the nurse should insert an NG tube to relieve gastric distention. The nurse should not apply abdominal pressure. Gastric distention should be relieved because it can interfere with adequate lung inflation.
Nursing process step: Intervention

58. The pathophysiology involved in myocardial contusion is related to which of the following?
A. Penetrating injuries of the myocardium
B. Bleeding into and direct injury to the myocardium
C. Occlusion of coronary vessels
D. All of the above

CORRECT ANSWER—**B.** *Rationales:* Myocardial contusion is caused by blunt trauma to the myocardium and not penetrating injuries. The pathophysiology relates to bleeding into the myocardium as well as direct injury to the muscle, not occlusion of coronary vessels.
Nursing process step: Analysis

59. Cardiac output is a product of what?
A. Heart rate times central venous pressure
B. Heart rate times systemic vascular resistance
C. Heart rate times stroke volume
D. Heart rate times cardiac index

CORRECT ANSWER—**C.** *Rationales:* Cardiac output is a product of heart rate times stroke volume. It is measured in liters per minute. The normal value is 4 to 6 L per minute.
Nursing process step: Assessment

60. Which of the following statements concerning unstable angina is not true?
A. It occurs more frequently at rest.
B. It is relieved with usual doses of sublingual nitroglycerin.
C. It is chest pain of increasing duration.
D. It is associated with reversible depression of ST segments.

CORRECT ANSWER—B. *Rationales:* Unstable angina is usually not relieved with sublingual nitroglycerin. The other statements are true. Patients with unstable angina require hospitalization.
Nursing process step: Assessment

61. Which of the following is not an action of lidocaine (Xylocaine)?
A. Decreases automaticity
B. Increases fibrillation threshold
C. Decreases fibrillation threshold
D. Suppresses ischemic tissue conduction

CORRECT ANSWER—C. *Rationales:* Lidocaine increases the fibrillation threshold and makes the myocardium less susceptible to fibrillation. This is why it is used to treat ventricular ectopy. The fibrillation threshold should not be decreased.
Nursing process step: Evaluation

62. For the nurse to hear S_3 and S_4, which is the best position for the patient?
A. Left lateral position
B. Supine position
C. High Fowler's position
D. Right lateral position

CORRECT ANSWER—A. *Rationales:* S_3 and S_4 are best heard when the patient is in the left lateral position. The bell of the stethoscope should be placed at the point of maximal impulse. S_3 is known as a ventricular gallop, and S_4 is known as an atrial gallop.
Nursing process step: Assessment

63. Which of the following is the primary nursing diagnosis for a patient with an aortic aneurysm?
A. Anxiety
B. Decreased cardiac output
C. Altered tissue perfusion
D. Fluid volume deficit

CORRECT ANSWER—B. *Rationales:* A patient with an aortic aneurysm may have decreased cardiac output related to fluid volume deficit if dissection or rupture of the aneurysm occurs. Decreased cardiac output would lead to anxiety and altered tissue perfusion. The primary problem is decreased cardiac output.
Nursing process step: Analysis

64. Which of the following is the primary nursing diagnosis for a patient experiencing angina?
A. Decreased cardiac output
B. Pain
C. Anxiety
D. Altered tissue perfusion

CORRECT ANSWER—D. *Rationales:* Angina is caused by altered tissue perfusion to the myocardium, resulting in ischemia. Treatment is aimed at reversing ischemia. Pain and anxiety should also be addressed. A patient with angina may or may not have a decreased cardiac output.
Nursing process step: Analysis

65. Appropriate interventions for a patient complaining of syncope include which of the following?
A. Obtaining orthostatic vital signs
B. Obtaining an ECG
C. Obtaining a home medication list
D. All of the above

CORRECT ANSWER—D. *Rationales:* All of the interventions are appropriate for a patient with syncope. Orthostatic vital signs reveal orthostatic hypotension, which may be the result of medications or hypovolemia. Syncope may also be related to cardiac arrhythmias.
Nursing process step: Intervention

66. A patient in ventricular tachycardia arrives at the emergency department. Which of the following should the emergency nurse do first?
A. Perform a precordial thump
B. Defibrillate at 200 joules
C. Assess the patient
D. Administer lidocaine (Xylocaine) 1 mg/kg I.V.

CORRECT ANSWER—C. *Rationales:* The nurse should first assess the patient. A patient in ventricular tachycardia may be hemodynamically stable for hours to days. Options A and B are not appropriate for patients with a pulse. Lidocaine may be appropriate if the patient is hemodynamically stable.
Nursing process step: Intervention

67. Which of the following drugs should the nurse anticipate giving to a patient suffering from acute myocardial infarction?
A. Morphine
B. Sodium bicarbonate
C. Atropine
D. Adenosine (Adenocard)

CORRECT ANSWER—A. *Rationales:* A patient with acute myocardial infarction may receive morphine to decrease pain, anxiety, and myocardial oxygen consumption. Sodium bicarbonate is not indicated for this patient. Atropine is given only for symptomatic bradycardias. Adenosine is given to patients with supraventricular tachycardias.
Nursing process step: Intervention

68. Which of the following characterizes complete atrioventricular (AV) block?
A. The atria and ventricles beat independently of one another.
B. The PR interval is greater than 0.20 second.
C. There is a cyclical prolongation of the PR interval.
D. The PR interval is greater than 0.20 second and consistent with periodic failure of the ventricle to respond.

CORRECT ANSWER—A. *Rationales:* In complete AV block, there is no association between the atria and the ventricles. Option B describes a first-degree AV block. Option C describes Mobitz Type I or Wenckebach. Option D describes Mobitz Type II block.
Nursing process step: Assessment

DISASTER MANAGEMENT

Disaster Management

1. What is an event that involves less than 100 victims called?
   A. Multiple-patient incident
   B. Multiple-casualty incident
   C. Mass-casualty incident
   D. Mass-patient incident

CORRECT ANSWER—B. *Rationales:* The triage classification of disasters occurs in three tiers. The first is a multiple-patient incident, which is a common occurrence that involves fewer than 10 casualties. The next is a multiple-casualty incident, which involves air, train, and bus crashes; fires; natural occurrences (hurricanes and tornadoes); and radiation or biochemical accidents. Casualties number 100 or fewer. A multiple-casualty incident strains the existing emergency medical system but does not overwhelm the components. A mass-casualty incident is the least common. It occurs with major earthquakes, explosions, structural failures, and large-scale fires. Casualties number more than 100. There are many deaths and injuries; property damage is extensive as well. The emergency medical system and health care facilities are overwhelmed.
Nursing process step: Assessment

2. Which of the following is one of the four key components of an emergency preparedness program?
   A. Mitigation and prevention
   B. Analysis
   C. Intervention
   D. Reassimilation

CORRECT ANSWER—**A.** *Rationales:* Analysis, intervention, and reassimilation are not part of the four key components of an emergency preparedness program. The four components include:
1. Mitigation and prevention: These components are crucial in helping to curtail or severely limit a disaster's severity.
2. Planning: Having emergency preparedness plans in place that have been practiced, critiqued, and periodically updated is crucial. Such plans help assure that emergency medical systems and health care facilities can respond to a disaster.
3. Response: The ability to respond to disasters with adequate staff, a mix of personnel, sufficient supplies, and a clear chain of command is paramount to the implementation of any emergency preparedness plan.
4. Recovery: This phase assesses the number of casualties, types of treatment, utilization of resources, and disposition of the incident. Overall response is evaluated and recommendations are made. The economic impact of the disaster is assessed, and all workers should receive critical incident stress debriefing.
Nursing process step: Planning/Intervention

3. Which of the following hospital departments provides the crucial interface during a disaster?
   A. Administration
   B. Emergency department
   C. Morgue
   D. Operating room

CORRECT ANSWER—**B.** *Rationales:* The emergency department is the interface between the hospital and the disaster scene and is the institution's first "clinical domino" to sustain the burden of patient care. How the staff performs during the initial disaster response has an effect throughout the hospital. Administration's role is to support the emergency department by setting up command operations and securing adequate staff to care for incoming casualties. The morgue's role is to hold casualties triaged as unsalvageable or dead on arrival. The operating room is the second most critical area for handling incoming casualties; many of the victims may need surgical intervention.
Nursing process step: Analysis

4. Which of the following agencies is responsible for disaster management in the United States?
A. Federal Emergency Management Agency (FEMA)
B. National Disaster Medical System (NDMS)
C. Disaster Medical Assistance Teams (DMATs)
D. Federal Bureau of Investigation

CORRECT ANSWER—A. *Rationales:* FEMA is responsible for disaster management at all levels of the government. The NDMS assists in the treatment and evacuation of patients at disaster scenes. It also provides a national network of hospitals that have agreed to accept patients in a national emergency or disaster. DMATs consist of nurses, doctors, and ancillary personnel who respond to assist in the disaster area as part of NDMS.
Nursing process step: Planning/intervention

5. The Joint Commission on Accreditation of Healthcare Organizations (JCAHO) has explicit requirements for hospital disaster preparedness. Which of the following is part of those requirements?
A. A description of the hospital's role in community-wide emergency preparedness planning
B. Evidence of staff education and training in disaster preparedness responsibilities
C. Evidence of semiannual disaster plan implementation either through drills or in actual disaster situations
D. All of the above

CORRECT ANSWER—D. *Rationales:* JCAHO requires each hospital to describe its role in the community-wide emergency preparedness plan. Each hospital must also be able to show evidence of staff education and training and of semiannual disaster plan implementation.
Nursing process step: Evaluation

6. After a disaster, the nurse caring for survivors may experience stress reactions that are both expected and normal. Which of the following is not an example of immediate stress?
A. Anxiety
B. Frustration and anger
C. Physical symptoms
D. Alcohol and drug use

CORRECT ANSWER—D. *Rationales:* The use of alcohol and drugs is considered a delayed reaction to the stress of a disaster. Anxiety manifests itself almost immediately after the staff learns of a disaster. Frustration and anger occur as the victims arrive and the staff deals with the pain and suffering of innocent casualties. This emotion is intensified if the disaster was caused deliberately.
Nursing process step: Evaluation

7. Which of the following is not considered part of the four levels of a disaster response?
A. Local emergency medical service response
B. Hospital response
C. Federal Emergency Management Agency (FEMA) response
D. Multiple-casualty response

CORRECT ANSWER—D. *Rationales:* Multiple-casualty response is not a disaster response. The four levels of disaster response are as follows:
• Level I is the hospital response—The hospital gears itself to handle the incoming casualties.
• Level II is the local emergency medical service response—Emergency medical technicians, fire-fighters, and law enforcement officers arrive at the scene to assess the disaster, secure the scene for evacuation of casualties, rescue casualties, and perform field triage.
• Level III is the National Disaster Management System (NDMS) response—NDMS assesses the need for additional personnel in the disaster area and provides relief as needed.
• Level IV is the FEMA response—FEMA provides additional resources, usually funding and governmental assistance (for example, national guard deployment).
Nursing process step: Planning/Intervention

8. Which of the following statements is true concerning immediate mass evacuation?
A. It involves the evacuation of people from a geographical area in response to a potential disaster.
B. Some sudden, unexpected event has occurred that immediately threatens the health and safety of a population.
C. Residents living in a disaster area need to evacuate but may have a few hours to retrieve personal property.
D. This type of evacuation is orderly and allows time for warning the population of potential disaster; the population is given updated information if the situation worsens as well as instructions for evacuating.

CORRECT ANSWER—B. *Rationales:* Immediate evacuation occurs without advance warning and requires the population to leave belongings and property behind. A potential mass evacuation involves the evacuation of people from a geographical area when the threat of disaster exists. Those living in the area may have a few hours to gather personal belongings. Evacuation is orderly and allows time for warning the population of potential disaster; the population is given updated information if the situation worsens as well as instructions for evacuating.
Nursing process step: Planning/Intervention

9. Which of the following is not taken into consideration when developing an emergency department disaster plan?
A. How the plan will be activated
B. Who will be in charge of managing incoming casualties
C. Which patient classification system will be used to triage casualties
D. How the "walking wounded" will be transported to hospitals from the disaster scene

CORRECT ANSWER—D. *Rationales:* How the plan will be activated, who will be in charge of the incoming casualties, and which classification system will be used to triage casualties should be considered when developing an emergency department disaster plan. Casualty transportation is handled by the community disaster plan and emergency medical services.
Nursing process step: Planning/Intervention

10. Which of the following is part of the four phases of mass evacuation after a disaster?
A. Prewarning phase
B. Withdrawal phase
C. Rebuilding phase
D. Nourishment phase

CORRECT ANSWER—B. *Rationales:* The four phases of mass evacuation developed by the Disaster Research Center of Ohio State University are as follows:
• Warning—Accurate, authoritative information is broadcast. People will not evacuate if they do not perceive a risk or if they receive conflicting information. All announcements should explain why evacuation is needed, when it is to occur, and where people should go.
• Withdrawal—In this phase, evacuation must occur and must be done in an orderly manner. Studies have shown that most evacuees leave in an orderly manner in their own transportation.
• Shelter—Evacuees are moved to an area of maximum protection. Shelters should be identified before a disaster, and community residents should know the locations of the shelters.
• Return—Of the four phases, this is the most chaotic and has not been well developed. In this phase, evacuees attempt to return to their homes or businesses. In most situations, many safety concerns have not yet been addressed. As a result, this phase leads to secondary injury from unstable structures or disease from unsanitary conditions.
Nursing process step: Assessment

11. Which of the following is an example of a natural disaster?
A. Hurricane Hugo in 1989
B. The Oklahoma City bombing of 1995
C. The Bhopal, India gas leak of 1984
D. The Kansas City Hyatt Regency skywalk collapse of 1981

CORRECT ANSWER—A. *Rationales:* Natural disasters arise from forces of nature, such as earthquakes, hurricanes, floods, and tornadoes. Natural disasters create a heavy toll of death, suffering, and destruction. The Oklahoma City bombing, the gas leak in India, and the collapse in Kansas City were all man-made disasters.
Nursing process step: Assessment

12. Which of the following is a true statement about disaster committee organization?
A. The selection of committee members must be based on their ability to take action and produce results
B. The committee should have a statement of philosophy
C. Each committee member should have defined roles and responsibilities.
D. All of the above are correct

CORRECT ANSWER—D. *Rationales:* Members of a disaster committee must be chosen for their ability to take action and produce results. Each member should have defined roles and responsibilities. The committee should have a statement of philosophy that all members can uphold.
Nursing process step: Planning/Intervention

13. Which of the following is essential in the development of a disaster plan?

    A. Organizing a disaster committee

    B. Having only verbal authority for the initiation of the disaster plan

    C. Eliminating the command center for the hospital disaster plan

    D. Holding biannual disaster drills

CORRECT ANSWER—A. *Rationales:* Essential elements for disaster plan development include having an organized disaster committee, authority to develop and initiate the plan, and a disaster control (or command) center in the hospital. On-scene medical teams, although integrated effectively into some plans, are not essential elements of the hospital disaster plan.

Nursing process step: Analysis

14. Which of the following statements about disaster drills is not true?

    A. They provide excellent feedback about how staff will perform in an actual disaster.

    B. They provide an opportunity to educate the staff about emergency preparedness.

    C. They allow the disaster committee to evaluate the disaster plan.

    D. They provide a valuable mechanism for disaster plan feedback.

CORRECT ANSWER—A. *Rationales:* There is no way to know how staff will perform in an actual disaster. Drills are best suited to educating staff, evaluating the plan, critiquing the drill and making modifications, and developing interagency relationships. All these elements prepare the committee and hospital staff for an actual disaster.

Nursing process step: Assessment

15. Which of the following is not a disaster drill?

    A. Tabletop exercise

    B. Functional exercise

    C. Full-scale exercise

    D. Participatory exercise

CORRECT ANSWER—D. *Rationales:* A participatory exercise is not a disaster drill. Tabletop exercises, which are done on paper, provide a simulated disaster without time constraints. Key disaster-response personnel have an opportunity to evaluate the plan and resolve issues in a nonthreatening manner. A functional exercise evaluates one or more complex activities in the plan. These scaled-down simulated disasters focus on a few aspects of the plan. A full-scale exercise evaluates all major aspects of the preparedness program. This type of drill involves the use of personnel, supplies, and equipment to simulate as closely as possible an actual disaster.

Nursing process step: Assessment

ENVIRONMENTAL EMERGENCIES

Environmental Emergencies

1. Which of the following interventions would be inappropriate for a patient with partial-thickness burns over 20% of the body surface area?
A. Remove restrictive clothing and jewelry.
B. Assess for tetanus prophylaxis.
C. Debride all blisters.
D. Do not shave eyebrows if burn involves the face.

CORRECT ANSWER—C. *Rationales:* Blisters should be left intact because they are a natural barrier to infection. Restrictive clothing and jewelry should be removed before edema develops. Patients with burns should receive appropriate tetanus prophylaxis. Eyebrows should not be shaved because they may not grow back.
Nursing process step: Intervention

2. Which of the following statements about frostbite is true?
A. Frostbite is reversible.
B. The emergency nurse should vigorously rub the affected area.
C. Frostbite is often accompanied by hypothermia.
D. The emergency nurse should immerse the affected area in hot (120° to 130° F [48.8° to 54.4° C]) water.

CORRECT ANSWER—C. *Rationales:* Frostbite occurs from overexposure to cold. It is often accompanied by hypothermia, which may need to be addressed first. Once frostbite has occurred, it is not reversible; however, surrounding tissues should be protected from injury. The affected area should not be rubbed; ice crystals have formed within the tissues, and rubbing would damage the tissue further. The affected area should be immersed in warm water (100° to 110° F [37.7° to 43.3° C]).
Nursing process step: Assessment

3. A patient arrives in the emergency department after a scuba diving trip with friends. He complains of these symptoms: shortness of breath, chest pain, and vertigo. He is coughing up pink, frothy sputum. The emergency nurse should assist the patient to which position?
A. High Fowler's
B. Right lateral decubitus
C. Trendelenburg in the left lateral decubitus
D. Semi-Fowler's

CORRECT ANSWER—C. *Rationales:* The patient is experiencing an air embolism caused by failure to exhale on ascent. He should be placed in Trendelenburg in the left lateral decubitus position to avoid a cerebral embolus.
Nursing process step: Intervention

4. A patient has a core temperature of 90° F (32.2° C). The emergency nurse should expect this patient to have which of these reactions?
   A. Shivering and cold, pale skin
   B. Apnea
   C. Muscle rigidity, no shivering
   D. None of the above

CORRECT ANSWER—**C.** *Rationales:* A patient with a core body temperature of 90° F (32.2° C) usually does not shiver. Shivering is present at higher temperatures. Patients generally do not become apneic until their core body temperature reaches 77° F (25° C).
Nursing process step: Assessment

5. Which of the following interventions is inappropriate for a patient with severe burns?
   A. Administration of I.M. narcotics
   B. Administration of humidified oxygen
   C. Aggressive fluid resuscitation
   D. All of the above

CORRECT ANSWER—**A.** *Rationales:* A burn patient should not receive I.M. or S.C. injections because of erratic drug uptake related to decreased peripheral circulation and fluid volume changes. Administration of humidified oxygen is appropriate for any trauma patient. This is particularly important in the severely burned patient if upper airway damage is suspected. Appropriate fluid resuscitation is essential to prevent hypovolemic shock.
Nursing process step: Intervention

6. A 2-year-old child is brought to the emergency department after being found submerged in a neighborhood pool. The child is unconscious with a pulse of 60 beats/minute and respirations of 4 breaths/minute. Breathing is being assisted with a bag-valve-mask device. What should be the first action of the emergency nurse?
   A. Administer epinephrine (Adrenalin)
   B. Assist with intubation
   C. Begin an intraosseous infusion
   D. Obtain a cervical spine film

CORRECT ANSWER—**B.** *Rationales:* Airway, breathing, and circulation are always first priority actions. Therefore, the emergency department nurse should first assist with intubation. Once the airway is stabilized, I.V. access can be attempted; if unsuccessful, the intraosseous route can be established. Epinephrine is the drug of choice in a child with refractory shock. An infusion of 1 mg in 500 ml of D5W should be started and titrated to effect. Once the patient is stabilized, a cervical spine film can be obtained.
Nursing process step: Intervention

7. Which patient should be referred to a burn center?
   A. A 54-year-old with full-thickness burns over 10% of the body surface area (BSA)
   B. A 30-year-old with partial-thickness burns over 15% of the BSA
   C. A 40-year-old with partial- and full-thickness burns over 15% of the BSA
   D. An 8-year-old with partial- and full-thickness burns over 5% of the BSA

CORRECT ANSWER—**A.** *Rationales:* Guidelines developed by the American Burn Association and the American College of Surgeons state that certain categories of burn victims should be referred to a burn center. Categories include full-thickness burns greater than 10% of the BSA in patients under age 10 or over age 50; partial- and full-thickness burns greater than 20% of the BSA in other age-groups; deep partial- and full-thickness burns that involve the face, hands, feet, genitalia, perineum, and overlying major joints; full-thickness burns greater than 5% of the BSA in any age-group.
Nursing process step: Assessment

8. A patient arrives in the emergency department after suffering chemical burns to his body while at work. Which of the following is the first priority of care for this patient?
A. Remove his clothes and irrigate the burns with copious amounts of water
B. Begin two large-bore I.V. lines and infuse lactated Ringer's solution
C. Contact the poison control center for specific instructions
D. Determine the type of chemical involved

CORRECT ANSWER—**A.** *Rationales:* The most important intervention is to wash off the chemical with copious amounts of water to prevent further tissue damage. Most chemicals are safely removed in this manner. The nurse should not attempt to neutralize the chemical; neutralizing may generate heat and cause further tissue damage. Once the burn has been irrigated, determine the type of chemical involved and contact the poison control center for additional instructions. Line placement and infusion of lactated Ringer's solution may also be helpful at this time.
Nursing process step: Intervention

9. Fluid resuscitation in the burn victim may be deemed effective if which of the following happens?
A. Central venous pressure is decreased
B. Urine output is 30 to 50 ml/hour
C. Electrolyte balance is achieved
D. Level of consciousness is improved

CORRECT ANSWER—**B.** *Rationales:* The best way to judge effectiveness of fluid resuscitation is to monitor urine output. Adequate fluid volume should result in a normal, not decreased, central venous pressure. Electrolyte balance is important but may not be achieved early in the resuscitation phase. Level of consciousness in the burn patient may be affected by many things, including concomitant injuries and narcotic administration.
Nursing process step: Evaluation

10. A patient is diagnosed with heat exhaustion. The emergency nurse should expect the patient to exhibit which of the following symptoms?
A. Tachycardia, hypotension, and hot, dry skin
B. Core body temperature of 105.6° F (40.9° C)
C. Headache, nausea, and dizziness
D. All of the above

CORRECT ANSWER—**C.** *Rationales:* A patient with heat exhaustion exhibits profuse sweating, headache, nausea, and dizziness. Blood pressure, heart rate, and respirations are usually normal, and the temperature is only mildly elevated. A patient with tachycardia, hypotension, and hot, dry skin with a temperature of 105.6° F is suffering from heatstroke.
Nursing process step: Assessment

11. Which of the following statements regarding decompression sickness (the "bends") is not true?
A. A diver at great depths for long periods may experience decompression sickness if he ascends rapidly.
B. The gas that is a problem in decompression sickness is oxygen.
C. Extremes of water temperature and poor physical condition are factors that increase the severity of this condition.
D. The treatment of choice for decompression sickness is recompression.

CORRECT ANSWER—**B.** *Rationales:* Nitrogen is dissolved in solution because a diver at great depths for long periods is breathing nitrogen at greater pressures than normal. However, the "bends" can occur at depths less than 33 feet. Ascending rapidly does not allow time for the nitrogen to reabsorb and bubbles form, causing decompression sickness. Options C and D are correct.
Nursing process step: Evaluation

12. A patient arrives at the emergency department after suffering a burn injury. The area is described as white and leathery with no blisters. Which is the best classification for this burn?
- A. First-degree burn
- B. Second-degree burn (partial thickness)
- C. Third-degree burn (full thickness)
- D. Fourth-degree burn (deep full thickness)

CORRECT ANSWER—C. *Rationales:* First-degree burns are superficial and involve the epidermis only. There is local pain and redness but no blistering. Second-degree burns appear red and moist with blister formation and are painful. Third-degree burns may appear white, red, or black and are dry and leathery with no blisters. There may be little pain with third-degree burns because the nerve endings have been destroyed. Fourth-degree burns involve muscle and bone tissue.
Nursing process step: Assessment

13. A patient with suspected burn inhalation injury is tested for carboxyhemoglobin. Which of the following is the normal carboxyhemoglobin level?
- A. Less than 5%
- B. 5% to 10%
- C. 10% to 20%
- D. 20% to 40%

CORRECT ANSWER—A. *Rationales:* In nonsmokers, less than 5% is a normal carboxyhemoglobin level. Smokers may have carboxyhemoglobin levels of 5% to 10%. Higher levels are considered abnormal. At levels of 20%, a patient may experience mild headache. As levels approach 40%, the patient may exhibit dizziness, confusion, nausea, vomiting, and loss of consciousness. Levels of 60% to 80% may result in death.
Nursing process step: Assessment

14. Which of the following is the primary cause of hypovolemia in a burn patient?
- A. Increased capillary permeability
- B. Blood loss
- C. Neurogenic shock
- D. All of the above

CORRECT ANSWER—A. *Rationales:* Capillary damage leads to increased capillary permeability. Fluid shifts into the interstitial spaces, and this leads to hypovolemia. Aggressive fluid resuscitation should be implemented. Options B and C may occur if there are concurrent injuries, but they are not the primary causes of hypovolemia.
Nursing process step: Evaluation

15. Which of the following is the most appropriate nursing diagnosis for a victim of near drowning?
- A. Impaired gas exchange
- B. Fluid volume excess
- C. Fluid volume deficit
- D. Ineffective breathing pattern

CORRECT ANSWER—A. *Rationales:* Impaired gas exchange is the primary problem in near-drowning victims. The inflammatory reaction to fluid in the lungs leads to plasma-rich exudate in the alveolus, and large areas of atelectasis are present. Breathing patterns may also be ineffective. Altered fluid volume may be a concern later in treatment.
Nursing process step: Analysis

16. Why are alkali burns more serious than acid burns?
  A. They are generally full thickness.
  B. They produce liquefaction necrosis.
  C. They produce coagulation necrosis.
  D. They cause extensive damage to fascia and muscle.

CORRECT ANSWER—**B.** *Rationales:* Alkali burns cause liquefaction necrosis and loosening of tissues, conditions that increase the spread of the offending agent. Treatment includes irrigation with copious amounts of water for at least 30 minutes to prevent further tissue damage. Acid burns cause coagulation necrosis. Extensive damage to fascia and muscle is likely to occur with electrical burns.
Nursing process step: Analysis

17. Which of the following is not a reason children have a better survival rate than adults in drowning accidents?
  A. Children experience a higher incidence of laryngospasm.
  B. Children become hypothermic more rapidly than adults.
  C. Children are more susceptible to the diving reflex.
  D. Children have a relatively larger surface area.

CORRECT ANSWER—**A.** *Rationales:* Children become hypothermic more rapidly than adults because of their relatively larger surface area and smaller amount of subcutaneous fat. They are also more susceptible to the diving reflex, which induces bradycardia and redistributes blood flow to the heart and brain.
Nursing process step: Evaluation

18. An adult weighing 88 kg is brought to the emergency department after sustaining a thermal injury. Burns are partial and full thickness over 38% of the body surface area. According to the Parkland formula, what would this patient's fluid requirements be for the first 24 hours after injury?
  A. 3,344 ml
  B. 13,376 ml
  C. 6,688 ml
  D. 18,796 ml

CORRECT ANSWER—**B.** *Rationales:* The Parkland formula is as follows: 4 ml of lactated Ringer's solution × kg of body weight × % of total body surface burned. In this example, 4 ml × 88 kg × 38% = 13,376 ml of lactated Ringer's solution. One-half the total volume should be administered in the first 8 hours after injury, one-quarter in the second 8 hours, and one-quarter in the remaining 8 hours. The nurse should remember to calculate the time from the time of injury.
Nursing process step: Intervention

MAXILLOFACIAL EMERGENCIES

CHAPTER 5

Maxillofacial Emergencies

1. Which of the following is not indicated for a patient with a nasal fracture?
A. Pain medication
B. Tetanus prophylaxis
C. Antibiotic therapy
D. Topical cocaine anesthetization

CORRECT ANSWER—D. *Rationales:* The administration of pain medication, tetanus prophylaxis, and antibiotics are all appropriate interventions because nasal fractures should be treated like open fractures. Topical cocaine is used for the treatment of epistaxis or foreign-body extraction.
Nursing process step: Intervention

2. A patient who has recently been involved in an altercation arrives in the emergency department. A zygomatic fracture is suspected. The nurse should check for anesthesia or hyperesthesia from infraorbital nerve damage in all the following areas except:
A. Upper jaw
B. Cheek
C. Nose
D. Upper lip

CORRECT ANSWER—A. *Rationales:* The cheek, nose, and upper lip are all supplied by the infraorbital nerve as it exits through the zygoma. The mandible is supplied by a branch of the facial nerve.
Nursing process step: Assessment

3. A patient with multiple traumas—a right fractured femur, right clavicle fracture, and right-sided pneumothorax—is suspected of having a zygomatic fracture. The doctor orders a Waters' view X-ray to obtain a definitive diagnosis of the zygomatic fracture. Why should the nurse question this X-ray view?
A. It requires a supine position with forward flexion of the neck.
B. It requires a right lateral position with hyperextension of the neck.
C. It requires a prone position with hyperextension of the neck.
D. It requires a left lateral position with flexion of the neck.

CORRECT ANSWER—C. *Rationales:* The Waters' view requires the patient to lie prone with hyperextension of the neck. This patient would not be able to safely assume the position because of the multiple injuries. Supine position with forward flexion of the neck represents a submentovertex view that could be used if cervical spine injury were ruled out. A right lateral position with hyperextension of the neck and a left lateral position with flexion of the neck are not positions of either view.
Nursing process step: Assessment

Questions 4 through 6 refer to the following information:
A patient has congestion, green purulent nasal drainage, headache, and fever. The patient is dirty and unkempt, smells of smoke, and has no home address except "the streets of L.A.," from which the patient has recently moved. The patient has no significant medical history.

4. Considering the patient's social history and general appearance, which of the following predisposing factors may be significant to a diagnosis of sinusitis?
A. Dental abscesses
B. Cocaine use
C. Smoking
D. All of the above

CORRECT ANSWER—D. *Rationales:* Dental abscesses, cocaine use, and smoking all are significant predisposing factors to a diagnosis of sinusitis. Others include foreign bodies in the nose, allergic rhinitis, use of nasogastric tubes, and air pollution.
Nursing process step: Assessment

5. Other evidence that supports a diagnosis of sinusitis includes all of the following except:
A. Conjunctivitis
B. Periorbital edema
C. Paresthesia of the cheek
D. Opacification to transillumination

CORRECT ANSWER—C. *Rationales:* Conjunctivitis, periorbital edema, and opacification to transillumination all indicate sinusitis. Paresthesia of the cheek is present with a zygomatic fracture.
Nursing process step: Assessment

6. Which of the following statements expresses a clear understanding of the patient's discharge instructions?
A. "I need to spray one time in each nostril with the decongestant."
B. "I'll buy an ice pack to use."
C. "I'll only use this spray (decongestant) for 3 days."
D. "When I feel better, I can stop the antibiotics."

CORRECT ANSWER—C. *Rationales:* Decongestants should be used only for about 3 days. If used for an extended period, a rebound occurs and may cause severe nasal congestion when the drug is discontinued. Two sprays are recommended: one to shrink the mucosa so the second spray (dose) can reach the upper turbinate and sinus ostia. Heat treatment is preferred to cold applications. Antibiotics should be taken for the full course of therapy. Discontinuing early may cause the infection to return.
Nursing process step: Evaluation

7. Cocaine (4%) is used in the treatment of epistaxis for which of the following purposes?
A. To reduce vomiting
B. To reduce anxiety
C. To constrict vessels
D. To dilate vessels

CORRECT ANSWER—C. *Rationales:* Cocaine on a saturated pledget that's inserted into the nares assists in epistaxis treatment by anesthetizing the area. It also constricts blood vessels and thereby decreases bleeding and improves visualization of the area. Reducing vomiting and anxiety and dilating vessels are not effects of cocaine.
Nursing process step: Planning/Intervention

8. All of the following infectious processes can cause significant airway obstruction, necessitating incision and drainage and, possibly, acute airway intervention except:
A. Epiglottitis
B. Peritonsillar abscess
C. Retropharyngeal abscess
D. Ludwig's angina

CORRECT ANSWER—A. *Rationales:* Epiglottitis, an acute bacterial infection, causes swelling of the epiglottis and subsequent airway obstruction. It is treated with antibiotics, intubation, or cricothyrotomy. Peritonsillar abscess and retropharyngeal abscess are complications of acute suppurative tonsillitis. Symptoms include a septic appearance, fever, drooling, foul breath, and a muffled voice. Patients with these abscesses require close airway monitoring, incisions, and drainage. Ludwig's angina presents with high fever, dyspnea, and elevation of the tongue and floor of the mouth. It's caused by streptococcal bacilli and results in a bilateral boardlike swelling of the neck. Sudden airway obstruction can occur; incision and drainage may be required. **Nursing process step:** Planning/Intervention

9. Which of the following medical history information would not be important in the assessment of a patient with epistaxis?
A. Hypertension
B. Arteriosclerotic heart disease
C. Arthritis
D. Chronic obstructive pulmonary disease

CORRECT ANSWER—D. *Rationales:* Hypertension may be a cause of epistaxis. Arteriosclerotic heart disease may predispose a patient to a decreased ability to withstand mild hypovolemia or an increased autonomic stimulation to the heart. Medications used to treat arthritis may increase a patient's hemostatic abnormalities. Chronic obstructive pulmonary disease would not be of concern regarding a nosebleed. **Nursing process step:** Assessment

10. A patient arrives in the emergency department with obvious facial injuries. The patient has a laceration and swelling over the left eye and pain and ecchymosis on the left side of the face. The patient can close the eyes tightly, wrinkle the forehead, and elevate the upper lip. Sensation to touch on the left side is absent. Which of the following cranial nerves may be damaged?
A. Oculomotor
B. Trochlear
C. Trigeminal
D. Facial

CORRECT ANSWER—C. *Rationales:* The trigeminal nerve provides facial sensation and jaw movements. These tests assess trigeminal nerve injury: pain, touch, hot and cold sensations, biting, and the ability to open the mouth against resistance. The facial nerve has three branches that deal with facial expression and taste (anterior two-thirds of the tongue). The zygomatic branch provides the ability to close the eyes tightly; the temporal branch provides the ability to elevate the brows and wrinkle the forehead; and the buccal branch provides the ability to wrinkle the nose, whistle, and elevate the upper lip. The oculomotor and trochlear nerves elicit movement of the eyeball as well as the pupillary response. **Nursing process step:** Assessment

11. Which of the following discharge instructions would not be appropriate for a patient with a diagnosis of trigeminal neuralgia?
A. Avoid cold drinks
B. Gently wash the face
C. Instill artificial tears
D. Use analgesics as ordered

CORRECT ANSWER—**C.** *Rationales:* Instilling artificial tears is an appropriate intervention for Bell's palsy, in which the eyelid is unable to close and injury and damage to the eye are potential problems. Trigeminal neuralgia causes severe, intermittent facial pain that can be elicited by stimulating a trigger zone on the face. Avoiding cold drinks, cold wind, and swimming in cold water as well as gentle washing of the face assists in decreased stimulation of the trigger zone. The patient needs to understand that analgesic medications are indicated until the problem resolves.
Nursing process step: Planning/Intervention

12. Which of the following nursing diagnoses are appropriate for a patient with Ménière's disease?
A. Chronic pain
B. Sensory or perceptual alterations
C. Ineffective breathing pattern
D. Aspiration risk

CORRECT ANSWER—**B.** *Rationales:* Ménière's disease causes vertigo, loss of hearing, and a roaring or ringing in the ears. A patient with this diagnosis will have difficulty with sensory or perceptual changes. Chronic pain, ineffective breathing pattern, and aspiration risk do not reflect a diagnosis of Ménière's disease.
Nursing process step: Analysis

13. Which of the following best describes the proper application of a dressing after incision and drainage of an auricular hematoma?
A. Provide support for the pinna with gauze in, around, and behind it. Place a slit 4 × 4 behind the ear, cover the ear with fluffed gauze, and apply a fluff roll bandage or a conforming gauze bandage circumferentially.
B. No dressing is required; simply apply antibiotic ointment, and instruct the patient to keep the area clean and dry.
C. Place Vaseline gauze over the incision area. Cover the gauze with several 4 × 4's, and tape them in place.
D. Fill the ear canal and pinna with gauze. Cover the area with 4 × 4's, wrap with a conforming gauze bandage, then apply a fairly tight elastic bandage.

CORRECT ANSWER—**A.** *Rationales:* To reduce pain and cartilage necrosis, the nurse should support the pinna with gauze in, around, and behind it; cover the ear with fluffed gauze; and apply a fluff roll bandage or conforming gauze bandage circumferentially. The ear should be protected and well padded with a bulky dressing. A constrictive dressing causes more damage, and no dressing does not protect the ear itself or prevent bacterial invasion. Taping a dressing will not keep it in place or provide the needed bulkiness.
Nursing process step: Planning/Intervention

14. Fourteen days after an altercation, a patient is complaining of outer ear pain. The nurse notes necrotic areas of auricular cartilage, and a diagnosis of "cauliflower ear" is made. Evaluation shows that initial treatment of the patient's wounds should have included which of the following?
A. Instillation of antibiotic eardrops for 5 days
B. Incision and drainage or aspiration of auricular hematoma
C. Omission of tetanus toxoid prophylaxis regimen
D. Application of ice packs to the affected ear

CORRECT ANSWER—B. *Rationales:* A hematoma to the pinna must be drained by either aspiration or incision. The outer ear cartilage is avascular and receives its nutrients from the perichondrial vessels. Disruption of this supply by a hematoma between the perichondrium and cartilage can cause necrosis and the resultant "cauliflower ear." The use of antibiotic drops is unnecessary for this injury. Tetanus prophylaxis relates to the prevention of tetanus only. Cold packs may reduce swelling, but if they are used inappropriately, they may further decrease blood supply. Cold packs alone are not sufficient to reduce the hematoma and its subsequent complications.
Nursing process step: Evaluation

15. A patient with the following symptoms is admitted to the emergency department: gingival pain, fever, chills, fatigue, bleeding gums, and foul breath odor. The diagnosis is trench mouth, or necrotizing ulcerative gingivitis. Which of the following is another term for this disease?
A. Vincent's angina
B. Ludwig's angina
C. Prinzmetal's angina
D. Variant angina

CORRECT ANSWER—A. *Rationales:* Vincent's angina is another name for necrotizing ulcerative gingivitis, caused by infectious organisms. Ludwig's angina is a generalized septic cellulitis surrounding the submandibular gland, beneath the jaw, and around the floor of the mouth. Prinzmetal's angina and variant angina relate to coronary artery spasm.
Nursing process step: Assessment

Questions 16 and 17 refer to the following information:
About 6 hours after being knocked down by another player who was running toward him in a basketball game, a patient arrives in the emergency department. Before this, the patient was hit in the upper chest area by a thrown ball. He complains of dysphagia and hemoptysis, and the nurse notes that he seems slightly hoarse. He appears to be in moderate respiratory distress with occasional inspiratory stridor that is worsening. Crepitus is noted in the throat area.

---

16. Which of the following is not likely to be the cause of the patient's primary problem of ineffective airway clearance?
A. Edema
B. Foreign body
C. Hemorrhage
D. Fracture

CORRECT ANSWER—B. *Rationales:* Ineffective airway clearance is the most important nursing diagnosis next to impaired gas exchange related to a fractured larynx, which is described above. The airway obstruction is caused by edema, hemorrhage, or the fracture itself. There is no indication in the symptomatology or assessment that might indicate the presence of a foreign body.
Nursing process step: Analysis

17. The patient continues to worsen, and an emergency needle cricothyroidotomy is performed. Which of the following is a true statement regarding this procedure?

A. Aspiration of sanguineous fluid confirms placement of the cannula in the trachea.

B. A 20G I.V. catheter should be used for insertion.

C. This method of ventilation can be used for up to 6 hours.

D. A #3 French endotracheal (ET) tube adaptor fits on the end for use with a bag-valve-mask device.

CORRECT ANSWER—**D.** *Rationales:* Aspiration of air, not sanguineous fluid, as the trachea is entered confirms that the cannula is in the correct place. A large-gauge needle (12G or 14G is recommended) should be used for cricothyroidotomy to assist respirations effectively. This is an emergency procedure; after the patient is stabilized, endotracheal intubation or a tracheostomy should be attempted. An adaptor can be removed from a #3 French ET tube and fits snugly into the hub of the cannula for use with a bag-valve-mask device.

Nursing process step: Planning/Intervention

18. Children are more prone to acute otitis media because the eustachian tube in children has which of these properties?

A. More tortuous

B. Vertical lying

C. Shorter

D. Contains positive pressure

CORRECT ANSWER—**C.** *Rationales:* The eustachian tube in children is short and lies in a horizontal plane that prevents secretions from draining into the nasopharynx. It also has a negative pressure from the middle ear that allows aspiration of nasopharyngeal secretions into the middle ear. The tube is not tortuous.

Nursing process step: Analysis

19. Treatment for a patient with external otitis media should include which of the following?

A. Instructions for decongestant

B. Insertion of an antibiotic-soaked wick

C. Performance of myringotomy

D. Application of cool compresses

CORRECT ANSWER—**B.** *Rationales:* The usual treatment for acute external otitis is the insertion of a wick soaked in antibiotic solution or ointment. Other treatments may include culture of any purulent drainage, analgesics, abscess incision and drainage, and application of hot compresses. Decongestants and myringotomy (incision of tympanic membrane) are possible treatments for acute otitis media.

Nursing process step: Planning/Intervention

20. Nifedipine (Procardia) is ordered on a patient with severe epistaxis. What should the nurse do to evaluate its efficacy?
   A. Connect the patient to a cardiac monitor.
   B. Monitor respiratory effectiveness and rate.
   C. Order a prothrombin time in 1 hour.
   D. Perform and document serial blood pressures.

CORRECT ANSWER—D. *Rationales:* Nifedipine is given to reduce hypertension. It works by inhibiting calcium ion influx across cardiac and smooth muscle cells, decreasing myocardial contractility and oxygen demand. It may also dilate coronary arteries. Serial blood pressures are necessary to evaluate its effectiveness and to make sure that hypotension does not occur. Connecting the patient to a cardiac monitor and monitoring the patient's respiratory status are not necessary because nifedipine does not affect cardiac rhythm or depress the respiratory system. A prothrombin time would be necessary to evaluate the effectiveness of warfarin sodium (Coumadin) therapy.
Nursing process step: Evaluation

21. All except which of the following may be appropriate treatments for postextraction bleeding?
   A. Using oil of cloves at area of injury
   B. Administering Surgicel to the site
   C. Using a wet teabag over the socket
   D. Applying a pressure pack to the hemorrhagic area

CORRECT ANSWER—A. *Rationales:* Possible treatment regimens for postextraction bleeding include the administration of Surgicel, Gelfoam, or thrombin; the application of a pressure pack; and the use of a wet teabag, which may produce hemostasis from the tannic acid. Oil of cloves, another home remedy, is used for analgesia.
Nursing process step: Planning/Intervention

22. After a motorcycle crash, a patient is brought to the emergency department. The patient has a fractured right humerus, a large laceration to the right lower leg and, possibly, a head injury. At present, the Glasgow Coma Scale is 8. Two avulsed teeth are located in the patient's mouth. All except which of the following are appropriate placements for the avulsed teeth to protect them for reimplantation?
   A. In saline solution
   B. In between the patient's gum and lip
   C. In Hank's solution
   D. In a container of milk

CORRECT ANSWER—B. *Rationales:* Avulsed teeth can be protected for reimplantation in saline solution, Hank's solution, or milk. A tooth placed in Hank's balanced salt solution can remain viable for up to 24 hours. This solution rehydrates the periodontal ligament cells and renourishes cellular nutrients. The teeth can also be saved by placing them between the patient's gum and lip, if the patient is able to perform this. The patient described is not fully conscious (Glasgow of 8); therefore, this would not be an appropriate action.
Nursing process step: Planning/Intervention

23. All except which of the following statements indicate an understanding of Ménière's disease?
A. "I need to remove excess furniture in my home."
B. "I'll be glad when this is over so it never happens again."
C. "I need to stand up slowly when I get up from a chair."
D. "I may need to have someone with me whenever I go out."

CORRECT ANSWER—**B.** *Rationales:* Ménière's disease is a dysfunction of the labyrinth and causes vertigo, tinnitus, and unilateral hearing loss. These symptoms occur suddenly and last from a few minutes to several hours with recurrences over several weeks or months. Therefore, removing excess furniture from the home, standing up slowly when getting out of a chair, and having someone accompany the patient outside the house would help the patient with safety related to the symptomatology. The belief that it will not occur again is incorrect.
Nursing process step: Evaluation

24. A patient complaining of swelling to the neck and shortness of breath is admitted to the emergency department. Vital signs are blood pressure 140/88 mm Hg, pulse 98 beats/minute, respirations 32 breaths/minute, temperature 102° F (38.9° C), and pulse oximetry 95% (on room air). When examining the patient, the nurse notices that the patient's tongue is elevated. Which of the following is a priority nursing diagnosis for this patient?
A. Fluid volume excess
B. Ineffective airway clearance
C. Altered oral mucous membrane
D. Pain related to infectious process

CORRECT ANSWER—**B.** *Rationales:* This patient's most urgent problem is a potential obstruction of the airway from edema secondary to an infectious process, Ludwig's angina. The swelling is caused by edema, not a fluid volume excess. Altered oral mucous membrane and pain can be problems, but neither reflects the priority nursing diagnosis.
Nursing process step: Analysis

25. Areas to avoid when using lidocaine with epinephrine for local anesthetic purposes include which of the following?
A. Pinna
B. Eyebrow
C. Scalp
D. Vermilion border

CORRECT ANSWER—**A.** *Rationales:* Lidocaine with epinephrine should not be used on the tip of the nose and the ears because those areas lack good peripheral circulation and epinephrine has a constricting effect. All other facial areas are considered appropriate for use with epinephrine.
Nursing process step: Planning/Intervention

26. Which of the following indicates the proper position for a patient during reduction of a dislocated temporomandibular joint?
A. Fowler's
B. Trendelenburg's
C. Reverse Trendelenburg's
D. Flat supine

CORRECT ANSWER—**A.** *Rationales:* For reduction of a temporomandibular joint, the doctor should be above the patient and the patient should be in Fowler's position (upright position) with good back support. Constant downward pressure enables the mandible to slide backward into proper alignment. The other positions do not allow for the proper movement and pressure needed to reduce the joint.
Nursing process step: Planning/Intervention

27. All except which of the following are likely to have a nursing diagnosis of "potential ineffective airway clearance"?
  A. Mandibular fracture
  B. LeFort II fracture
  C. Ludwig's angina
  D. Zygomatic fracture

CORRECT ANSWER—D. *Rationales:* A zygomatic fracture does not normally cause an edematous or hemorrhagic airway problem. It is also anatomically farther away from the airway. Both a mandibular fracture and a LeFort II maxillary fracture can cause airway obstruction from hemorrhage or edema formation and bony disturbance. Ludwig's angina causes edema related to the inflammatory process.
Nursing process step: Analysis

28. Which of the following treatments would be appropriate for the nursing diagnosis of altered tissue perfusion?
  A. Incision and drainage of a septal hematoma
  B. Insertion of nasopharyngeal airway
  C. Oral suctioning of the pharynx
  D. Debridement of devitalized tissue

CORRECT ANSWER—A. *Rationales:* A septal hematoma must be drained to prevent tissue necrosis and destruction of cartilage from a disruption of the nutrient supply. Insertion of a nasopharyngeal airway and oral suctioning relate to ineffective airway clearance. Wound debridement is treatment for the nursing diagnosis of impaired skin integrity.
Nursing process step: Analysis

29. After reduction of a dislocated temporomandibular joint, the patient will have which of the following responses?
  A. Spasms of the masseter muscle
  B. Full range of motion of the temporomandibular joint
  C. Severe pain for a period of time
  D. Numbness from the injection of lidocaine (Xylocaine)

CORRECT ANSWER—B. *Rationales:* After reduction, a patient with a dislocated temporomandibular joint will have pain relief and full range of motion. Spasms of the masseter muscle occur before reduction. Lidocaine is not used in reduction.
Nursing process step: Evaluation

30. What injury does not normally have cerebrospinal fluid leak as objective data?
  A. LeFort I
  B. LeFort II
  C. LeFort III
  D. Mandible fracture

CORRECT ANSWER—A. *Rationales:* A LeFort I fracture involves the area immediately inferior to the nose and above the lip. LeFort II and LeFort III fractures involve more facial structures and are prone to cerebrospinal fluid leaks. A mandibular fracture can cause cerebrospinal fluid otorrhea, especially if the condyles are fractured.
Nursing process step: Assessment

31. A patient with a LeFort II fracture is transferred to the emergency department. The nurse will look for free-floating movement in which of the following?
A. Unilateral periorbital area
B. Nose and dental arch
C. Teeth and lower maxilla
D. All facial bones

CORRECT ANSWER—B. *Rationales:* A LeFort II fracture involves a pyramidal fracture that includes the central portion of the maxilla across the superior nasal area. It may also involve the orbit. This produces a free-floating nose and dental arch. Free-floating movement of the unilateral periorbital area does not describe a clinical situation. The free-floating movement of the teeth and maxilla describes a LeFort I fracture and the free-floating movement of all the facial bones describes a LeFort III fracture.
Nursing process step: Assessment

32. Which of the following statements from a patient discharged after postextraction bleeding indicates an understanding of instructions?
A. "I need to rinse my mouth three times a day with hydrogen peroxide until the bleeding stops completely."
B. "I need to drink warm tea and coffee several times a day while bleeding is present."
C. "I can have foods like ice cream, macaroni, and cooked oatmeal for the next several days."
D. "I can have any type of liquids, especially those I can use a straw with."

CORRECT ANSWER—C. *Rationales:* After postextraction bleeding, a patient should be instructed to eat only soft foods for several days. The patient also needs to understand that the oral cavity should not be rinsed until bleeding has stopped. The patient should avoid warm or hot liquids and should not drink through a straw. The patient should use ice packs intermittently.
Nursing process step: Evaluation

33. Which of the following products would be indicated for posterior epistaxis?
A. Merocel nasal tampon
B. 16G indwelling urinary catheter
C. Nasostat nasal balloon
D. Gelfoam hemostatic agent

CORRECT ANSWER—B. *Rationales:* A 16F indwelling urinary catheter can be used to control bleeding and provide hemostasis for a posterior nosebleed. It is inserted into the nares and into the posterior nasal passage, inflated, and pulled against the nasopharynx. Other choices include gauze packs connected to a string, the Merocel posterior pack, and the Epistat (a double-ballooned catheter). The Merocel nasal tampon is inserted into the anterior nares and swells with blood and nasal secretions, then it exerts gentle pressure on the inside of the nares. The Nasostat nasal balloon is placed into the affected nares and inflated with 15 to 20 cc of air (normal saline is inserted if bleeding stops). Gelfoam is an absorbable hemostatic agent that stimulates coagulation. The Merocel nasal tampon, the Nasostat nasal balloon, and the Gelfoam hemostatic agent are used for anterior epistaxis.
Nursing process step: Planning/Intervention

MEDICAL EMERGENCIES AND COMMUNICABLE DISEASES

CHAPTER 6

Medical Emergencies and Communicable Diseases

1. The signs and symptoms associated with diphtheria include which of the following?

A. High fever, cervical adenopathy, and a beefy red pharynx

B. Sore throat, fever, lymphedema, fatigue, and an enlarged spleen

C. Fever and enlarged cervical nodes with a gray membrane attached to the pharynx

D. Sore throat, voice changes, dysphagia, and white lesions in the pharynx

CORRECT ANSWER—C. *Rationales:* Option C strongly indicates a diagnosis of diphtheria, especially in the patient who has an incomplete or questionable immunization status. Option A is associated with a diagnosis of group A streptococcal infections. Option B is commonly found in the patient diagnosed with infectious mononucleosis. Option D is more likely with thrush or streptococcal infection.
Nursing process step: Assessment

2. Hepatitis A is least likely to be transmitted through which of the following?

A. Sexual contact

B. Oral-fecal route

C. Contaminated food, shellfish, or milk products

D. Blood

CORRECT ANSWER—D. *Rationales:* Blood is the primary mode of transmission for hepatitis B and C. The primary mode of transmission for hepatitis A is through fecal contamination of food or water. Hepatitis A is also commonly transmitted through sexual contact with people previously diagnosed with hepatitis A.
Nursing process step: Assessment

3. A patient has diffuse urticaria, facial swelling, and mild respiratory distress after eating at a friend's house. What is the nurse's priority in caring for this patient?

A. Administer epinephrine (Adrenalin), 0.3 ml of a 1:1,000 solution S.C.

B. Obtain vital signs

C. Deliver high-flow oxygen

D. Initiate I.V. access

CORRECT ANSWER:—C. *Rationales:* The priority in treating a medical emergency is establishing or maintaining an airway and supplementing respiratory effort. Options A, B, and D are also appropriate interventions for a patient having an allergic or anaphylactic reaction. These interventions should follow airway and breathing interventions.
Nursing process step: Intervention

4. To prevent transmission of hepatitis, the health care worker should do all except which of the following?
   A. Wash hands after every patient contact.
   B. Obtain a single hepatitis B virus (HBV) vaccine immunization before exposure.
   C. Place all patients with hepatitis A on enteric precautions.
   D. Avoid recapping needles.

CORRECT ANSWER—**B.** *Rationales:* A single dose of the vaccine HBV alone does not give an employee active immunity. The employee should obtain a series of three HBV vaccines in this order: The second and third doses should be obtained 1 and 6 months after the first dose. Universal precautions and handwashing should be practiced during the treatment of all patients. Because transmission of hepatitis A is primarily through the fecal route, enteric precautions should be initiated. Recapping needles greatly increases the employee's risk of getting unintentional puncture wounds.
Nursing process step: Intervention

5. Clinical manifestations of acquired immunodeficiency syndrome (AIDS) include all except which of the following?
   A. Sore throat
   B. Trismus
   C. Kaposi's sarcoma
   D. Dementia

CORRECT ANSWER—**B.** *Rationales:* Trismus is not a symptom of AIDS. Trismus, present in a patient with tetany, is marked by painful spasms of the masticatory muscles. Options A, C, and D are common developments of AIDS-related diseases. A sore throat suggests oral candidiasis. Kaposi's sarcoma, the most common neoplasm found in a patient with AIDS, appears as blue to violet lesions. Dementia occurs from cortical atrophy.
Nursing process step: Assessment

6. Toxic effects of zidovudine (Retrovir) may be indicated by which of the following laboratory results?
   A. Platelet count: 300,000 mm^3
   B. White blood cell (WBC) count: 2.9×10^3/mm^3
   C. Hematocrit: 44%
   D. Potassium level: 5 mEq/L

CORRECT ANSWER—**B.** *Rationales:* The toxic effects of zidovudine result in reduced WBC count, bone marrow suppression, anemia, and low platelet count. The normal platelet range is 100,000 to 500,000 per mm^3. Hematocrit, an indicator of anemia, is normal in the range of 36% to 50%. Potassium levels, normally 3.5 to 5.5 mEq/L, are unaffected by zidovudine.
Nursing process step: Evaluation

7. Laboratory findings on the cerebrospinal fluid of a patient diagnosed with meningitis show all except which of the following?
   A. Elevated protein level
   B. Elevated glucose level
   C. Purulent appearance
   D. Leukocytes

CORRECT ANSWER—B. *Rationales:* The glucose level in a patient diagnosed with bacterial meningitis is decreased. It may be normal in viral meningitis. An elevated protein level is seen in most cases of meningitis. Protein levels are higher in bacterial meningitis than in viral meningitis. Generally, cerebrospinal fluid is purulent or turbid. Trauma during a lumbar puncture may cause the sample to appear bloody. In bacterial meningitis, the cells that are identified in a positive cerebrospinal fluid sample are predominantly polymorphonuclear leukocytes; in viral meningitis, they are lymphocytes.
Nursing process step: Analysis

8. Signs of meningitis include which of the following?
   A. Cullen's sign
   B. Koplik's spots
   C. Kernig's sign
   D. A and C

CORRECT ANSWER—C. *Rationales:* In Kernig's sign, the patient is in the supine position with knees flexed; a leg is flexed then at the hip so that the thigh is brought to a position perpendicular to the trunk. An attempt is then made to extend the knee. If meningeal irritation is present, the knee cannot be extended and attempts to extend the knee result in pain. Other common symptoms include stiff neck, headache, and fever. Cullen's sign is the bluish discoloration of the periumbilical skin due to intraperitoneal hemorrhage. Koplik's spots are reddened areas with grayish blue centers that are found on the buccal mucosa of a patient with measles.
Nursing process step: Assessment

9. Diuretics are indicated as part of the treatment regimen for edema and hypertension. Which of the following is one of the most potent types of loop diuretic?
   A. Mannitol (Osmitrol)
   B. Furosemide (Lasix)
   C. Hydrochlorothiazide (HydroDIURIL)
   D. Spironolactone (Aldactone)

CORRECT ANSWER—B. *Rationales:* Furosemide acts by blocking the reabsorption of sodium chloride, which causes a significant diuresis of isotonic urine. Loop diuretics also cause the renal vasculature to vasodilate, which increases their effect. Mannitol is an osmotic diuretic, which, when present, exerts an osmotic effect, causing water diuresis. Hydrochlorothiazide inhibits the reabsorption of sodium in the loop of Henle. One of the potassium-sparing diuretics, spironolactone promotes potassium reabsorption and sodium secretion, which produces a mild diuretic effect.
Nursing process step: Intervention

10. A patient on diuretic therapy is instructed to eat foods that are high in potassium. The selection of which of the following foods indicates the need for further patient education?
    A. Potatoes
    B. Honey
    C. Beef
    D. Cheese

CORRECT ANSWER—B. *Rationales:* Excellent sources of potassium are cheese, beans, potatoes, broccoli, milk, and beef. Honey has a moderate amount of iron but has inappreciable amounts of potassium.
Nursing process step: Evaluation

Questions 11 through 13 refer to the following information:
 A patient in severe respiratory distress is brought to the emergency department. On arrival, the patient's vital signs are temperature 101° F rectally, pulse 114 beats/minute, respirations 36 breaths/minute and labored, and blood pressure 100/58 mm Hg. The patient demonstrates the use of accessory muscles and is unable to speak in full sentences. Oxygen is administered at 15 L by way of a nonrebreather mask; a chest X-ray is ordered. Noninvasive monitoring reveals sinus tachycardia and a pulse oximetry reading of 94%. Thirty minutes later, family members arrive and inform the staff of the patient's recent complaints of cough, night sweats, weight loss, and blood-tinged sputum. Respiratory isolation is initiated, and the patient is evaluated for a probable diagnosis of tuberculosis.

---

11. The use of isoniazid (Laniazid) is contraindicated in which of these patients?
    A. Patients diagnosed with coronary artery disease
    B. Patients receiving diuretic therapy
    C. Patients taking phenytoin (Dilantin)
    D. Patients with glaucoma

CORRECT ANSWER—C. *Rationales:* Isoniazid is contraindicated in patients who take phenytoin. Isoniazid can decrease the excretion of phenytoin or may enhance its effects. To avoid phenytoin intoxication, adjustments to the anticonvulsant should be initiated. Options A, B, and D are not documented reactions to isoniazid.
Nursing process step: Evaluation

12. Which of the following demonstrates proper administration of the tuberculin skin test?
    A. Administration of the purified protein derivative (PPD) through a 21G steel needle
    B. Administration of 5 tuberculin units in adult patients and 2 tuberculin units in pediatric patients
    C. An immediate wheal 6 to 10 mm in diameter at the site of injection
    D. Follow-up appointment to record test results within 24 hours

CORRECT ANSWER—C. *Rationales:* Injection of the tuberculin test should result in a wheal about 6 to 10 mm in diameter. If no wheal appears, the injection was probably too deep. Another injection should be repeated at least 5 mm away from the initial site. PPD administration should be through a short (½") 26G or 27G needle. The amount of PPD injection does not vary from 5 tuberculin units, regardless of the age or weight of the patient. Reading the tuberculin skin test at the end of 24 hours results in an inaccurate diagnosis. The tuberculin skin tests are tests of delayed hypersensitivity and should be read in 48 to 72 hours.
Nursing process step: Intervention

13. The education of a patient diagnosed with tuberculosis should include which of the following?

A. Stating that the patient will no longer be infectious after being on chemotherapy for 2 to 4 weeks.

B. Informing the patient that sputum smears will remain positive for 3 to 5 months

C. Educating the patient about potential side effects of prescribed medications

D. All of the above

CORRECT ANSWER—D. *Rationales:* Options A, B, and C are examples of information that should be given to a patient diagnosed with tuberculosis. Additionally, the patient should be aware of potential complications, such as hemorrhage and pleurisy. The patient should be taught proper methods of controlling transmission of the disease: washing hands, covering nose and mouth when coughing, and properly disposing of used tissues.

Nursing process step: Intervention

14. Pheochromocytoma is most commonly found in patients of which of the following age-groups?

A. Over age 65

B. Between ages 20 and 30

C. Between ages 30 and 60

D. Under age 10

CORRECT ANSWER—C. *Rationales:* Pheochromocytoma is a neoplasm that is associated with hyperfunction of the adrenal medulla. Although any age-group can be affected, the disease primarily occurs in people between ages 30 and 60. It seldom occurs in patients over age 65. Common symptoms include sustained hypertension, visual disturbances, headaches, hyperglycemia, and excessive perspiration.

Nursing process step: Analysis

15. Excessive weight gain, moon face, muscle wasting, truncal obesity, and the appearance of a "buffalo hump" in the neck and supraclavicular area are manifestations of which diagnosis?

A. Addison's disease

B. Syndrome of inappropriate antidiuretic hormone

C. Graves' disease

D. Cushing's syndrome

CORRECT ANSWER—D. *Rationales:* The symptoms described are common manifestations of Cushing's syndrome, a disorder of increased levels of glucocorticoids and ACTH (adrenocorticotropic hormone). Addison's disease presents with hyperpigmentation, changes in sexual characteristics, and dehydration from sodium and fluid volume deficit. Syndrome of inappropriate antidiuretic hormone results in emotional and behavioral changes, hostility, anorexia, nausea, and weight gain. Graves' disease, a result of hyperthyroidism, is evidenced by proptosis (forcing of the eyes to a more forward position), fluid accumulation, tremors, and goiters.

Nursing process step: Assessment

Questions 16 through 18 refer to the following information:
 A patient with a history of insulin-dependent diabetes mellitus arrives at the triage desk. Subjective data include complaints of blurred vision, abdominal pain, excessive thirst, and vomiting. The patient has flushed skin, decreased skin turgor, and a sweet, acetone breath odor. Vital signs reveal temperature of 100° F (37.8° C) rectally, pulse 116 beats/minute, respirations 28 breaths/minute and slightly labored, and blood pressure 100/64 mm Hg when the patient is lying down. The patient is diagnosed with diabetic ketoacidosis.

16. Initial nursing intervention for a patient diagnosed with diabetic ketoacidosis should include which of the following?
  A. Establish I.V. D$_5$W at a rate of 500 ml/hour
  B. Administer NaHCO$_3$ (sodium bicarbonate) I.V.
  C. Administer regular insulin I.V. or S.C.
  D. Administer potassium 50 mEq in 250 ml of normal saline

CORRECT ANSWER—C. *Rationales:* Regular insulin should be administered I.V. or S.C. and followed by an insulin drip to increase glucose use and decrease lipolysis. Hourly glucose levels should be obtained to monitor patient response to interventions. The rate of insulin administration should be slowed as glucose levels near 200 to 300 mg/dl. Infusing additional dextrose products during diabetic ketoacidosis will result in a worsening of the patient's condition. I.V. replacement should initially be an infusion of isotonic saline. This will rehydrate the patient, who is usually volume depleted. After hypovolemia and hyperglycemia have been addressed, the solution should be changed to D$_5$W and half-normal saline. Although NaHCO$_3$ is indicated for the correction of acidosis, it should not be initiated until decreased pH is confirmed by arterial blood gas analysis. If the patient's pH is less than 7.0, NaHCO$_3$ should be administered according to doctor's orders until NaHCO$_3$ levels are adjusted. Potassium replacement is not always indicated in the treatment of diabetic ketoacidosis. Initially, potassium measurements can range from low to high. Whenever levels are abnormal, cardiac monitoring should be done to observe for hypokalemia or hyperkalemia. Potassium replacement should not be initiated until urine output is established. If the patient is suffering from acute renal failure, potassium replacement could quickly produce toxic levels. **Nursing process step:** Intervention

17. Based on a diagnosis of diabetic ketoacidosis, the nurse should expect which of the following blood gas values at room air (FIO$_2$ of .21)?

A. pH, 7.14; PaO$_2$, 70 mm Hg; PaCO$_2$, 58 mm Hg; and HCO$_3$-, 26 mEq/L

B. pH, 7.50; PaO$_2$, 100 mm Hg; PaCO$_2$, 36 mm Hg; and HCO$_3$-, 30.5 mEq/L

C. pH, 7.56; PaO$_2$, 90 mm Hg; PaCO$_2$, 16 mm Hg; and HCO$_3$-, 24 mEq/L

D. pH, 7.12; PaO$_2$, 100 mm Hg; PaCO$_2$, 35 mm Hg; and HCO$_3$-, 12.5 mEq/L

CORRECT ANSWER—D. *Rationales:* Metabolic acidosis is a diagnostic finding in a patient with diabetic ketoacidosis. Arterial blood gas analysis indicates a pH below 7.35 (normal range is 7.35 to 7.45), a condition that indicates acidosis. The respiratory component (PaCO$_2$) is normal (normal range is 35 to 45 mEq/L), and the metabolic component (HCO$_3$-) is low (normal range 22 to 26 mEq/L). Option A reveals respiratory acidosis because the PaCO$_2$ is greater than 45 mm Hg and the pH is less than 7.35. Option B reveals metabolic alkalosis, as indicated by a pH greater than 7.45, an HCO$_3$- level greater than 26 mEq/L, and a normal PaCO$_2$. Option C indicates respiratory alkalosis because the pH is above 7.45 and the PaCO$_2$ is low. The HCO$_3$-, which is the metabolic component, is normal.
Nursing process step: Assessment

18. Which of the following respiratory patterns is associated with a diagnosis of diabetic ketoacidosis?

A. Cheyne-Stokes

B. Kussmaul's

C. Apneustic

D. Biot's

CORRECT ANSWER—B. *Rationales:* Frequently seen in diabetic ketoacidosis patients, Kussmaul's respiration is a hyperventilation that attempts to correct the respiratory component of metabolic acidosis through deep respirations. Cheyne-Stokes respiration, a pattern associated with brain injury, is characterized by periods of apnea lasting for 10 to 60 seconds, followed by increasing depth and frequency of respirations. Apneustic breathing indicates lower pontine injury. The respiratory cycle consists of a prolonged inspiratory phase followed by apnea. Biot's respiration is a variation of Cheyne-Stokes respiration in which periods of apnea alternate irregularly with periods of breath of equal depth.
Nursing process step: Assessment

19. Which of the following statements is not true about the administration of dextrose in a patient with confirmed hypoglycemia?
A. Administration of 50% dextrose should be delivered with a slow I.V. push
B. It is not necessary to ensure I.V. placement before administration
C. In the alcohol-dependent patient, thiamine (vitamin B1) should be administered before dextrose.
D. Hypoglycemic neonates should receive a 10% concentration of dextrose

CORRECT ANSWER—B. *Rationales:* Because dextrose can sclerose subcutaneous tissues, the nurse must make sure that the I.V. catheter is in the vein. Dextrose is administered in a 50-ml dose, given in a slow I.V. push and followed by a continuous infusion. Administering dextrose to an alcohol-dependent patient who is deficient in thiamine can precipitate Korsakoff's syndrome or Wernicke's encephalopathy; thiamine is necessary for carbohydrate metabolism. When used to treat hypoglycemia, dextrose should be given in these concentrations: adults 50%, children 25%, and neonates 10%.
Nursing process step: Intervention

20. What might be the approximate blood alcohol level of an intoxicated patient who has seizures, impaired deep tendon reflexes, hypoventilation, and nystagmus?
A. 100 to 249 mg/dl
B. 250 to 299 mg/ dl
C. 300 to 499 mg/dl
D. 500 mg/dl

CORRECT ANSWER—C. *Rationales:* A blood alcohol level of 100 to 249 mg/dl is associated with slurred speech, ataxia, decreased reaction time, and decreased inhibitions; 250 to 299 mg/dl, sedated affect, muscle incoordination, decreased level of responsiveness, nausea, and vomiting; 300 to 499 mg/dl, impaired deep tendon reflexes, comatose state, seizures, nystagmus, and hypoventilatory efforts; 500 mg/dl and above, respiratory or cardiac arrest.
Nursing process step: Assessment

21. As a result of thiamine deficiency, patients with alcoholism may develop which of the following conditions?
A. Wernicke-Korsakoff syndrome
B. Delirium tremens
C. Vincent's angina
D. Achalasia

CORRECT ANSWER—A. *Rationales:* Wernicke-Korsakoff syndrome occurs from nutritional deficit and reduced absorption of thiamine. Wernicke's encephalopathy progresses to the degenerative brain lesions of Korsakoff's psychosis. The syndrome presents with confusion, nystagmus, ataxia, memory loss, and dementia. Delirium tremens may occur 2 to 5 days after the last drink. It is characterized by disorientation, hallucinations, and gross tremors. Vincent's infection is a necrotic ulcerative inflammation of the gums that may result from inadequate diet and sleep, alcoholism, and infectious diseases. Achalasia is a condition in which there is an absence of peristalsis in the esophagus and in which the esophageal sphincter fails to relax after swallowing.
Nursing process step: Analysis

22. Which of the following statements about administering insulin is not true?
A. All insulin may be administered through the I.V. route.
B. NPH insulin action peaks 8 to 12 hours after injection.
C. The appearance of regular insulin is clear.
D. Protamine zinc is a long-acting insulin.

CORRECT ANSWER—**A.** *Rationales:* Only regular insulin may be administered through the I.V. route. All other insulins (NPH, Lente) can only be administered S.C. NPH, an intermediate-acting insulin, peaks in 8 to 12 hours and lasts for 18 to 24 hours. Regular insulin, crystalline zinc insulin, and globin zinc insulin are clear; the other types are cloudy. Protamine zinc peaks in 14 to 20 hours, and ultralente peaks in 10 to 30 hours.
Nursing process step: Evaluation

23. Which of the following are major side effects of thyroid replacement?
A. Nervousness and tremors
B. Muscle and joint discomfort
C. Obesity
D. Adversity to cold

CORRECT ANSWER—**A.** *Rationales:* Nervousness and tremors reflect the hypermetabolic effect of thyroid replacement medications. Options B and D are clinical manifestations of hypothyroidism. Thyroid hormones alone or in combination with other medicines have been used to treat obesity.
Nursing process step: Evaluation

24. Which of the following are symptoms of psychogenic polydipsia?
A. Increased specific gravity
B. Elevated serum sodium level
C. Behavioral changes, confusion
D. Hypoventilation

CORRECT ANSWER—**C.** *Rationales:* Because brain cells are extremely sensitive to increases in cellular water, mental changes are the first observed symptoms. The dilution of body fluids causes the specific gravity of urine to be significantly decreased. Serum sodium levels are critically depressed in water intoxication (116 mEq/L). Vital signs reflect hyperventilation, slow bounding pulses, increased systolic blood pressure, and decreased diastolic pressure.
Nursing process step: Assessment

25. A patient presents with complaints of fever (105.4° F [40.8° C]) and rapid pulse (168 beats/minute). Patient history reveals that the patient is on levothyroxine sodium (Synthroid). Based on this information, the nurse should suspect which of the following?
A. Graves' disease
B. Myxedema coma
C. Thyroid storm
D. Subacute thyroiditis

CORRECT ANSWER—**C.** *Rationales:* Thyroid storm is hyperthyroidism that is exaggerated by stress or infection. It is manifested by fever and increased pulse rate. Other symptoms include hypotension, vomiting, hyperreflexia, and extreme irritability. Graves' disease is characterized by hyperthyroidism, diffuse goiter, and exophthalmos. Myxedema coma represents a severe form of hypothyroidism and is manifested by coma, hypothermia, and hyponatremia. Subacute thyroiditis is a self-limiting inflammation of the thyroid gland from a viral infection.
Nursing process step: Assessment

26. What does a positive Chvostek's sign indicate?
   A. Hypocalcemia
   B. Hyponatremia
   C. Hypokalemia
   D. Hypermagnesemia

CORRECT ANSWER—**A.** *Rationales:* Chvostek's sign is elicited by tapping the patient's face lightly over the facial nerve, just below the temple. A calcium deficit is suggested if the facial muscles twitch. Hyponatremia is identified by the symptoms of weight loss, abdominal cramping, muscle weakness, headache, and postural hypotension. Hypokalemia presents with paralytic ileus and muscle weakness. Hypermagnesemia is marked by loss of deep tendon reflexes, coma, and cardiac arrest.
Nursing process step: Analysis

27. Signs and symptoms of dehydration include all except which of the following?
   A. Increased hematocrit
   B. Tachycardia
   C. Decreased body temperature
   D. Oliguria

CORRECT ANSWER—**C.** *Rationales:* Body temperature increases in a patient with water deficit because there is less water available for thermoregulation. Signs and symptoms of dehydration include flushed and dry skin, dry mucosa, decreased blood pressure, increased pulse rate, elevated blood urea nitrogen level and hematocrit, abnormal electrolyte levels, thirst, weight loss, and decreased urine output.
Nursing process step: Assessment

28. What is the primary treatment for a patient diagnosed with hypernatremia?
   A. Administer sodium polystyrene sulfonate (Kayexalate)
   B. Replace fluid
   C. Administer diuretics
   D. Administer activated charcoal

CORRECT ANSWER—**B.** *Rationales:* The primary treatment for a patient with hypernatremia is fluid replacement. The choice of fluid should be determined by the cause of the imbalance. If the patient is hypovolemic, fluid replacement should begin with normal saline and proceed to half-normal saline. If the cause of the hypernatremia is pure water loss, the fluid of choice is D_5W. Administering Kayexalate, which contains up to 10 g of sodium, will increase the serum sodium level. Hypernatremia is associated with using diuretics. Activated charcoal is ineffective in absorbing sodium and other small electrolytes.
Nursing process step: Intervention

Questions 29 through 31 refer to the following information:
A black male child weighing 18 kg is brought by his mother for evaluation. The mother states that the child is inconsolable. The child's rectal temperature is 102.8° F (39.3° C). Nursing assessment reveals swollen hands, primarily over the joints, and icteric sclera.

---

29. Based on the information above, the child is evaluated for which of the following potential diagnoses?
  A. Meningitis
  B. Hepatitis
  C. Discoid lupus
  D. Sickle cell disease

CORRECT ANSWER—D. *Rationales:* Sickle cell disease is an inherited disorder that primarily affects West African and African-American blacks. Children generally do not show sickled cells until late in the first year of life. The pain is caused by localized bone marrow necrosis that often affects the long bones, spine, pelvis, and chest. Children primarily complain of pain in their hands or feet; the pain is usually accompanied by swelling. A diagnosis of meningitis is not consistent with findings of joint swelling and jaundice. Signs of meningitis include fever, petechial rash, nuchal rigidity, and irritability. Hepatitis is manifested by low-grade fever, jaundice, clay-colored stools, concentrated urine, and hepatomegaly. Discoid lupus affects the connective tissue of the skin. It is identified by malar erythema (butterfly rash), arthralgia, fever, and changes in behavior.
Nursing process step: Analysis

30. The 18-kg child continues to be febrile, so an antipyretic is ordered. The nurse should administer which of the following drugs?
  A. Acetaminophen (Tylenol), 80 mg
  B. Ibuprofen (Motrin), 180 mg
  C. Aspirin (salicylate), five chewable children's aspirin (1 tablet = 81 mg)
  D. Ketorolac (Toradol), 10 mg

CORRECT ANSWER—B. *Rationales:* The standard dose for children's ibuprofen is 10 mg/kg (18 kg × 10 mg = 180 mg). Acetaminophen 80 mg is below the recommended dose. For a child weighing 18 kg, the dose should be about 240 mg. Each children's aspirin contains 81 mg of medication, so five tablets would equal 405 mg, which is 75% more than recommended. Aspirin is not recommended for children or teenagers with chickenpox or flu symptoms because of the risk of their developing Reye's syndrome. Ketorolac is not for children.
Nursing process step: Intervention

31. The parents of a child diagnosed with sickle cell disease should be instructed to do which of the following?
A. Apply cold to the affected areas to reduce the child's discomfort.
B. Restrict the child's fluid intake during crisis situations.
C. Avoid areas of low oxygen concentration (high-altitude areas)
D. Encourage exercise to reduce the likelihood of crisis.

CORRECT ANSWER—C. *Rationales:* Areas of low oxygen (high altitude) should be avoided because they may precipitate sickle cell crisis. Applying warm compresses reduces discomfort in the affected area; cold may add to discomfort by impairing circulation. Fluids to rehydrate cells should be encouraged. Strenuous exercise, emotional stress, cigarette smoking, and alcohol can induce crisis situations.
Nursing process step: Intervention

32. A patient with heatstroke may develop which of the following?
A. Hyperkalemia
B. Respiratory alkalosis
C. Metabolic acidosis
D. All of the above

CORRECT ANSWER—D. *Rationales:* Hyperkalemia may indicate damage to muscle cells and may result in renal failure. Hyperventilation may result in respiratory alkalosis. Metabolic acidosis may occur from decreased tissue perfusion.
Nursing process step: Assessment

33. A patient with a tar burn is brought to the emergency department. What is the best method for removing tar?
A. Softening it with warm compresses
B. Peeling it off the skin after administering analgesia
C. Flushing the area with cool water and peeling off the tar
D. Removing it with an acetone-based product

CORRECT ANSWER—B. *Rationales:* The tar should be flushed with cool water and peeled off the skin. If any tar remains, it may be dissolved with mineral oil. The other options are not appropriate.
Nursing process step: Intervention

GENITOURINARY AND GYNECOLOGIC EMERGENCIES

CHAPTER 7

Genitourinary and Gynecologic Emergencies

1. A patient enters the emergency department and complains of nausea, vomiting, restlessness, and severe right-sided lower back pain with sudden onset 1 hour ago. The patient appears slightly pale and is diaphoretic. Vital signs are blood pressure 140/92 mm Hg, pulse 120 beats/minute, respirations 32 breaths/minute, temperature 98° F. Subjective data supporting a diagnosis of renal calculi would include which of the following?
   A. History of mild flu symptoms last week
   B. Coffee-ground vomitus
   C. Dark, scant urine output
   D. Pain radiating to the right upper quadrant

CORRECT ANSWER—C. *Rationales:* Most patients with renal calculi have blood in their urine from the stone's passing. The urine is dark, tests Hemoccult positive, and usually is scant. Option B refers to an upper GI bleed. Option D refers to cholecystitis. Option A is not a precipitating factor relating to renal calculi.
Nursing process step: Assessment

2. Which of the following laboratory values support a diagnosis of pyelonephritis?
   A. Myoglobinuria
   B. Ketonuria
   C. Pyuria
   D. Low white blood cell count

CORRECT ANSWER—C. *Rationales:* Pyelonephritis is diagnosed by the presence of leukocytosis, hematuria, pyuria, and bacteriuria. The patient presents with fever, chills, and flank pain. Because there is often a septic picture, the white blood cell count is more likely to be elevated, not low as indicated in option D. Ketonuria indicates a diabetic state.
Nursing process step: Assessment

Questions 3 through 6 refer to the following information:
A 27-year-old paraplegic with a pounding, severe headache is admitted to the emergency department. Vital signs are blood pressure 240/110 mm Hg, pulse 60 beats/minute, respirations 28 breaths/minute, and temperature 99° F (37.2° C). The patient seems anxious. An indwelling urinary catheter was inserted 30 minutes ago, and 100 ml of urine is in the bag. The patient also has three decubiti in varying stages.

3. Which of the following indicates a priority medication for this patient?
  A. Nifedipine (Procardia)
  B. Meperidine (Demerol)
  C. Verapamil (Calan)
  D. Heparin sodium (Liquaemin Sodium)

CORRECT ANSWER—**A.** *Rationales:* Autonomic dysreflexia is a potentially life-threatening emergent situation that occurs in quadriplegics and high-cord-lesion (above T-6) paraplegics. The priority is to lower the blood pressure by using nifedipine. Lowering the blood pressure should eliminate the headache. Meperidine would not lower blood pressure. Verapamil is contraindicated because it is used to treat supraventricular tachycardia. Heparin sodium should not be used because there is a potential for a cerebral or subarachnoid bleed from hypertension.
Nursing process step: Planning/Intervention

4. What is another symptom that might occur in this patient?
  A. Flushing of skin below the lesion
  B. Pale, cool skin above the cord lesion
  C. Diaphoresis above the cord lesion
  D. Increased temperature below the cord lesion

CORRECT ANSWER—**C.** *Rationales:* Autonomic dysreflexia occurs as a result of autonomic responses to stimuli. Autonomic dysreflexia then causes an increase in sympathetic responses above the splanchnic outflow level. The increase in turn causes cutaneous vasodilation above the cord lesion (flushing and excessive sweating) and cutaneous vasoconstriction below the lesion (pallor, coolness). Thus, options A, B, and D are incorrect.
Nursing process step: Assessment

5. Potential precipitating factors of this disorder include all except which of the following?
  A. Rectal impaction
  B. Skin lesions
  C. Catheter manipulation
  D. Bladder distention

CORRECT ANSWER—**D.** *Rationales:* The most common cause of autonomic dysreflexia is bladder distention, but this patient had an indwelling urinary catheter inserted 30 minutes before admission. Urine return was 100 ml. This indicates that the bladder has been drained. The second most common cause of this condition is rectal distention from an impaction. Other causes include catheterization and catheter manipulation; cleansing enemas; acute abdominal or genitourinary pathology; skin lesions, such as decubiti and ingrown toenails; temperature extremes; and the delivery process.
Nursing process step: Evaluation

6. All except which of the following are appropriate potential nursing diagnoses for this patient?
  A. Altered cerebral tissue perfusion
  B. Ineffective thermoregulation
  C. Fluid volume excess
  D. Increased cardiac output

CORRECT ANSWER—**A.** *Rationales:* Hypertension can lead to seizures, cerebral bleed, subarachnoid hemorrhage, and hypertensive encephalopathy. It can also cause retinal hemorrhages and respiratory distress. It does not disrupt thermoregulation or cause fluid volume excess. Bradycardia can lead to decreased cardiac output.
Nursing process step: Analysis

7. Which of the following is an appropriate intervention for a patient with a kidney stone?
   A. I.V. fluids at a keep-vein-open (KVO) rate
   B. Narcotic analgesics, preferably I.V.
   C. Indwelling urinary catheter, gravity drainage
   D. Nasogastric (NG) tube, low suction

CORRECT ANSWER—**B.** *Rationales:* The rule of therapy for a patient with a kidney stone is hydration and analgesia. Usually narcotics are required to control the pain. The I.M. route may be used, but I.V. is preferred. I.V. fluids are provided to hydrate the patient and help flush out the stone. Option A only provides for a KVO rate; a faster rate is necessary to accomplish the goals. An indwelling urinary catheter and an NG tube are usually unnecessary.
Nursing process step: Planning/Intervention

8. Possible causes of priapism include all except which of the following?
   A. Spinal cord injury
   B. Leukemia
   C. Bacterial infection
   D. Sickle cell disease

CORRECT ANSWER—**C.** *Rationales:* Bacterial infections are not a cause of priapism. Causes of priapism (a prolonged and painful penile erection that is usually not associated with sexual desire) include spinal cord injury, leukemia, and sickle cell disease. Other causes are psychotropic drugs, multiple sclerosis, prolonged sexual stimulation, penile or urethral tumor, anticoagulant therapy, and treatments for impotence.
Nursing process step: Assessment

9. A patient with scrotal pain that has been present for 2 days is admitted to the emergency department. Which of the following results would indicate a diagnosis of epididymitis rather than testicular torsion?
   A. Hypoperfusion on testicular scan
   B. Leukopenia on complete blood count
   C. Bacteriuria on urinalysis
   D. Elevated creatinine level on electrolyte study

CORRECT ANSWER—**C.** *Rationales:* Epididymitis is suggested by hyperperfusion on testicular scan, an elevated white blood cell count, and the presence of bacteria in the urine. An elevated creatinine level is an indicator of renal, not scrotal, disease.
Nursing process step: Assessment

10. Which of the following orthostatic readings would be of concern for a patient suspected of hemorrhage?

A. Lying: blood pressure 120/64 mm Hg, heart rate 82 beats/minute. Sitting: blood pressure 114/60 mm Hg, heart rate 86 beats/minute. Standing: blood pressure 132/84 mm Hg, heart rate 92 beats/minute

B. Lying: blood pressure 92/40 mm Hg, heart rate 64 beats/minute. Sitting: blood pressure 94/60 mm Hg, heart rate 72 beats/minute. Standing: blood pressure 86/54 mm Hg, heart rate 78 beats/minute

C. Lying: blood pressure 128/52 mm Hg, heart rate 74 beats/minute. Sitting: blood pressure 96/48 mm Hg, heart rate 94 beats/minute. Standing: blood pressure 72/40 mm Hg, heart rate 120 beats/minute

D. Lying: blood pressure 116/80 mm Hg, heart rate 76 beats/minute. Sitting: blood pressure 120/76 mm Hg, heart rate 82 beats/minute. Standing: blood pressure 130/64 mm Hg, heart rate 88 beats/minute

CORRECT ANSWER—C. *Rationales:* Orthostatic hypotension can be a sign of hemorrhage and a precursor to hypovolemic shock. It is a good test to use in the early phases of hemorrhage, when other symptomatology may be absent (a negative orthostatic test does not rule out the possibility of bleeding). An increase in the pulse of 20 beats/minute or a systolic drop of 10 to 20 mm Hg is a positive indicator of occult blood loss. Some experts say a drop in systolic blood pressure of 25 mm Hg or a drop in diastolic of 10 mm Hg is positive. Option C has both of these present. The other options do not represent positive orthostatics.
Nursing process step: Evaluation

11. Which of the following is an appropriate nursing diagnosis for a patient with renal calculi?
A. Altered tissue perfusion
B. Functional incontinence
C. High risk for infection
D. Decreased cardiac output

CORRECT ANSWER—C. *Rationales:* Infection can occur with renal calculi from urine stasis caused by the obstruction. Options A and D are not appropriate for this diagnosis, and retention of urine usually occurs rather than incontinence.
Nursing process step: Analysis

12. All except which of the following are possible complications from an ovarian cyst?
A. Adhesions
B. Peritonitis
C. Ischemic ovary
D. Mittelschmerz

CORRECT ANSWER—D. *Rationales:* An ovarian cyst can cause adhesions and peritonitis from leakage of cystic contents. An ovary can become ischemic from torsion that occurs when a cyst is twisted on its pedicle. Mittelschmerz occurs in the form of abdominal pain at ovulation. It needs to be considered in the differential diagnosis of an ovarian cyst.
Nursing process step: Evaluation

13. A patient is taken to surgery and a large ovarian endometrioma (chocolate cyst) is found and removed. Which of the following nursing diagnoses best typifies the priority concern with this particular type of cyst?
A. Fluid volume deficit
B. Pain
C. Body image disturbance
D. Altered tissue perfusion

CORRECT ANSWER—A. *Rationales:* A chocolate cyst is one in which endometrial tissue locates on the ovary and cyclically bleeds at each monthly menstrual cycle. The cyst contains blood and blood clots. If the cyst ruptures, there is danger of hypovolemic shock and fluid volume deficit. Although pain may be present, it is not the most significant problem for this patient. Body image disturbance should not be a priority problem either. Specific tissue perfusion is not altered in this problem.
Nursing process step: Analysis

14. Which of the following is an appropriate measure to be taken when collecting a gonococcal specimen?
A. The agar plate should be cool to the touch.
B. The specimen must be kept in an anaerobic environment.
C. Sterile saline should be used to cover the specimens in the test tube.
D. The fixative agent should be applied immediately after the specimen is placed.

CORRECT ANSWER—B. *Rationales:* Gonococcal growth is encouraged in an anaerobic environment. Carbon dioxide pellets should be broken once the plate is in a closed plastic bag. The plate should also be warmed for growth to occur. Specimens collected and placed in a test tube of normal saline are for trichomonas study. A fixative agent is used for *Chlamydia* detection (Pap smears).
Nursing process step: Planning/Intervention

15. In the treatment of genital herpes lesions, oral acyclovir (Zovirax) is the drug of choice. It works by accomplishing all except which of the following?
A. Providing bactericidal functions
B. Relieving local and systemic pain
C. Diminishing the interval of viral shedding
D. Decreasing the formation of new lesions

CORRECT ANSWER—A. *Rationales:* Herpes is a viral, not a bacterial, infection (although a secondary bacterial infection can occur) and acyclovir is not a bactericide. Acyclovir relieves systemic pain, diminishes the interval of viral shedding, and decreases the formation of new lesions.
Nursing process step: Planning/Intervention

16. Which of the following is an ovarian cyst that often contains hair and teeth?
A. Corpus luteum
B. Teratoma
C. Endometrioma
D. Chocolate cyst

CORRECT ANSWER—B. *Rationales:* A teratoma, or dermoid cyst, is produced from all three germ layers and often contains hair and teeth, although it can contain tissue from any body structure. Teratoma cysts usually occur during active reproductive years. A corpus luteum cyst is caused by cystic changes in an ovary from hemorrhage in a mature corpus luteum. It can cause bleeding and hemorrhage. An ovarian endometrioma is a chocolate cyst and occurs when endometrial tissue in an ovary cyclically bleeds with monthly periods and collects blood and blood clots. Hemorrhage is a major concern.
Nursing process step: Assessment

17. Which of the following is a true statement regarding treatment regimens for herpetic lesions?
A. Systemic antibiotics are not necessary.
B. Topical acyclovir (Zovirax) assists with pain relief.
C. Oral acyclovir (Zovirax) should be taken continuously.
D. The use of condoms allows immediate return of sexual relations.

CORRECT ANSWER—**B.** *Rationales:* Topical acyclovir only relieves pain and itching. Unlike oral acyclovir, it does not help prevent new lesions and reduce the duration of viral shedding. Systemic antibiotics may be necessary to treat secondary infections caused by scratching the lesions. Oral acyclovir should be taken from the onset of prodromal symptoms for 5 days. Lesions may occur in areas left uncovered by condoms, such as the base of the penis and around the labia. Sexual activity should cease from the onset of prodromal symptoms until lesions are healed.
Nursing process step: Evaluation

18. A hydatidiform mole shows which of the following human chorionic gonadotropin levels?
A. Zero
B. Very low
C. Very high
D. Normal for gestational age

CORRECT ANSWER—**C.** *Rationales:* A hydatidiform mole or gestational trophoblastic tumor demonstrates an extremely elevated human chorionic gonadotropin level. Other signs include snowstorm pattern on ultrasound, early preeclampsia, absence of fetal heart tones, bleeding or spotting, and enlarged uterus.
Nursing process step: Assessment

Questions 19 through 21 refer to the following information:
After an alleged sexual assault, a female patient enters the emergency department. She is tearful and withdrawn. No external injuries are found.

---

19. Which of the following test results provides information that is important immediately post assault for treatment purposes?
A. Negative serologic test for syphilis
B. Complete blood count within normal limits
C. Positive Rh factor
D. Negative pregnancy test

CORRECT ANSWER—**D.** *Rationales:* Treatment for patients who have been sexually assaulted include the use of prophylactic antibiotic therapy. Cultures and tests for syphilis will not be finished for several days, so antibiotics may be routinely started before receiving test results. A complete blood count does not provide vital information for this patient. It might be useful if trauma were relevant to the situation and hypovolemia was suspected. The positive Rh factor does not require treatment. It is important to know if the patient was pregnant before the attack so that pregnancy prevention medication can be started, if appropriate. Ovral (ethinyl estradiol and norgestrel) may be used but must be given within 72 hours to prevent pregnancy.
Nursing process step: Planning/Intervention

20. When evidence is collected, what should be done with the patient's clothing?
A. Shaken out carefully to look for hidden evidence
B. Returned to the patient after determining no evidence is present
C. Placed in a plastic bag and labeled with the patient's name.
D. Placed in a paper bag and sealed with evidence tape

CORRECT ANSWER—D. *Rationales:* Evidence obtained in a rape exam, including the clothing, should be placed in a paper bag and secured with evidence tape to ensure that no tampering occurs. The patient's clothing should be carefully removed but not shaken out; microscopic evidence may be lost. All clothing should be given to the police; it is their responsibility to determine if evidence is present. Clothing should not be placed in plastic bags, which cause mildewing and moisture retention. Both conditions can cause loss of evidence. All evidence collected should be labeled with the patient's name, site of collection, date and time of collection, and the name of the person collecting the evidence.
Nursing process step: Planning/Intervention

21. Which of the following should not be collected during the rape exam?
A. Fingernail scraping and clippings
B. Pubic hair
C. Saliva specimen
D. Upper thigh scrapings

CORRECT ANSWER—D. *Rationales:* As a rule, any potential foreign material, such as suspected semen, blood, or saliva, should be collected with a cotton swab moistened with saline, not scraping. However, evidence under fingernails must be obtained by scraping or clipping. Options A, B, and C are all part of the routine evidence collection.
Nursing process step: Planning/Intervention

22. A male patient has been involved in a motorcycle crash. He presents with abdominal pain and an inability to void. Guarding is present with slight abdominal rigidity. He has a laceration across the upper thigh and blood at the meatus. A gentle pelvic rock invokes pain. Vital signs are blood pressure 108/62 mm Hg, pulse 116 beats/minute, respirations 32 breaths/minute, temperature 99° F (37.2° C), and pulse oximetry 96% (room air). Which of the following interventions are appropriate at this time?
A. Insert an indwelling urinary catheter
B. Perform a peritoneal lavage
C. Complete a retrograde urethrogram
D. Complete a cystogram

CORRECT ANSWER—C. *Rationales:* The absence of urine production and blood at the meatus indicate a ruptured urethra. A retrograde urethrogram can be used to determine injury. The nurse should not insert an indwelling urinary catheter before urologic consultation. A peritoneal lavage requires the use of an indwelling urinary catheter, so it cannot be done until urethral injury has been ruled out. A cystogram may be necessary, but again, an indwelling urinary catheter is needed for this diagnostic tool.
Nursing process step: Assessment

23. A patient has abdominal pain, guarding, increased pulse rate, decreased blood pressure, and anuria. A pelvic rock elicits pain, and a large laceration is noted across the upper left thigh. Possible nursing diagnoses for this patient include all except which of the following?
   A. Decreased cardiac output
   B. Impaired skin integrity
   C. Urine retention
   D. Infection

CORRECT ANSWER—C. *Rationales:* This patient shows signs of a pelvic fracture and ruptured bladder. Urine retention is not the problem if the bladder is ruptured. The combined injuries can create decreased cardiac output from hypovolemia and impaired skin integrity and infection from the laceration. The patient may also have peritonitis and urethral injury and may need a catheter.
Nursing process step: Analysis

24. A trauma patient with a diagnosis of a ruptured bladder has two large-bore I.V. lines, oxygen, a nasogastric tube, and an indwelling urinary catheter in place. Initial vital signs were blood pressure 120/54 mm Hg, pulse 120 beats/minute, respirations 32 breaths/minute, pulse oximetry 95% (room air), and temperature 98.2° F (36.8° C). Which of the following might indicate impending hypovolemic shock?
   A. Pulse of 100 beats/minute
   B. Restlessness
   C. Blood pressure 106/64 mm Hg
   D. Request for pain relief

CORRECT ANSWER—B. *Rationales:* Restlessness is often the first sign of impending hypovolemic shock or hypoxia. A pulse rate of 100 beats/minute is actually a decrease compared with the original 120 beats/minute, and the blood pressure is close to the initial reading. Requests for pain relief are normal for a trauma patient.
Nursing process step: Evaluation

25. Which of the following would be further evidence of a urethral injury in a patient during a rectal exam?
   A. A low-riding prostate
   B. The presence of a boggy mass
   C. Absent sphincter tone
   D. A positive Hemoccult

CORRECT ANSWER—B. *Rationales:* When the urethra is ruptured, a hematoma or collection of blood separates the two sections of urethra. This may feel like a boggy mass on rectal exam. Because of the rupture and hematoma, the prostate becomes high-riding. A palpable prostate gland usually indicates a nonurethral injury. Absent sphincter tone would refer to a spinal cord injury. The presence of blood would probably correlate with a GI bleed or colon injury.
Nursing process step: Assessment

26. After falling 8 feet and landing on his buttocks, a patient is brought to the emergency department. Along with possible spinal compression fractures, what signs may be present indicating possible genitourinary trauma?
   A. Bruit at the second lumbar vertebra
   B. Suprapubic pain on palpation
   C. Slowly escalating hypertension
   D. Decreased or absent bowel sounds

CORRECT ANSWER—A. *Rationales:* A contrecoup injury can occur to the kidney after a fall that exerts force from above the kidney. The force tears the renal pedicle and causes a bruit that can be auscultated at the first or second lumbar vertebra. Suprapubic pain would accompany a bladder injury, not a vascular disruption. Sometimes hypertension occurs after an injury has been repaired. Decreased or absent bowel sounds would occur with an abdominal insult that created an ileus.
Nursing process step: Assessment

27. Which of the following vaginal infections does not require treatment of sexual partners?
   A. *Neisseria gonorrhoea*
   B. *Candida albicans*
   C. *Trichomonas vaginalis*
   D. *Chlamydia trachomatis*

CORRECT ANSWER—**B.** *Rationales: Candida* is treated with Mycostatin (nystatin) and does not require sexual partner treatment. Options A, C, and D are sexually transmitted diseases that necessitate partner treatment.
Nursing process step: Planning/Intervention

28. Which of the following diluents is best to use when giving an I.M. injection of ceftriaxone (Rocephin)?
   A. Sterile water
   B. Dextrose in water
   C. Sterile saline
   D. 1% lidocaine

CORRECT ANSWER—**D.** *Rationales:* Because injections of ceftriaxone cause discomfort, 1% lidocaine is recommended as the diluent of choice. Sterile water, dextrose in water, and sterile saline can be used, but they will increase discomfort.
Nursing process step: Planning/Intervention

29. For mothers with chlamydial infections, cesarean section is often the delivery method of choice because it decreases the infant's chances of contracting which condition?
   A. Blindness
   B. Hepatitis
   C. Pneumonia
   D. Encephalitis

CORRECT ANSWER—**C.** *Rationales:* A mother infected with *Chlamydia* can pass the organisms to her infant during its passage through the cervix. Potential complications for the infant include conjunctivitis and chlamydia pneumonia. Blindness, hepatitis, and encephalitis are not passed by *Chlamydia*.
Nursing process step: Planning/Intervention

30. Which of the following interventions is useful in dealing with the nursing diagnosis of decreased cardiac output in a pregnant patient with vaginal bleeding?
   A. Perform vaginal exam on all pregnant patients
   B. Initiate I.V. Pitocin (oxytocin) drip
   C. Infuse D$_5$W with wide open rate
   D. Insert indwelling urinary catheter for ultrasound exam

CORRECT ANSWER—**B.** *Rationales:* A Pitocin drip can encourage the uterus to clamp down and decrease bleeding. Pelvic exams should not be done routinely on pregnant patients past 20 weeks' gestation. It is vital to rule out placenta previa. Hypovolemic patients should not receive D$_5$W; it can cause a reflex diuresis instead of improving circulatory volume. An ultrasound, requiring insertion of an indwelling urinary catheter is an important diagnostic tool, but is not a treatment regimen.
Nursing process step: Intervention

NEUROLOGIC EMERGENCIES

Neurologic Emergencies

1. Damage to which area of the brain results in receptive aphasia?
  A. Parietal lobe
  B. Occipital lobe
  C. Temporal lobe
  D. Frontal lobe

CORRECT ANSWER—C. *Rationales:* The temporal lobe contains the auditory association area. If the area is damaged in the dominant hemisphere, the patient hears words but does not know their meaning. Damage to the parietal lobe affects the patient's ability to identify special relationships with the environment. When damaged, the occipital lobe affects visual associations. The patient can visualize objects but cannot identify them. The frontal lobe acts as a storage area for memory.
Nursing process step: Analysis

2. During neurosurgical evaluation of an unresponsive patient, the doctor evaluates the oculocephalic reflex (doll's eye phenomenon). When the head is rotated to the left, the patient's eyes also move to the left. What does this finding indicate?
  A. No abnormality
  B. Damage to cranial nerve I
  C. Damage to the fovea
  D. A lesion at the pontine (midbrain level of the brain stem)

CORRECT ANSWER—D. *Rationales:* In an unconscious patient, evaluation of brain stem function can be done by testing the oculocephalic reflex. When the patient's head is rotated, the eyes should move in a direction that is opposite the head movement. Evaluation of this reflex is contraindicated in a patient with suspected cervical spine injury. Cranial nerve I is the olfactory nerve. Damage to this nerve results in the inability to identify odors. The fovea is the center of the retina's macula, the area of greatest visual acuity.
Nursing process step: Assessment

3. During a neurologic exam, the patient cannot raise the eyebrows or close the eyes tightly against resistance. Which cranial nerve might be damaged?
  A. Cranial nerve VII
  B. Cranial nerve V
  C. Cranial nerve II
  D. Cranial nerve XII

CORRECT ANSWER—A. *Rationales:* The facial nerve, cranial nerve VII, controls facial expression and taste in the anterior two thirds of the tongue. Cranial nerve V, the trigeminal nerve, controls jaw movement and facial sensation. Cranial nerve II, the optic nerve, allows the patient to blink and perceive light. Cranial nerve XII, the hypoglossal nerve, controls movement of the tongue .
Nursing process step: Assessment

Questions 4 through 6 refer to the following information:
M.J. is found lying supine on the sidewalk and is brought to the emergency department for evaluation. The odor of ethanol is present. M.J. complains of head and neck pain and does not recall events leading up to his arrival in the emergency department. On arrival, M.J. is tested and has a Glasgow Coma Scale of 14. A hematoma is palpated to the occipital and frontal skull areas. M.J. denies significant past medical history and is not taking any medications. Vital signs show blood pressure 160/88 mm Hg, pulse 108 beats/minute, respirations 18 breaths/minute and regular, and temperature 98.8° F (37.1° C).

4. What is the priority intervention for this patient?
  A. Perform a complete head-to-toe assessment
  B. Apply cervical immobilization
  C. Administer narcotic analgesics for complaints of discomfort
  D. Obtain a specimen to determine the blood alcohol level

CORRECT ANSWER—B. *Rationales:* Immobilization of the head and neck reduces the risk of further damage to the cervical spine. All patients with suspected head and neck trauma should be immobilized until all seven cervical vertebrae are cleared by X-ray visualization. A complete head-to-toe assessment (secondary survey) should be performed after airway, breathing, and circulation are assessed; the cervical spine is immobilized; and the patient is evaluated for potential life-threatening injuries (primary survey). Administering narcotic analgesics to a patient with altered mental status or head injuries is not a priority intervention. The effect of narcotics on the nervous system may obscure the clinical course of patients with head injuries. Narcotics can also increase respiratory depression and hypotension in patients with head injury. Obtaining a specimen for blood alcohol level helps to determine whether the amount of alcohol the patient has consumed corresponds with the level of consciousness. Although this is useful information, it is not a priority intervention.
Nursing process step: Intervention

5. Thirty minutes after admission to the emergency department, the nurse performs a repeat neurologic exam. M.J. does not follow commands, but after several attempts by the nurse to apply noxious stimuli, he opens his eyes and moves the nurse's hand. M.J. utters a one-word response to the nurse. The nurse determines that the Glasgow Coma Scale should be which of the following?

A. 12
B. 7
C. 10
D. 15

CORRECT ANSWER—C. *Rationales:* The patient is given 5 points for purposeful movement to pain (motor), 3 points for inappropriate words (verbal), and 2 points for eye opening in response to painful stimuli. The total score is 10.
Nursing process step: Evaluation

6. Which of the following signs and symptoms may indicate the presence of a spinal cord injury?

A. Hypertension with tachycardia
B. Numbness and tingling in the extremities
C. Cloudy cerebrospinal fluid
D. Exophthalmos

CORRECT ANSWER—B. *Rationales:* A patient with possible spinal cord injury often complains of numbness and tingling in the extremities or an inability to detect sensation. A patient with injury to the spinal cord often becomes bradycardic and hypotensive. Cloudy cerebrospinal fluid is associated with bacterial infections, such as meningitis. Exophthalmos is an abnormal protrusion of the eyeball. It is associated with orbital tumors, thyroid disorders, and orbital cellulitis.
Nursing process step: Assessment

7. An ovoid-shaped pupil indicates which of these conditions?

A. Traumatic orbital injury
B. Intracranial hypertension
C. History of cataract surgery
D. Pontine hemorrhage

CORRECT ANSWER—B. *Rationales:* An ovoid pupil is a sign of increased intracranial pressure. It is the midpoint between a normally round pupil and a fully dilated and fixed pupil. Traumatic orbital injury results in a jagged-appearing pupil. A keyhole-shaped pupil is common in patients who have had an iridectomy as part of cataract surgery. Pontine hemorrhage causes the pupil to be pinpoint.
Nursing process step: Assessment

8. Pharmacologic aids are ordered for a combative patient with head injuries. The patient, who is awaiting a diagnostic computed tomographic scan, responds to noxious stimuli only when his Ramsey score reaches what level?
A. 1
B. 3
C. 5
D. 15

CORRECT ANSWER—C. *Rationales:* The Modified Ramsey Score for Sedation measures the level of sedation achieved with pharmacologic agents. A Ramsey score of 5 suggests that the patient responds only to noxious stimuli. A patient who is anxious, agitated, or restless has a Ramsey score of 1. A patient who is cooperative, tranquil, and oriented has a score of 2. A patient who responds to voice and verbal commands has a Ramsey score of 3. A patient who responds to gentle shaking scores a 4. A patient who shows no response to noxious stimuli is considered a 6 on the scale.
Nursing process step: Evaluation

9. In an adult patient with head injuries, which of the following medications should be administered before sedating the patient with succinylcholine (Anectine)?
A. Atropine
B. Ketamine (Ketalar)
C. Lidocaine (Xylocaine)
D. Meperidine (Demerol)

CORRECT ANSWER—C. *Rationales:* Succinylcholine is a neuromuscular blocking agent that can increase intracranial pressure in patients with head injuries. Administering 1 mg/kg of lidocaine provides intracranial pressure control. Atropine is the premedication of choice for children receiving succinylcholine because it decreases the bradycardia that occurs with succinylcholine administration. Ketamine and meperidine are contraindicated in head-injured patients because they increase intracranial pressure.
Nursing process step: Intervention

10. A patient with an intracranial pressure reading of 8 mm Hg exhibits which of these clinical manifestations?
A. Widening pulse pressure
B. Hyperthermia
C. Cheyne-Stokes respirations
D. None of the above

CORRECT ANSWER—D. *Rationales:* Normal intracranial pressure should be less than 10 mm Hg when measured at the foramen of Monro. An intracranial pressure reading of 8 mm Hg is considered within normal limits. Widening pulse pressure, hyperthermia, and Cheyne-Stokes respirations are signs of increased intracranial pressure.
Nursing process step: Assessment

11. Which of the following interventions reduces the risk of complications in a patient with head injury?
A. Frequent suctioning of the airway
B. Administering meperidine (Demerol) for pain
C. Maintaining the patient in Trendelenburg position
D. Administering mannitol (Osmitrol)

CORRECT ANSWER—D. *Rationales:* Mannitol is an osmotic diuretic that decreases intracranial pressure. Suctioning the patient's airway should be minimized to prevent increased intracranial pressure. Meperidine should be used cautiously in a patient with head injury or increased intracranial pressure; the drug's respiratory depressant effects are considerably enhanced in these situations. Patients with head injury should have their heads elevated 30 degrees to promote venous drainage. Placing a patient in Trendelenburg position obstructs venous return from the brain and increases intracranial pressure.
Nursing process step: Intervention

12. Early symptoms of multiple sclerosis include all except which of the following?
A. Diplopia
B. Scotomas
C. Blindness
D. Paralysis

CORRECT ANSWER—D. *Rationales:* Paralysis is a late symptom of multiple sclerosis. Motor symptoms initially present as weakness and then progress to paralysis. Included in the early signs and symptoms of multiple sclerosis are diplopia (blurred vision), scotomas (spots before the eyes), tremor, blindness, weakness, fatigue, bowel and bladder incontinence, and emotional instability.
Nursing process step: Assessment

13. P.B. is brought by ambulance to the emergency department. The patient's chief complaint is lethargy. Two days ago, the patient had been in a high-speed motor vehicle crash and had refused care. Since that time, the patient has complained of headaches and drowsiness. Her friend states that she is now difficult to wake up. Assessment reveals a right pupil that is fixed and dilated with papilledema present. The Glasgow Coma Scale is 8. What signs does the patient exhibit?
A. Subdural hematoma
B. Epidural hematoma
C. Diffuse axonal injury
D. Postconcussion syndrome

CORRECT ANSWER—A. *Rationales:* A subdural hematoma occurring between the dura mater and the arachnoid layer of the meninges is bleeding. The bleeding causes direct pressure to the surface of the brain. Signs and symptoms appear within 48 hours (acute) and can be delayed as long as several months (chronic). Symptoms of an epidural hematoma include a history of momentary loss of consciousness that is followed by a lucid period. After that, the patient's mental status deteriorates. The clinical manifestations of a diffuse axonal injury are immediate and prolonged coma with decorticate or decerebrate posturing. Manifestations of postconcussion syndrome include headache, dizziness, irritability, poor judgment, and insomnia.
Nursing process step: Analysis

14. Which area of the brain controls the respiratory and cardiac systems?
A. Medulla
B. Frontal lobe
C. Diencephalon
D. Hypothalamus

CORRECT ANSWER—**A.** *Rationales:* The medulla controls the rate and depth of respirations, the arterioles, and blood pressure. Severe injury to this area generally results in death. The medulla also controls yawning, coughing, vomiting, and hiccoughing. The frontal lobe of the cerebrum controls personality, judgment, thought, and logic. The diencephalon contains the thalamus, which is the sensory pathway between the spinal cord and the cortex of the brain. The hypothalamus regulates body temperature, heart rate, appetite, and sleep.
Nursing process step: Evaluation

15. Which of the following is a delayed sign of a basilar skull fracture?
A. Battle's sign
B. Headache
C. Decreased level of consciousness
D. Respiratory irregularities

CORRECT ANSWER—**A.** *Rationales:* All the options listed are symptoms of a basilar skull fracture. Battle's sign, a later manifestation, may not become evident until 12 to 24 hours after injury.
Nursing process step: Assessment

16. Which of the following head injuries results in a collection of blood between the skull and the dura mater?
A. Subdural hematoma
B. Subarachnoid hemorrhage
C. Epidural hematoma
D. Contusion

CORRECT ANSWER—**C.** *Rationales:* An epidural hematoma results from blood collecting between the skull and the dura mater. A subdural hematoma is frequently caused by trauma or violent shaking and results in a collection of venous blood between the dura mater and the arachnoid mater. A subarachnoid hemorrhage is a collection of blood between the pia mater and the arachnoid membrane. A contusion is a bruise on the surface of the brain.
Nursing process step: Evaluation

Questions 17 through 19 refer to the following information:
A mother brings her 1-year-old child to the emergency department and complains that the child is "not acting right" since falling down the stairs 2 hours ago. The child is dirty and wearing clothing that is inappropriate for the cold weather. The child cries when the head and neck are palpated. During the exam, the child is inconsolable and bruises at various stages of healing are noted on the buttocks and back. As the doctor enters the room, the child begins seizing.

17. Based on the history above, the child is evaluated for which of the following conditions?
   A. Coagulation disorder
   B. Meningitis
   C. Subarachnoid hemorrhage
   D. Leukemia

CORRECT ANSWER—C. *Rationales:* The child has classic signs of a subarachnoid hemorrhage. A subarachnoid hemorrhage is caused by arterial disruption that leads to the collection of blood between the pia mater and the arachnoid membrane. This injury is frequently associated with child abuse. A patient with a history of coagulation or hematologic disorders may present with ecchymoses, petechiae (in platelet disorders), or purpura. However, when assessing any patient, the history, psychological findings, and patient's appearance must also be considered. It is important to determine if the signs and symptoms are consistent with the patient history. Meningitis is associated with lethargy, irritability, fever, seizures, and headache. Petechiae and purpura present in meningococcemia. Again, it is important to determine if the signs and symptoms are consistent with the patient history.
Nursing process step: Assessment

18. What is the immediate intervention for this patient?
   A. Administer lorazepam (Ativan) I.V.
   B. Administer oxygen by way of a nonrebreather mask at 15 L/minute
   C. Establish I.V. access
   D. Immobilize the cervical spine

CORRECT ANSWER—D. *Rationales:* Based on the history of falling down stairs, the cervical spine must be stabilized to prevent injury to the spinal cord until no cervical fracture is seen on the X-ray. Airway, breathing, and circulation are the next priority during rapid primary assessment. Lorazepam is effective in controlling seizure activity and may be administered either I.M. or I.V. The priority in the seizing patient with suspected cervical spine injury is to prevent further insult to the cervical spine. After the cervical spine is immobilized, the patient should be provided supplemental oxygen if respiratory effort becomes insufficient. The postictal patient should be maintained in the side-lying position to prevent aspiration or occlusion of the airway by the tongue. After immobilizing the cervical spine and doing a rapid primary survey, the nurse should establish I.V. access to facilitate pharmacologic interventions.
Nursing process step: Intervention

19. Which would be an ominous sign in this child?
   A. Heart rate of 60 beats/minute
   B. Respiratory rate of 30 breaths/minute
   C. Capillary refill at 3 seconds
   D. Positive Babinski reflex

CORRECT ANSWER—A. *Rationales:* The normal heart rate for a 1-year-old child ranges from 90 to 120 beats/minute. Bradycardia is a sign of increasing intracranial pressure. Normally, respirations for a child this age range from 20 to 30 breaths/minute. Capillary refill less than or equal to 3 seconds is a normal finding. After 2 years of age or after the child is walking, the Babinski reflex is an abnormal finding.
Nursing process step: Assessment

20. While caring for the patient with a ventriculostomy, the nurse notices that the intracranial pressure is 30 mm Hg. The nurse assesses the patient and the intracranial pressure monitor and determines that the drain is open. Immediate interventions should include which of the following?
   A. Hyperventilate the patient with 100% oxygen
   B. Lower the head of the bed to the Trendelenburg position
   C. Close the stopcock on the ventriculostomy to prevent drainage of spinal fluid
   D. All of the above

CORRECT ANSWER—A. *Rationales:* Hyperventilating the patient with 100% oxygen causes vasoconstriction, which reduces cerebral blood volume. Lowering the head of the bed would increase the pressure on the brain. Ideally, the head of the bed should be maintained at 30 degrees, and hyperextension, flexion, and rotation of the head should be avoided. Closing the stopcock on the ventriculostomy causes the intracranial pressure to rise because there is no longer an outlet for cerebrospinal fluid.
Nursing process step: Intervention

21. A patient involved in a 20-foot fall is determined to have a fracture with spinal cord transection at the level of C-6. This injury results in which of the following findings?
   A. Quadriplegia with diaphragmatic breathing and gross arm movements
   B. Quadriplegia with loss of respiratory function
   C. Paraplegia with variable loss of intercostal and abdominal muscle use
   D. Bowel and bladder dysfunction

CORRECT ANSWER—A. *Rationales:* A patient with an injury at the level of C-6 has quadriplegia with diaphragmatic breathing and gross arm movements. The patient may also suffer from hypotension and an atonic bladder. An injury at the level of C-2 results in total loss of respiratory function and movement from the shoulders down. Paraplegia with loss of portions of intercostal and abdominal muscles is indicative of injury at T-1 to L-2. An injury below L-2 results in mixed motor sensory loss and bowel and bladder dysfunction.
Nursing process step: Assessment

22. When administering a loading dose of phenytoin (Dilantin), it is important to remember which of the following?
A. Therapeutic blood levels should be between 20 and 30 mg/ml
B. Rapid administration of phenytoin can lead to cardiac arrhythmias
C. Phenytoin is normally mixed in dextrose in water solution
D. Phenytoin potentiates the action of digitalis glycosides

CORRECT ANSWER—B. *Rationales:* When phenytoin is administered I.V., it should not be given faster than 50 mg/minute because it can depress the myocardium and lead to arrhythmias and cardiac arrest. Therapeutic blood levels should range from 10 to 20 mg/ml. Mixing phenytoin in any solution other than normal saline can cause the drug to precipitate into crystals. Phenytoin inhibits the action of digitalis glycosides and corticosteroids. It does, however, potentiate the actions of propranolol (Inderal), methotrexate (Mexate), and antihypertensives.
Nursing process step: Intervention

23. Discharge instructions for a patient taking phenytoin (Dilantin) should include which of the following?
A. Missed doses of phenytoin can easily be made up without adverse effects
B. Routine blood studies may be necessary to evaluate anemia, which is a side effect that occurs with the use of phenytoin
C. Status epilepticus can be precipitated by abrupt anticonvulsant withdrawal
D. All of the above

CORRECT ANSWER—D. *Rationales:* Because of the slow absorption of phenytoin from the GI tract, daily drug routines can be easily adjusted when a dose is forgotten. The most common cause of seizures in patients taking phenytoin is discontinuing the medication. Patients should anticipate being on anticonvulsants for the rest of their lives.
Nursing process step: Intervention

24. Guillain-Barré syndrome is characterized by which of the following statements?
A. Most common in children and in young adults under age 18
B. Demyelination of the cranial and spinal nerves
C. Slow and insidious onset of symptoms
D. Paralysis of the lower extremities exclusively

CORRECT ANSWER—B. *Rationales:* Guillain-Barré syndrome is distinguished from other forms of polyneuritis by its acute onset and rapid progression. It is classified as a neuritis because it causes demyelination of the spinal cord, peripheral nerves, root ganglia, and nerve roots. The disease manifests itself by sudden onset of lower-extremity weakness that rapidly progresses to the arms, trunk, and face. It primarily affects people between the ages of 30 and 50.
Nursing process step: Analysis

25. Clinical manifestations of Parkinson's disease do not include which of the following?
A. Pill-rolling movement when at rest
B. Bradykinesia
C. Rigidity
D. Alopecia

CORRECT ANSWER—D. *Rationales:* Alopecia is not a manifestation of Parkinson's disease. The symptom that most often characterizes this disease is a faint tremor that slowly progresses in intensity. As the patient's muscle tone becomes more rigid, the gait takes on a shuffling appearance. The patient's face is masklike and the speech is slow and monotone. It is common for the patient to develop dysphagia and drooling. The patient's judgment becomes impaired even though actual intelligence remains unaffected.
Nursing process step: Assessment

26. Which of these medicines is commonly used to treat the symptoms of Parkinson's disease?
A. Trihexyphenidyl hydrochloride (Artane)
B. Reserpine (Serpalan)
C. Haloperidol (Haldol)
D. Prochlorperazine (Compazine)

CORRECT ANSWER—A. *Rationales:* Trihexyphenidyl hydrochloride is an anticholinergic that primarily acts to reduce muscle rigidity. The use of dopamine-blocking drugs has been linked to pharmacologically increased parkinsonism. Dopamine and acetylcholine are neurotransmitters that act on the input nuclei to the basal ganglia. When dopamine (an inhibitor) is reduced, acetylcholine (an excitatory neurotransmitter) becomes predominant and precipitates tremor.
Nursing process step: Intervention

27. Many patients with myasthenia gravis are treated with anticholinesterase drugs. What is the antidote for anticholinesterase toxicity?
A. Vitamin K analogue (AquaMEPHYTON)
B. Atropine sulfate
C. Physostigmine salicylate (Antilirium)
D. Pyridostigmine bromide (Mestinon)

CORRECT ANSWER—B. *Rationales:* Atropine sulfate is the antidote for anticholinesterase toxicity and should be available to patients on this pharmacologic routine. It corrects the extreme bradycardia that can be associated with the use of anticholinesterase-type drugs. Vitamin K analogue is the antidote for warfarin (Coumadin) ingestion. Physostigmine salicylate and pyridostigmine bromide are anticholinesterase drugs that are used to treat myasthenia gravis.
Nursing process step: Intervention

28. A 28-year-old woman presents to the emergency department with blurred vision and drooping of the right eyelid. She also complains of intermittent episodes of muscle weakness and that her neck doesn't feel strong enough at times to support her head. She tires when eating and must take frequent breaks during a meal. Several times, she has had to close her mouth using her hand because "the muscles in my face feel so weak." What is the probable diagnosis for this patient?
A. Myasthenia gravis
B. Bell's palsy
C. Trigeminal neuralgia
D. Glioblastoma

CORRECT ANSWER—A. *Rationales:* Myasthenia gravis affects two to three times more women than men until age 40. This disease may result from a defect at the myoneural junction. The primary symptom is weakness of voluntary muscles, especially those of the face. This weakness may temporarily improve with short periods of rest. Bell's palsy is an inflammatory reaction involving the facial nerves. It presents as ipsilateral facial paresis. Trigeminal neuralgia is characterized by sudden episodes of ipsilateral facial pain. Glioblastomas are intracranial tumors that present with symptoms of increased intracranial pressure and focal deficits.
Nursing process step: Analysis

29. Which of these tests is frequently used to diagnose myasthenia gravis?
A. Lumbar puncture
B. Tensilon test
C. Allen's test
D. Magnetic resonance imaging

CORRECT ANSWER—B. *Rationales:* In the Tensilon test, edrophonium chloride is administered by I.V. infusion to a patient exhibiting signs of muscle weakness. Significant improvement in the patient's muscle tone indicates a positive diagnosis for myasthenia gravis. This effect lasts for about 4 to 5 minutes. A lumbar puncture is frequently performed to assist in diagnosing meningitis. Allen's test is performed to evaluate the circulatory function of the ulnar artery. Magnetic resonance imaging is effective in detecting degenerative central nervous system diseases, malignant tumors, and oxygen-deprived tissue. None of these findings are associated with myasthenia gravis.
Nursing process step: Evaluation

30. Medications that reduce the spasticity and tremors associated with multiple sclerosis include all except which of the following?
A. Diazepam (Valium)
B. Baclofen (Lioresal)
C. Isoniazid (INH)
D. Cyclophosphamide (Cytoxan)

CORRECT ANSWER—D. *Rationales:* Cytoxan is used in immunosuppressive therapy that can occasionally induce a year-long remission of symptoms. Diazepam, baclofen, and isoniazid are associated with medical management of the patient with multiple sclerosis. Diazepam and baclofen are primarily effective in decreasing the spasms and stiffness associated with the disease. Isoniazid decreases the presenting tremor.
Nursing process step: Intervention

31. Alzheimer's disease is characterized by profound impairment of cognitive functions. Which of the following is the cause of this disorder?
A. Destruction of motor cells in the anterior gray horns and pyramidal tracts
B. Metabolic disorders
C. Cerebral atrophy and cellular degeneration
D. Degeneration of the basal ganglia

CORRECT ANSWER—C. *Rationales:* Alzheimer's disease is a neurologic and degenerative disorder that is the result of cerebral atrophy and cellular degeneration. Predominating symptoms are mental status changes, increased anxiety, forgetfulness and, eventually, the inability to recognize significant others and to perform activities of daily living. Destruction of motor cells in the anterior gray horns and pyramidal tracts can result in the symptoms associated with amyotropic lateral sclerosis (Lou Gehrig's disease). Metabolic disorders may cause altered cognitive function but can be reversed by correction of the underlying problem. Degeneration of the basal ganglia is usually associated with Parkinson's disease.
Nursing process step: Evaluation

32. A nurse determines the following nursing diagnosis for a patient with encephalitis: altered cerebral tissue perfusion related to cerebral edema and increased intracranial pressure. Based on this nursing diagnosis, which interventions are appropriate in caring for this patient?
A. Maintain the head of the bed in a flat position
B. Avoid Valsalva's maneuver
C. Maintain intracranial pressure at 20 mm Hg
D. Encourage isometric exercises while bedridden to prevent muscle atrophy

CORRECT ANSWER—B. *Rationales:* Valsalva's maneuver is contraindicated for a patient with increased intracranial pressure. The patient with increased intracranial pressure should have the head of the bed maintained at 15 to 30 degrees to promote venous return. Having the bed flat or in Trendelenburg position increases the flow of blood to the head and, as a result, increases intracranial pressure. An intracranial reading of 20 mm Hg is abnormally high. The normal range for intracranial pressure is less than 15 mm Hg. Isometric exercises should be avoided because they raise systemic blood pressure, which in turn raises intracranial pressure.
Nursing process step: Intervention

Questions 33 through 35 refer to the following information:
A woman with complaints of seeing "zigzagging lines" in her visual field after waking this morning presents to the emergency department. She now complains of a right temporal headache that is accompanied by nausea. The patient denies injury and does not have a significant medical history. She covers her head with the blanket because "the light hurts my eyes."

33. Based on the symptoms above, the patient is evaluated for which of the following conditions?
   A. Sinusitis
   B. Meningitis
   C. Migraine
   D. Trigeminal neuralgia

CORRECT ANSWER—C. *Rationales:* The patient is experiencing a migraine headache. Migraines are more prevalent in women than in men, and there is usually a familial tendency. Migraines are divided into three phases: aura (visual disturbances, confusion, paresthesia), which precedes the headache and lasts from 15 to 30 minutes; headache, which is characterized by a throbbing pain that often begins as unilateral and progresses to bilateral and is accompanied by nausea or vomiting; and postheadache, which is accompanied by scalp tenderness and muscular aching of the neck. Sinusitis is described as pain or pressure over the maxillary or frontal sinus areas. The pain can be reproduced by palpation. Meningitis presents with symptoms of fever, headache, severe neck discomfort, and irritability. Often there is an altered level of consciousness. Trigeminal neuralgia is characterized by ipsilateral facial pain from the side of the mouth to the ear, eye, or nostril on the same side.
Nursing process step: Assessment

34. Which of the following medications would the patient receive as prophylactic treatment for her migraine headache?
   A. Clonidine hydrochloride (Catapres)
   B. Promethazine hydrochloride (Phenergan)
   C. Codeine sulfate
   D. Diphenhydramine (Benadryl)

CORRECT ANSWER—A. *Rationales:* Clonidine hydrochloride is used in the prophylactic treatment of migraine headaches, especially those precipitated by dietary factors. It causes the blood vessels to be less responsive to vasoconstriction or vasodilation. Promethazine hydrochloride is used to control the nausea and vomiting associated with a migraine headache. Codeine sulfate can be given for the pain of a full-blown migraine. Diphenhydramine is useful in treating cluster headaches.
Nursing process step: Intervention

35. The patient is prescribed ergotamine tartrate (Cafergot) for treatment of her headache. The drug has a cumulative effect that increases the risk of drug overdose. Clinical manifestations of ergotamine overdose (ergotism) include which of these symptoms?

A. Altered mental status
B. Hypertension and tachycardia
C. Numbness and tingling in the toes and fingers
D. Ataxia

CORRECT ANSWER—C. *Rationales:* Symptoms of ergotamine overdose are in response to intense arterial vasoconstriction, which produces signs and symptoms of peripheral vascular ischemia. In addition to numbness of fingers and toes, the patient may experience muscle pain and weakness, gangrene, and blindness. Altered mental status, hypertension, tachycardia, and ataxia are not associated with ergotamine tartrate overdose.
Nursing process step: Assessment

36. What is the immediate action in establishing an airway in a patient with suspected neck injury?

A. Insert a nasopharyngeal airway
B. Prepare for blind orotracheal intubation
C. Perform the jaw thrust/chin lift maneuver
D. Conduct head tilt maneuvers

CORRECT ANSWER—C. *Rationales:* The preferred method of opening the airway in a patient with a suspected neck injury is the jaw thrust/chin lift maneuver. Options A and B are appropriate methods to maintain or establish an open airway. The head tilt causes the neck to hyperextend, which causes further damage in a patient with a cervical spine injury.
Nursing process step: Intervention

37. Appropriate interventions for a patient having a seizure include all except which of the following?

A. Administer oxygen
B. Administer I.V. diazepam (Valium)
C. Insert a tongue blade into the mouth
D. Turn the head or body to one side

CORRECT ANSWER—C. *Rationales:* Inserting a wooden tongue blade into the mouth of a patient having a seizure puts the patient at risk for oral injury from splinters. The patient is also at risk for aspiration of the foreign body. Administering oxygen and diazepam and turning the patient's head or body to one side are appropriate interventions. Additionally, suction should be available and side rails should be padded and raised to protect the patient from self-injury.
Nursing process step: Intervention

38. A patient arrives by ambulance for evaluation of seizure activity. The person had been arguing with her employer when she suddenly fell to the ground. The nurse hears screaming and observes violent flinging of all extremities. There is no evidence of incontinence or tongue biting. Prehospital providers state that this episode has lasted for 40 minutes. Based on this information, the patient is diagnosed with which of the following conditions?
A. Pseudoseizures
B. Petit mal seizures
C. Grand mal seizures
D. Jacksonian seizures

CORRECT ANSWER—A. *Rationales:* Emotional upset usually precedes a pseudoseizure, which generally lasts longer than a true seizure. In a true seizure, screams can be heard at the onset of the event, and repetitive, consistent movement of the extremities can be observed. Petit mal seizures, also known as absence seizures, are manifested by an absence of consciousness for 5 to 10 seconds. Grand mal seizures present with the following pattern: aura, cry, loss of consciousness, fall, tonic-clonic movement, and incontinence. Jacksonian seizures present with convulsive movements that begin in the fingers and progress to the hand, wrist, and forearm and eventually lead to a grand mal event.
Nursing process step: Assessment

39. Phenytoin (Dilantin) is ineffective in the treatment of which of the following seizure classifications?
A. Status epilepticus
B. Petit mal
C. Psychomotor
D. Grand mal

CORRECT ANSWER—B. *Rationales:* Phenytoin is not effective in the treatment of petit mal seizures. Petit mal seizures are treated with trimethadione (Tridione), clonazepam (Clonopin), ethosuximide (Zarontin), and valproic acid (Depakene). Phenytoin is effective in the treatment of grand mal, psychomotor, and focal seizures.
Nursing process step: Intervention

40. Temporary periods of cerebral ischemia may result in which of the following conditions?
A. Transient ischemic attacks
B. Hypercapneic encephalopathy
C. Disequilibriun syndrome
D. Transtentorial herniation

CORRECT ANSWER—A. *Rationales:* Transient ischemic attacks are temporary episodes of neurologic dysfunction in response to brief episodes of cerebral ischemia. Most commonly, a transient ischemic attack presents as weakness of the lower face and upper and lower extremities as well as dysphagia, which may occur multiple times during the day. Between each attack, neurologic findings are normal. Hypercapneic encephalopathy is seen in patients with problems associated with chronic respiratory acidosis. Disequilibrium syndrome is an acute complication of peritoneal dialysis or hemodialysis. Transtentorial herniation occurs as a result of downward pressure from edema in the parietal or frontal lobes.
Nursing process step: Analysis

41. Which drug class is most commonly used in the treatment of cerebrovascular accident (CVA)?
A. Thrombolytics
B. Neuroleptics
C. Anticoagulants
D. Vasopressors

CORRECT ANSWER—C. *Rationales:* Antiplatelet agents and antithrombotics are primarily used in anticoagulation at the tissue level. They include aspirin, heparin, and warfarin. Thrombolytics are part of a new drug therapy that dissolves clots by fibrinolysis (urokinase, tissue plasminogen activator, streptokinase). Neuroleptics, which are antipsychotics, are not indicated in CVA. Vasopressors elevate blood pressure and increase oxygen demands, which are contraindicated in the patient with CVA.
Nursing process step: Intervention

42. What is the treatment for a warfarin sodium (Coumadin) overdose?
A. Vitamin K (AquaMEPHYTON)
B. Protamine sulfate
C. Acetylcysteine (Mucomyst)
D. Atropine

CORRECT ANSWER—A. *Rationales:* Vitamin K is used to treat warfarin sodium overdose. Resumption of warfarin therapy reverses the effect of vitamin K. Protamine sulfate is the reversing agent for heparin overdose. Acetylcysteine is used in the treatment of acetaminophen (Tylenol) overdose. Atropine is used in the treatment of bradycardia.
Nursing process step: Intervention

43. What is the term for difficulty in transforming sound into patterns of understandable speech?
A. Receptive aphasia
B. Dysphagia
C. Expressive aphasia
D. Apraxia

CORRECT ANSWER—C. *Rationales:* Expressive aphasia is indicative of stroke syndrome on the left side (right-sided hemiplegia). Receptive aphasia is an impaired ability to understand spoken words. Dysphagia refers to difficulty in swallowing, which occurs when injury affects the vertebrobasilar region. Apraxia is the inability to perform a learned movement, such as using a comb, brushing one's teeth, and waving good-bye.
Nursing process step: Analysis

44. Brain tumors of the frontal lobe result in which of the following symptoms?
A. Jacksonian seizures
B. Personality changes
C. Visual hallucinations
D. Loss of right-left discrimination

CORRECT ANSWER—B. *Rationales:* The frontal lobe provides storage of memory, thought expression, and word formation. In addition to personality changes, a person with a brain tumor of the frontal lobe exhibits indifference to bodily functions and inappropriate affects. Jacksonian seizures are indicative of tumors in the precentral gyrus area. Visual hallucinations are manifested in temporal lobe abnormalities. The loss of right-left discrimination is caused by disturbances in the parietal lobe.
Nursing process step: Assessment

45. Which of the following is one of the most malignant and rapidly growing form of brain tumor?
   A. Astrocytoma
   B. Meningioma
   C. Neuroma
   D. Glioblastoma

CORRECT ANSWER—**D.** *Rationales:* The glioblastoma and medullablastoma are two of the most malignant and rapidly growing brain tumors. They are difficult to excise and can cause death within months. An astrocytoma is a slower growing form of glioma. A meningioma is benign and frequently encapsulated. A neuroma is an extremely slow growing tumor that arises from any of the cranial nerves.
Nursing process step: Evaluation

46. Children under age 8 are most likely to injure which portion of the vertebral column?
   A. C-6 to C-7
   B. C-1 to C-3
   C. C-5 to C-6
   D. C-7 exclusively

CORRECT ANSWER—**B.** *Rationales:* When a young child is placed in a safety restraint seat facing the front of the car, the risk of cervical fracture at the C-1 to C-3 level increases because of the fulcrum effect as the child's head whips forward in an accident. For several reasons, a child's cervical spine is more susceptible to injury than an adult's. A child's vertebral bodies are wedged anteriorly and tend to slide forward with flexion; the neck ligaments of children are more lax; the neck muscles of children are weaker; upper cervical spine facets are flatter. Options A, C, and D are more common injuries in older children and adults.
Nursing process step: Analysis

47. What are the signs and symptoms of a subdural hematoma in a child younger than age 2?
   A. Bulging fontanels
   B. Hypovolemia
   C. Retinal hemorrhages
   D. All of the above

CORRECT ANSWER—**D.** *Rationales:* A child with a subdural hematoma exhibits bulging fontanels because the sutures separate as intracranial pressure increases. An increase in intracranial pressure also causes retinal hemorrhages. Hypovolemia may occur if a large amount of blood has been lost because of bleeding from a subdural hematoma.
Nursing process step: Assessment

48. Before applying Crutchfield tongs, the nurse should tell the patient about which of the following?
A. There will be numbness in the extremities after application of the tongs
B. X-rays will be taken after each addition of weight to the traction setup
C. The traction and weights should rest against the foot of the bed to prevent unnecessary movement
D. The Crutchfield tong application will be done under general anesthesia

CORRECT ANSWER—B. *Rationales:* X-rays are taken after the addition of each weight to evaluate progress in reducing cervical spine injury. Neurologic status should be reevaluated at that time; there should be no worsening of neurologic deficit as a result of traction. The traction and weight should suspend freely to prevent interference with traction. The application of Crutchfield tongs can be accomplished under local anesthetic.
Nursing process step: Intervention

49. Clinical symptoms of autonomic dysreflexia include headache, profuse sweating, piloerection (gooseflesh), hypertension, and bradycardia. This syndrome occurs in patients with injuries at or above which of the following levels?
A. S-5
B. L-1
C. T-6
D. T-12

CORRECT ANSWER—C. *Rationales:* Autonomic dysreflexia is most commonly associated with spinal cord injuries at or above the T-6 level. This serious hypertensive condition occurs during the rehabilitative phase of spinal cord injury. It is caused by noxious stimuli that create an exaggerated sympathetic response.
Nursing process step: Assessment

50. What is the outermost covering of the brain?
A. Pia mater
B. Galea aponeurotica
C. Dura mater
D. Arachnoid mater

CORRECT ANSWER—C. *Rationales:* The dura mater is a tough fibrous tissue that makes up the outermost covering of the brain. The pia mater is a delicate layer that adheres to the surface of the spinal cord and the brain. The galea aponeurotica is a dense, fibrous tissue that covers the skull and absorbs the forces of external trauma. The arachnoid mater is a fine fibrous layer that lies between the dura mater and the pia mater.
Nursing process step: Analysis

51. What is the function of cerebrospinal fluid?
A. Cushions the brain and spinal cord
B. Acts as an insulator to maintain a constant spinal fluid temperature
C. Acts as a barrier to bacteria
D. Produces cerebral neurotransmitters

CORRECT ANSWER—A. *Rationales:* Cerebrospinal fluid is primarily produced in the lateral ventricles of the brain. It acts as a shock absorber and cushions the spinal cord and brain against injury caused by sudden or extreme movement. Cerebrospinal fluid also functions in the removal of waste products from cerebral tissue. The other options are not functions of cerebrospinal fluid.
Nursing process step: Analysis

52. A patient on heparin sodium therapy should be instructed to look for which of these signs of overdose?
A. Constipation and severe abdominal pain
B. Visual hallucinations and disorientation
C. Hematuria and rectal bleeding
D. Tinnitus and dry mouth

CORRECT ANSWER—C. *Rationales:* The clinical manifestations of heparin overdose are hematuria, rectal bleeding, epistaxis, petechial formation, and easy bruising. Constipation, severe abdominal pain, visual hallucinations, tinnitus, and dry mouth are not associated with heparin sodium overdose.
Nursing process step: Assessment

53. Which of the following information should be included in the initial history of a patient being evaluated for seizures?
A. Recent falls or injury to the head
B. Ethanol use
C. Use of opioids
D. Compliance with taking medications

CORRECT ANSWER—A. *Rationales:* All the information should be included in the history of a patient with seizures; however, a history of falls or head injury, when accompanied by seizures, could indicate severe complications of head injury. These complications may include cerebral irritation or edema, epidural hematoma, and cerebral contusions and may require immediate attention.
Nursing process step: Assessment

54. When administering diazepam (Valium), the nurse should be aware of which life-threatening side effect?
A. Respiratory arrest
B. Syncope
C. Hypotension
D. Cardiac arrhythmias

CORRECT ANSWER—A. *Rationales:* Diazepam is a central nervous system depressant. It should be administered slowly with reassessment of the patient's vital signs, including respiratory status. Syncope, hypotension, and cardiac arrhythmias are adverse effects of diazepam, but are usually not life-threatening.
Nursing process step: Intervention

55. Which of the following should the initial treatment of a cluster headache include?
A. Lithium carbonate
B. Oxygen
C. Calcium channel blockers
D. Corticosteroids

CORRECT ANSWER—B. *Rationales:* All the medications listed are appropriate for treating cluster headaches. However, oxygen relieves headache symptoms in 90% of patients.
Nursing process step: Intervention

56. Diagnostic testing is performed on a patient with altered mental status. For which of the following findings would the nurse expect the patient to be comatose?
A. PO_2 between 30 and 50 mm Hg
B. Glasgow Coma Scale finding of 9
C. Decerebrate posturing
D. Midposition round pupils

CORRECT ANSWER—C. *Rationales:* Decerebrate posturing indicates a lesion at the level of the brain stem. This response is usually found in a comatose patient. The brain is extremely sensitive to hypoxia, and coma usually results when the PO_2 falls below 25 mm Hg. A Glasgow Coma Scale of 7 or less is associated with comatose states of unconsciousness. Midposition round pupils are a normal finding.
Nursing process step: Assessment

57. Which symptom is associated with a cluster headache?
A. Lacrimation
B. Fever
C. Aphasia
D. Epistaxis

CORRECT ANSWER—A. *Rationales:* A cluster headache is characterized by pain episodes that are grouped or clustered together for a few days or a few weeks with long periods of remission. Clinical manifestations include lacrimation, diaphoresis, temporal vessel swelling, nasal congestion, and flushed appearance.
Nursing process step: Assessment

Questions 58 through 60 refer to the following information:
A patient complaining of the "worst headache of my life" is brought to the emergency department. A friend states that the patient "isn't acting right" and has been vomiting throughout the morning. The patient is holding her head and complaining of photosensitivity. She has difficulty speaking. Vital signs taken at triage show that the patient is bradycardic with a heart rate of 54 beats/minute and hypertensive with a blood pressure of 182/120 mm Hg.

---

58. This patient exhibits symptoms for which of the following conditions?
A. Cerebrovascular accident
B. Ruptured cerebral aneurysm
C. Migraine headaches
D. Acoustic neuroma

CORRECT ANSWER—B. *Rationales:* Patients with cerebral aneurysms are asymptomatic until the time of bleeding. At the time of rupture, blood is forced into the subarachnoid space, causing symptoms of meningeal irritation, including nausea, vomiting, aphasia, photosensitivity, hypertension, and bradycardia. Symptoms of a cerebrovascular accident vary, depending on the location of the insult. There is often contralateral paralysis, aphasia, sensory impairment, and dysphagia. Migraine headaches are associated with aura, throbbing sensation, nausea, vomiting, and visual disturbances. Acoustic neuromas can be identified by vertigo, tinnitus, hearing loss, facial weakness, and hoarseness.
Nursing process step: Assessment

59. Nitroprusside (Nipride) is ordered to treat the patient's hypertension. What are the guidelines for administering nitroprusside?
A. Nitroprusside should be reconstituted with normal saline only
B. Once reconstituted, nitroprusside deteriorates in light
C. Nitroprusside overdose is treated with amyl nitrate inhalations
D. Options B and C

CORRECT ANSWER—D. *Rationales:* Nitroprusside solution should be wrapped in an opaque material promptly to protect it from light, which causes it to deteriorate. Nitroprusside overdose results in cyanide toxicity, which is treated with amyl nitrate inhalations. Nitroprusside should be administered or reconstituted with dextrose in water only.
Nursing process step: Intervention

60. What is the average dose of nitroprusside (Nipride) for adults and children?
A. 3 mcg/kg/minute
B. 5 mg/kg
C. 0.2 mcg/kg/minute
D. 10 mcg/kg/minute

CORRECT ANSWER—A. *Rationales:* The recommended average dose of nitroprusside is 3 mcg/kg/minute (range of 0.5 to 10.0 mcg/kg/minute). Nitroprusside can be increased in increments of 0.2 mcg/kg/minute. The maximum recommended dosage for nitroprusside is 10 mcg/kg/minute.
Nursing process step: Intervention

61. Which is the earliest indicator of change in a patient's neurologic status?
A. Pupillary reaction
B. Motor response
C. Capillary refill
D. Level of consciousness

CORRECT ANSWER—D. *Rationales:* The earliest indicator of neurologic status is the level of consciousness. A patient who exhibits altered mental status or decreased consciousness should be reevaluated by the nursing and medical staff. Changes in the reaction and shape of pupils is a late indicator of neurologic problems. Motor response appears as a delayed sign of neurologic status change. Capillary refill is an indicator of circulatory status.
Nursing process step: Assessment

62. What is the purpose of corticosteroid therapy in a patient diagnosed with a brain tumor?
A. To control petit mal seizures
B. To relieve symptoms of agitation
C. To reduce cerebral edema
D. To reduce pain

CORRECT ANSWER—C. *Rationales:* Corticosteroids reduce inflammation and cerebral edema and help prevent an increase in intracranial pressure. Anticonvulsants are used to control petit mal seizures. Antipsychotics and antianxiety drugs may be used sparingly to control agitation. Preferably, nonnarcotics are used to relieve pain. Narcotics may make it difficult to assess a patient's level of consciousness.
Nursing process step: Intervention

63. Which of the following is a contraindication for lumbar puncture?
A. Increased intracranial pressure
B. Warfarin sodium (Coumadin) therapy
C. Infection of the cutaneous or osseous areas at the lumbar puncture site
D. All of the above

CORRECT ANSWER—D. *Rationales:* Increased intracranial pressure, warfarin therapy, and infection of the cutaneous or osseous areas at the lumbar puncture site are contraindications to performing a lumbar puncture unless the benefits outweigh the risks. Performing a lumbar puncture on a patient with increased intracranial pressure may result in brain stem compression or herniation. A patient receiving anticoagulation therapy is at increased risk for hemorrhage. Performing a lumbar puncture at the site of infection increases the chance of introducing bacteria into the cerebrospinal fluid.
Nursing process step: Assessment

OBSTETRIC EMERGENCIES

Obstetric Emergencies

1. A woman complains of abdominal pain. Her last menstrual period was 8 weeks ago. Which type of pain is usually associated with a ruptured ectopic pregnancy?
A. Lower quadrant pain radiating to the shoulder
B. Sharp upper abdominal pain
C. Flank pain
D. Colicky, diffuse abdominal pain

CORRECT ANSWER—A. *Rationales:* Ectopic pregnancies that are leaking or have ruptured result in referred pain to the shoulder from blood irritating the diaphragm. Sharp upper abdominal pain is too high for pain caused by an ectopic pregnancy. Flank pain may be associated with kidney infection or kidney stones. Colicky, diffuse abdominal pain is more often associated with intestinal disorders.
Nursing process step: Assessment

2. A woman in her 34th week of pregnancy presents to the emergency department and complains of sudden onset of bright red vaginal bleeding. Her uterus is soft, and she is experiencing no pain. Fetal heart tones are 120 beats/minute. Based on the history above, the emergency nurse should suspect which of the following conditions?
A. Abruptio placentae
B. Preterm labor
C. Placenta previa
D. Threatened abortion

CORRECT ANSWER—C. *Rationales:* Placenta previa is associated with painless vaginal bleeding that occurs when the placenta, or a portion of the placenta, covers the cervical os. In abruptio placentae, the placenta tears away from the wall of the uterus before delivery; the patient usually has pain and a boardlike uterus. Preterm labor is associated with contractions and should not involve bright red bleeding. By definition, threatened abortion occurs during the first 20 weeks of gestation.
Nursing process step: Analysis

3. After a fall down a flight of stairs, a woman in her 38th week of pregnancy is brought to the emergency department. Unless contraindicated, she should be placed in which of the following positions during assessment?
   A. Trendelenburg
   B. Flat on back
   C. Left lateral recumbent
   D. Knee-chest

CORRECT ANSWER—C. *Rationales:* The left lateral recumbent position avoids compression of the inferior vena cava; compressing the vessel may result in decreased uterine blood flow, fetal hypoxia, and maternal hypotension. Trendelenburg or the flat position would compress this vessel. If a pregnant patient must lie flat on a backboard for cervical spine evaluation, a wedge may be placed under the right hip to avoid compressing the vessel. If the umbilical cord is prolapsed, the knee-chest position may be used to avoid compressing the cord.
Nursing process step: Intervention

4. Which intervention is considered inappropriate for a patient with placenta previa?
   A. Performing a pelvic exam to determine extent of dilatation
   B. Maintaining strict bed rest and observing for further bleeding
   C. Monitoring for signs of shock
   D. Preparing the patient for pelvic ultrasound

CORRECT ANSWER—A. *Rationales:* A pelvic exam should not be performed on a pregnant patient with vaginal bleeding. In cases of placenta previa, the exam could cause further bleeding and damage the placenta. Patients with placenta previa should be placed on bed rest and pad count and be monitored for signs of shock if bleeding is heavy and persists. A pelvic ultrasound is useful for detecting placenta previa. The nurse should fill the bladder by way of an indwelling urinary catheter rather than by mouth in the event a cesarean section is necessary. In most cases, patients with placenta previa stop bleeding with bed rest and pelvic rest.
Nursing process step: Intervention

5. A patient with pregnancy-induced hypertension probably exhibits which of the following symptoms?
   A. Proteinuria, headaches, vaginal bleeding
   B. Headaches, double vision, vaginal bleeding
   C. Proteinuria, headaches, double vision
   D. Proteinuria, double vision, uterine contractions

CORRECT ANSWER—C. *Rationales:* A patient with pregnancy-induced hypertension complains of headache, double vision, and sudden weight gain. A urine specimen reveals proteinuria. Vaginal bleeding and uterine contractions are not associated with pregnancy-induced hypertension.
Nursing process step: Assessment

6. A pregnant woman arrives in the emergency department and states, "My baby is coming." The emergency nurse sees a portion of the umbilical cord protruding from the vagina. Why should manual pressure be applied to the baby's head?

A. To slow the delivery process
B. To reinsert the umbilical cord
C. To relieve pressure on the umbilical cord
D. To rupture the membranes

CORRECT ANSWER—C. *Rationales:* Manual pressure is applied to the baby's head by gently pushing up with the fingers to relieve pressure on the umbilical cord. This intervention is effective if the cord begins to pulsate. The mother may also be placed in the knee-chest or Trendelenburg position to ensure blood flow to the baby. This intervention is not done to slow the delivery process. A prolapsed cord necessitates emergency cesarean section. The nurse should not attempt to reinsert the umbilical cord because this would further compromise blood flow. At this point, the membranes are probably ruptured.
Nursing process step: Evaluation

7. Which of the following is the primary nursing diagnosis for a patient with a ruptured ectopic pregnancy?

A. Anxiety
B. Pain
C. Fluid volume deficit
D. Anticipatory grieving

CORRECT ANSWER—C. *Rationales:* Ruptured ectopic pregnancy is associated with hemorrhage and requires immediate surgical intervention. The other options are correct but are not the primary nursing diagnosis. This patient is probably experiencing anxiety because this is a surgical emergency. Pain is also present and should be addressed as warranted. The patient with ruptured ectopic pregnancy may experience anticipatory grieving at the loss of her fetus.
Nursing process step: Analysis

8. A patient in her 34th week of pregnancy presents to the emergency department. Her blood pressure is 180/110 mm Hg, and she is complaining of headache and blurred vision. During treatment of this patient, the nurse should be prepared for which of the following complications?

A. Precipitous delivery
B. Vaginal bleeding
C. Cardiac arrhythmias
D. Seizure activity

CORRECT ANSWER—D. *Rationales:* These are symptoms of pregnancy-induced hypertension. This patient has a potential for seizure activity because of central nervous system irritability. Seizure precautions should be instituted. Precipitous delivery, vaginal bleeding, and cardiac arrhythmias are not complications of pregnancy-induced hypertension.
Nursing process step: Evaluation

9. A patient in her 15th week of pregnancy arrives in the emergency department. She is complaining of abdominal cramping and vaginal bleeding for the past 8 hours. She has passed several clots. What is the primary nursing diagnosis for this patient?
   A. Knowledge deficit
   B. Fluid volume deficit
   C. Anticipatory grieving
   D. Altered comfort and pain

CORRECT ANSWER—B. *Rationales:* If bleeding and clots are excessive, this patient may become hypovolemic. Pad count should be instituted. Although the other options are applicable to this patient, they are not the primary diagnosis.
Nursing process step: Analysis

10. Which of the following indicates imminent delivery?
   A. Need to bear down by the mother
   B. Rupture of membranes
   C. Loss of mucous plug
   D. None of the above

CORRECT ANSWER—A. *Rationales:* The desire to bear down or push usually indicates that delivery is near (especially in the multiparous mother). Other signs of imminent delivery are heavy bloody show and a bulging perineum. Rupture of membranes may occur before labor begins. Loss of the mucous plug is likely to occur at the beginning of labor.
Nursing process step: Assessment

11. A pregnant trauma patient should be assessed for which of the following conditions?
   A. Uterine contractions, vaginal bleeding or ruptured membranes, and fetal heart tones
   B. Uterine contractions and vaginal bleeding or ruptured membranes
   C. Fetal heart tones and fetal position
   D. All of the above

CORRECT ANSWER—A. *Rationales:* All pregnant trauma patients should be assessed for uterine contractions. A fetal monitor may be applied or the uterus may be palpated for tone. Observe for vaginal bleeding or ruptured membranes. Fetal heart tones should be part of the vital signs for all pregnant women and may be auscultated with a Doppler stethoscope after about 14 weeks' gestation. Normal fetal heart tones are 120 to 160 beats/minute. It is not necessary to assess for fetal position at this time.
Nursing process step: Assessment

12. During neonatal resuscitation immediately after delivery, chest compressions should be initiated when the heart rate falls below which of the following?
   A. 60 beats/minute
   B. 80 beats/minute
   C. 100 beats/minute
   D. 110 beats/minute

CORRECT ANSWER—A. *Rationales:* The normal neonatal heart rate is 120 to 160 beats/minute. Heart rates less than 60 beats/minute necessitate chest compressions and ventilatory support.
Nursing process step: Intervention

13. The emergency nurse should determine an Apgar score on the neonate at 1 minute and again at 5 minutes. The nurse assesses which of the following parameters?

A. Heart rate, muscle tone, reflexes, respiratory effort, color

B. Heart rate, temperature, reflexes, respiratory effort, color

C. Heart rate, muscle tone, weight, respiratory effort, color

D. Heart rate, muscle tone, reflexes, respiratory effort, swallowing ability

CORRECT ANSWER—A. *Rationales:* The Apgar score should be determined at 1 and 5 minutes. Heart rate, muscle tone, reflexes, respiratory effort, and color are assessed. A score of 7 to 10 is favorable.

Nursing process step: Assessment

14. Which is the most common risk factor for an ectopic pregnancy?

A. Pelvic inflammatory disease

B. Spontaneous abortion

C. Fertility difficulties

D. Multiple pregnancies

CORRECT ANSWER—A. *Rationales:* Ectopic pregnancies are most often related to scarring secondary to pelvic inflammatory disease. Spontaneous abortion and multiple pregnancies are not associated with this condition. Scarring from pelvic inflammatory disease may also result in fertility difficulties.

Nursing process step: Assessment

OCULAR EMERGENCIES

CHAPTER 10

Ocular Emergencies

1. Conjunctivitis may be caused by bacteria, viruses, allergens, and irritants. Which characteristics differentiate bacterial conjunctivitis from other types?

A. Subacute onset, severe pain, preauricular adenopathy

B. Recurrent onset, no pain, clear discharge

C. Acute onset, moderate pain, purulent discharge

D. Acute onset, mild pain, clear discharge

CORRECT ANSWER—C. *Rationales:* Bacterial conjunctivitis has an acute onset, moderate pain, copious purulent discharge, and preauricular adenopathy. Viral conjunctivitis has an acute or a subacute onset, mild to moderate pain, and moderate and seropurulent discharge; preauricular adenopathy is common. Allergic conjunctivitis has a recurrent onset, no pain, moderate clear discharge, and no preauricular adenopathy. Irritant conjunctivitis has acute onset, no pain to mild pain, minimal clear discharge and, rarely, preauricular adenopathy.
Nursing process step: Assessment

2. On evaluation of the effectiveness of therapy for conjunctivitis, which of the following findings indicates the need for further treatment?

A. Pain in eye is relieved

B. Preauricular adenopathy is decreased

C. Purulent discharge is resolved

D. Both eyes have purulent discharge

CORRECT ANSWER—D. *Rationales:* A patient who now has bilateral involvement needs further therapy. After effective treatment for conjunctivitis, eye pain should be relieved, the preauricular adenopathy should be decreased or resolved, and purulent discharge should be absent. Patient education on disease transmission and method for cleaning the eye is needed.
Nursing process step: Evaluation

3. What is the treatment of choice for a patient with iritis?

A. Instill topical decongestants, 1 drop three to four times daily

B. Instill prednisolone acetate (Pred-Forte) and tropicamide (Mydriacyl) to affected eye

C. Administer erythromycin (Ilotycin Ophthalmic Ointment)

D. Refer immediately to an ophthalmologist

CORRECT ANSWER—B. *Rationales:* Iritis is treated with prednisolone acetate to reduce inflammation (five times daily) and tropicamide to reduce ciliary muscle spasm (1 to 2 drops, repeated in 5 minutes if necessary). Topical decongestants and antibiotics are used in the treatment of conjunctivitis. Referral to an ophthalmologist is generally not necessary in the treatment of iritis.
Nursing process step: Intervention

4. Central retinal artery occlusion from a blockage of the artery by a thrombus or an embolus is a true ocular emergency. Which is the most definitive assessment finding?
A. Sudden unilateral loss of vision without pain
B. Pupil small but reactive
C. Decreased visual acuity with sudden onset of severe pain
D. Increased intraocular pressure

CORRECT ANSWER—A. *Rationales:* Central retinal artery occlusion presents with a sudden, painless unilateral loss of vision. Light perception is all that remains in the affected eye. The pupil is dilated and nonreactive. Glaucoma occurs with severe, sudden onset of pain; diminished vision; semidilated and nonreactive pupils; and increased intraocular pressure.
Nursing process step: Assessment

5. Which of the following is the most appropriate nursing diagnosis for a patient with central retinal artery occlusion?
A. Pain related to inflammatory process
B. Potential for infection related to injury
C. Impaired skin integrity related to laceration
D. Altered tissue perfusion to the optic nerve related to vascular blockage

CORRECT ANSWER—D. *Rationales:* Central retinal artery occlusion is vascular blockage to the optic nerve and leads to vision loss without pain. There is no laceration or infection potential for a patient with this disorder.
Nursing process step: Analysis/Nursing diagnosis

6. A patient is admitted complaining of pain, photophobia, and blurred vision after falling asleep with his contact lenses in place. Which of the following is the most appropriate intervention?
A. Apply a tight eye patch
B. Administer topical anesthetics
C. Irrigate the eye gently with sterile saline
D. Instill ophthalmic corticosteroid ointment

CORRECT ANSWER—C. *Rationales:* The most appropriate intervention is irrigation of the eye gently with sterile saline. The patient may require instillation of ophthalmic antibiotic ointment but should never contain a corticosteroid. This increases the chance of infection. Topical anesthetics may lead to irreversible corneal damage and should never be administered. After treatment, an eye bandage should be applied firmly but not tightly.
Nursing process step: Intervention

7. Severe cases of corneal abrasion present with which of the following conditions?
A. Loss of vision and excessive tearing
B. Corneal surface irregularity and loss of luster
C. Redness and purulent discharge
D. Pupil dilated and nonreactive

CORRECT ANSWER—B. *Rationales:* Severe corneal abrasions present with corneal surface irregularity and loss of luster. Tearing is common; however, vision is only blurred, not lost. Redness without purulent discharge is also a common finding. The pupils are of normal size and reactivity, unless eyedrops are used for examination and relief of severe pain.
Nursing process step: Assessment

Questions 8 through 11 refer to the following information:
A patient arrives in the emergency department, complains of pain, and states that something is in his right eye. He had been working under his car. Other significant findings include tearing and redness.

8. What important information should the nurse obtain before intervention?
   A. Allergies to medications
   B. List of current medications
   C. History of glaucoma
   D. All of the above

CORRECT ANSWER—D. *Rationales:* A patient with a lidocaine allergy may be allergic to the medications administered to anesthetize the eye. Many medications have cross-reactivity with drugs commonly used for the examination and treatment of eye injuries. Atropine is also often used for eye examination and can worsen glaucoma.
Nursing process step: Assessment

9. What is the priority in the care of this patient?
   A. Irrigate the eye with sterile normal saline
   B. Instill ophthalmic antibiotic ointment
   C. Anesthetize the cornea with proparacaine (Ophthaine)
   D. Manually remove foreign bodies before irrigation

CORRECT ANSWER—C. *Rationales:* The priority in caring for a patient with an extraocular foreign body is to relieve pain with an anesthetic, such as proparacaine or tetracaine (Pontocaine) solution. Anesthetizing the eye allows for a more comfortable inspection and irrigation with normal saline. Ophthalmic antibiotic ointments are used after the foreign body is removed. If the foreign body is not removed with irrigation, it should be removed manually.
Nursing process step: Intervention

10. Which is the most appropriate nursing diagnosis for this patient?
   A. Pain related to injury
   B. Ineffective individual coping
   C. Altered thought processes related to injury
   D. Fluid volume deficit related to injury

CORRECT ANSWER—A. *Rationales:* The most appropriate nursing diagnoses for a patient with an extraocular foreign body include pain related to injury, anxiety related to injury and treatment, knowledge deficit related to lack of education about or experience with eye injury, and self-care deficit. Options B, C, and D are not applicable to this patient.
Nursing process step: Analysis/Nursing diagnosis

11. The patient is given discharge instructions regarding an extraocular foreign body. Which of the following statements indicate an understanding of the discharge instructions?
   A. "I can save the topical anesthetic to use in the future"
   B. "I will need both eyes patched to prevent excessive eye movement"
   C. "I will need to see my doctor in a week"
   D. "I will be able to drive home as long as I am careful"

CORRECT ANSWER—B. *Rationales:* Consensual eye movement, which can result in increased injury, occurs if only the injured eye is patched. Even though topical anesthetics effectively eliminate pain, they should not be sent home with a patient because they can mask complications of the injury and increase eye damage. Because bilateral eye patching is usually performed, the patient cannot drive home.
Nursing process step: Evaluation

12. Signs and symptoms of retinal detachment include all except which of the following?
  A. Painless decrease in vision
  B. Curtain or veil over visual field
  C. Increased intraocular pressure
  D. Flashing lights

CORRECT ANSWER—**C.** *Rationales:* A patient with retinal detachment has a painless decrease in vision and indicates that vision is cloudy or smoky with flashing lights. The patient may also indicate that a curtain or veil is over the visual field. Intraocular pressure is normal or low.
Nursing process step: Assessment

13. Which is the most important intervention for a patient with retinal detachment?
  A. Admit to the hospital on strict bed rest
  B. Patch both eyes
  C. Refer to an ophthalmologist
  D. Prepare for emergent surgery

CORRECT ANSWER—**A.** *Rationale:* Immediate bed rest is necessary to prevent further injury. Both eyes should be patched and the patient should receive early referral to an ophthalmologist. If the macula is attached and central visual acuity is normal, the condition should be urgently treated by an ophthalmologist. Retinal reattachment can be accomplished by surgery only. If the macula is detached or threatened, surgery is urgent; prolonged detachment of the macula results in permanent loss of central vision.
Nursing process step: Intervention

14. Which is the initial intervention for a patient with a chemical burn of the eye?
  A. Patch the affected eye and call the ophthalmologist
  B. Administer a cycloplegic agent to reduce ciliary spasm
  C. Immediately instill a topical anesthetic then irrigate with copious amounts of normal saline
  D. Administer antibiotics to reduce the chance for infection

CORRECT ANSWER—**C.** *Rationales:* The initial intervention for a chemical burn is to instill a topical anesthetic immediately and then irrigate the eye with copious amounts of normal saline. Irrigation should be done for 5 to 10 minutes, and then the pH of the eye should be checked. Irrigation should be continued until the pH of the eye reaches 7.0. Double eversion of the eyelids should be performed to look for and remove material lodged in the cul-de-sac. A cycloplegic agent can then be used to reduce ciliary spasm, and an antibiotic ointment can be administered to reduce the risk of infection. Then the eye should be patched. Parenteral narcotic analgesia is often required for pain relief. An ophthalmologist should also be consulted.
Nursing process step: Intervention

15. Which of the following indicates successful treatment of a chemical burn to the eye?
A. Eye pH of 7.8
B. Evidence of corneal opacity
C. Evidence of decreased visual acuity
D. Relief of pain

CORRECT ANSWER—D. *Rationales:* Pain is a common complaint with chemical burns to the eye. The patient stating that the pain is relieved signifies successful treatment. The normal pH of the eye is 6.9 to 7.2. Improved vision would be indicated by normal visual acuity and no evidence of corneal opacity.
Nursing process step: Evaluation

16. A patient is admitted to the emergency department after blunt trauma to the right eye. The patient complains of blurred and blood-tinged vision. The nurse's assessment reveals blood in the eye. Which of the following is the most likely type of eye injury?
A. Hyphema
B. Retinal detachment
C. Globe rupture
D. Orbital fracture

CORRECT ANSWER—A. *Rationales:* The most frequent symptoms of hyphema include impaired visual acuity, blood visualized in the anterior chamber of the eye, and blood-tinged vision. Globe ruptures present with decreased visual acuity, shallow anterior chamber, irregularities in pupillary borders, and decreased intraocular pressure. In retinal detachment, the patient complains of smoky or cloudy vision, flashing lights, and a curtain or veil over the visual field. Orbital fractures produce alterations in extraocular movement of the affected eye, paresthesia of the lip, crepitus over the fracture site, and periorbital edema.
Nursing process step: Assessment

17. The threat of a secondary bleed occurring in 3 to 5 days is a significant risk in the patient with hyphema. Which is an indication of successful prevention of rebleeding?
A. Blood only in the inferior portion of the anterior chamber
B. Improved visual acuity
C. Decreased blurred vision
D. All of the above

CORRECT ANSWER—D. *Rationales:* Improved visual acuity, decreased blurred vision, and blood found only in the inferior portion of the anterior chamber are signs of improvement.
Nursing process step: Evaluation

18. A laceration of the eyelid commonly causes the inability to do which of the following?
A. Raise the upper lid
B. Close the affected eye
C. Look upward or downward with the affected eye
D. Look outward or inward with the affected eye

CORRECT ANSWER—A. *Rationales:* A deep laceration to the eyelid often involves the levator muscle. As a result, the patient cannot raise the upper lid of the affected eye. In addition, the eye is generally swollen shut, so extraocular movement, which should not be affected, cannot be assessed. Orbital fracture can cause loss of extraocular movement and result in an inability to look upward or downward with the affected eye.
Nursing process step: Assessment

19. After blunt trauma to the eye, a patient arrives in the emergency department. The patient exhibits abnormal extraocular movement, paresthesia of the lip, periorbital edema and ecchymosis, and subconjunctival hemorrhage. Which disorder is most consistent with these assessment findings?

A. Globe rupture
B. Orbital fracture
C. Retinal detachment
D. Eyelid laceration

CORRECT ANSWER—B. *Rationales:* Orbital fracture occurs after blunt trauma and causes crepitus at the fracture site, paresthesia of the lip, abnormal extraocular movements, subconjunctival hemorrhage, and periorbital edema and ecchymosis. A globe rupture presents with irregularity of pupillary borders, decreased visual acuity, decreased intraocular pressure, and shallow anterior chamber. An eyelid laceration has periorbital edema and bleeding. Retinal detachment has specific visual alterations that include flashes of light, floating black spots, and curtain-like defects that result in decreased peripheral vision.
Nursing process step: Assessment

20. Which intervention is appropriate for a patient with an orbital fracture?

A. Ice to the affected eye
B. Analgesics to relieve pain
C. Orbit and facial view X-rays
D. All of the above

CORRECT ANSWER—D. *Rationales:* Ice to the affected orbit decreases swelling. Analgesics relieve pain and reduce anxiety. X-rays should be done to verify the extent of fractures. An otolaryngologist and ophthalmologist should be consulted before the patient is discharged from the emergency department. Patients with orbital floor or rim fractures with no limitation of ocular mobility and without associated injury of the globe may be discharged from the emergency department and referred to an otolaryngologist to be seen in a few days.
Nursing process step: Intervention

Questions 21 and 22 refer to the following information:
After a fight that caused a penetrating injury to the right eye, a patient arrives in the emergency department. The patient has severe pain in the eye. A doctor diagnoses the problem as a globe rupture.

21. Which of the following signs or symptoms should the nurse expect to see?

A. Irregular pupillary borders
B. Normal visual acuity
C. Increased intraocular pressure
D. Redness and purulent drainage

CORRECT ANSWER—A. *Rationales:* A patient with a globe rupture usually has had a penetrating injury, and the foreign body can often be seen in the anterior chamber. The borders of the pupils are irregular. Other signs and symptoms include decreased visual acuity, shallow anterior chamber, and decreased intraocular pressure. Redness and purulent drainage from an eye usually means conjunctivitis.
Nursing process step: Assessment

22. When caring for this patient, the nurse should be sure to perform which intervention?
  A. Open the eye to search for a foreign body
  B. Position the patient in a supine position
  C. Patch the injured eye lightly
  D. Administer analgesics as prescribed

CORRECT ANSWER—D. *Rationales:* If a patient is believed to have a globe rupture, the eye should not be opened. The patient should be placed in semi-Fowler's position to maintain reduced intraocular pressure. Both eyes should be lightly patched to minimize consensual movement. Pain can be minimal to severe; therefore, the patient should be assessed and analgesics administered as needed. An ophthalmologist should be consulted.
Nursing process step: Intervention

23. Chemical burns constitute a true ocular emergency. Which assessment findings are consistent with a chemical burn?
  A. Corneal whitening
  B. Dilated, nonreactive pupils
  C. Redness and purulent discharge
  D. Corneal irregularity and luster

CORRECT ANSWER—A. *Rationales:* The most significant assessment finding in a chemical burn to the eye, especially an alkaline burn, is corneal whitening. There is pain and variable loss of vision. It is also difficult to define specific eye structures. There may be redness but no purulent discharge. A corneal abrasion presents with corneal irregularity and no corneal luster.
Nursing process step: Assessment

ORTHOPEDIC EMERGENCIES

Orthopedic Emergencies

1. Which of the following is the most appropriate nursing diagnosis for a patient with a strained ankle?
A. Impaired skin integrity
B. Impaired physical mobility related to pain and tissue damage
C. Fluid volume deficit risk
D. Body image disturbances

CORRECT ANSWER—B. *Rationales:* Ankle strains result in pain and damage to ligaments as well as altered physical mobility. Although the traumatic event that caused the strain may disrupt the skin, the manifestations of a strain do not include disruption of skin integrity. Risk for fluid volume deficit is an appropriate nursing diagnosis for a process that results in the loss of a large volume of fluid or blood. Disruptions in body image can occur if the patient's livelihood is altered because of the strain.
Nursing process step: Analysis/Nursing diagnosis

2. Which of the following nursing interventions is essential in caring for a patient with compartment syndrome?
A. Keeping the affected extremity below the level of the heart
B. Wrapping the affected extremity with a compression dressing to help decrease the swelling
C. Removing all external sources of pressure, such as clothing and jewelry
D. Starting an I.V. line in the affected extremity in anticipation of venogram studies

CORRECT ANSWER—C. *Rationales:* Nursing measures should include removing all clothing, jewelry, and external forms of pressure (such as pressure dressings or casts) to prevent constriction and additional tissue compromise. The extremity should be maintained at heart level (further elevation may increase circulatory compromise, whereas a dependent position may increase edema). A compression wrap, which increases tissue pressure, could further damage the affected extremity. There is no indication that diagnostic studies would require I.V. access in the affected extremity.
Nursing process step: Intervention

3. Which of the following injuries results from excessive stretching or tearing of a ligament?
   A. Strain
   B. Sprain
   C. Fracture
   D. Avulsion

CORRECT ANSWER—B. *Rationales:* A sprain results from excessive stretching or tearing of a ligament. A strain occurs from the overstretching of a tendon or muscle. A fracture is a break in the continuity of the bone as a result of excessive force. An avulsion is a full-thickness separation of the skin.
Nursing process step: Assessment

4. Excessive or continuous stress on a tendon results in which of the following conditions?
   A. Tinnitus
   B. Tendinitis
   C. Bursitis
   D. Nerve entrapment

CORRECT ANSWER—B. *Rationales:* Tendinitis is an inflammation of a tendon from excessive or continuous force. It commonly occurs in the shoulder (rotator cuff tendinitis), elbow (tennis elbow), knee (jumper's knee), or heel (Achilles tendinitis). Tinnitus is ringing in the ears. Bursitis is an inflammation of the bursa, or sac, that covers a bony prominence between bones, muscles, or tendons. Nerve entrapment results from the compression of a nerve, causing ischemia of that nerve.
Nursing process step: Assessment

Questions 5 through 7 refer to the following information:
After falling down four stairs, a patient presents to the emergency department and complains of right shoulder pain. He states that he has dislocated his right shoulder multiple times in the past and thinks that it is dislocated again.

---

5. Which of the following interventions should be avoided in the patient with a suspected shoulder dislocation?
   A. Immobilizing the shoulder to prevent further injury and relieve pain
   B. Applying ice
   C. Placing the patient in a traction splint to eliminate muscle spasms
   D. Determining neurovascular status distal to the injury

CORRECT ANSWER—C. *Rationales:* Traction splints, designed for use on lower extremities, are indicated only for treating femur and proximal tibia fractures; their use in upper-extremity trauma is contraindicated. Immobilizing the shoulder, applying ice, and determining the neurovascular status distal to the injury are all appropriate interventions for a dislocated shoulder.
Nursing process step: Intervention

6. Which of the following is not indicative of neurovascular compromise in a patient with a shoulder dislocation?
   A. Intense pain with movement of the joint
   B. Numbness of an extremity
   C. Inability to move the extremity
   D. Paresthesias of the extremity

CORRECT ANSWER—A. *Rationales:* Patients with a shoulder dislocation have pain with any movement of the joint. When there is neurovascular compromise, the patient experiences numbness, paresthesia, and the inability to move the extremity.
Nursing process step: Assessment

7. Which of the following is not an expected outcome for this patient?
  A. The patient states that the injured shoulder feels better
  B. The patient verbalizes the need to follow up with an orthopedic surgeon for fixation if the shoulder becomes dislocated again
  C. The patient verbalizes activities to avoid to prevent future dislocations
  D. The patient's facial expressions and body positioning demonstrate that he is calm and relaxed

CORRECT ANSWER—**B.** *Rationales:* With a history of repetitive dislocation, the patient should be evaluated by an orthopedic surgeon for possible joint fixation. The patient should be placed on restricted activity at least until follow-up is complete. The appearance of a calm, relaxed patient indicates that interventions of pain control, positioning, and education have been successful.
Nursing process step: Evaluation

8. Which of the following is a priority intervention in the patient experiencing fat embolism syndrome?
  A. Replacing fluids to maintain cardiac function
  B. Administering I.V. corticosteroids
  C. Administering high-flow oxygen by way of a nonrebreather mask
  D. Providing discharge planning and education

CORRECT ANSWER—**C.** *Rationales:* The priority nursing intervention for this syndrome is administering high-flow oxygen. Airway and breathing are always top-priority interventions. After administering oxygen, the priority interventions are mechanical ventilation, if indicated; fluid replacement; I.V. corticosteroids; and patient education.
Nursing process step: Intervention

Questions 9 through 11 refer to the following information:
After an assault, a patient presents to the emergency department. The patient complains of an injury to the left femur. There is an obvious deformity to the middle of the thigh and bone is protruding. The patient's left foot is pale and cool and palpable pulses are absent.

---

9. Which of the following is a priority intervention for this patient?
  A. Applying pneumatic antishock trousers to the patient and inflating the left leg compartment
  B. Attempting to push the bone back into the wound
  C. Administering oxygen at 2 liters per nasal cannula
  D. Applying firm in-line traction to the left leg, reassessing distal neurovascular status, and anticipating placement of a traction splint

CORRECT ANSWER—**D.** *Rationales:* Applying firm in-line traction to the left leg, reassessing the distal neurovascular status, and anticipating the placement of a traction splint are the priority interventions for a patient with an open femur fraction. The use of pneumatic antishock trousers is controversial, and their value for stabilizing femur fractures has not been proved. Protruding bone should not be pushed back into the wound. Administering oxygen to a patient with a femur fracture should be done at 10 to 15 L/minute by way of a nonrebreather mask.
Nursing process step: Intervention

10. Which of the following is a priority intervention when caring for an open wound?
A. Cleaning the wound with a solution of betadine and hydrogen peroxide
B. Covering the wound with a wet sterile dressing
C. Leaving the wound open to air
D. Setting up for immediate wound closure

CORRECT ANSWER—B. *Rationales:* A break in the skin near the site of a suspected fracture is considered an open fracture until proven otherwise. The proper care for this wound is covering it with a sterile dressing, getting wound cultures, and administering tetanus toxoid and antibiotics as ordered. The wound should not be cleaned or closed by way of a suture until an open fracture is ruled out.
Nursing process step: Intervention

11. An X-ray of the left femur shows a fracture that extends through the midshaft of the bone and multiple splintering fragments. What is this type of fracture called?
A. Compression fracture
B. Greenstick fracture
C. Comminuted fracture
D. Impacted fracture

CORRECT ANSWER—C. *Rationales:* A comminuted fracture typically is transverse the shaft of the bone and has multiple splintered bone fragments. A closed fracture implies that the skin integrity at or near the point of fracture is intact. A greenstick fracture occurs when the bone buckles or bends and the fracture line does not extend through the entire bone. An impacted fracture occurs when the distal and proximal portions of the fracture are wedged into each other. A compression fracture occurs when a severe force presses the bone together on itself.
Nursing process step: Analysis

12. Which of the following is not one of the 5Ps for assessing an extremity?
A. Pain
B. Pallor
C. Paresthesia
D. Purulence

CORRECT ANSWER—D. *Rationales:* The 5Ps in the neurovascular assessment of an injured extremity include pain, pallor, paresthesia, pulses, and paralysis. Purulence is not an assessment of neurovascular status; it is an indication of infection.
Nursing process step: Assessment

Questions 13 through 15 refer to the following information:
A patient arrives in the emergency department by private vehicle after an industrial accident that resulted in a midforearm amputation. The patient has a tourniquet in place, bleeding is minimal, and the amputated part is wrapped in a towel.

13. Which of the following interventions is a priority for this patient?

A. Caring for the severed part

B. Removing the tourniquet and controlling bleeding with other methods

C. Preparing the patient for reimplantation

D. Obtaining an X-ray of the extremity to rule out a fracture proximal to the point of amputation

CORRECT ANSWER—**B.** *Rationales:* A tourniquet is an intervention of last resort to control bleeding. Removing the tourniquet is crucial to preserving as much of the stump as possible for the best therapeutic outcome. Caring for the amputated part, preparing for possible reimplantation, and obtaining X-rays should follow. **Nursing process step:** Intervention

14. Which of the following is an appropriate intervention for the preservation of the amputated part?

A. Discard the amputated part if it has been severed longer than 30 minutes

B. Wrap the amputated part in a towel and moisten with cool tap water

C. Immerse the amputated part directly into a bath of ice and water

D. Anticipate the need to X-ray the severed part before reimplantation

CORRECT ANSWER—**D.** *Rationales:* Radiologic examination should be done to rule out fractures and foreign bodies. The severed part can be reimplanted many hours after amputation. It needs to be wrapped in gauze and moistened with sterile normal saline solution. Direct immersion of the amputated part results in tissue damage secondary to thermal injury. The appropriate intervention is to gently clean the amputated part to remove gross debris. Then the part should be wrapped in gauze soaked with normal saline and placed in a plastic bag. The bag should be sealed tightly, placed on ice, and monitored to ensure that the tissue does not freeze. **Nursing process step:** Intervention

15. Which of the following is a priority nursing diagnosis for the patient with an amputated extremity?

A. Impaired skin integrity related to effects of the injury

B. Anticipatory grieving related to the loss of a limb

C. Body image disturbance related to changes in the structure of a body part

D. Altered peripheral tissue perfusion related to injury and amputation

CORRECT ANSWER—**D.** *Rationales:* The priority diagnosis is altered peripheral tissue perfusion resulting from the loss of circulation secondary to amputation. All the nursing diagnoses listed are appropriate for a patient presenting to the emergency department after a traumatic amputation of an extremity. **Nursing process step:** Analysis

16. Which part of the body is most likely to develop compartment syndrome?

A. Upper arm

B. Lower arm

C. Upper leg

D. Joint spaces

CORRECT ANSWER—**B.** *Rationales:* Compartment syndrome is most likely to occur in the lower arm, hand, lower leg, and foot. These areas have limited ability to expand with increasing tissue pressures. **Nursing process step:** Analysis

17. Which of the following is not a factor in the development of compartment syndrome?
A. Injury of an extremity
B. Prolonged overuse of an extremity
C. Recent surgery in an extremity
D. Preexisting joint inflammation (arthritis, synovitis)

CORRECT ANSWER—D. *Rationales:* Common causes of compartment syndrome include injury to an extremity; prolonged overuse of an extremity; recent extremity surgery; use of casts, wraps, splints, or pneumatic antishock garments; circumferential taping of an extremity; and past medical conditions such as hemophilia, nephrotic syndrome, and nerve dysfunctions. Preexisting joint disease does not play a role in the development of compartment syndrome.
Nursing process step: Analysis

18. Which of the following is incorrect regarding a dislocated wrist?
A. It is usually caused by a fall onto outstretched hands
B. It is frequently associated with sporting mishaps
C. It may result in median nerve damage
D. It usually does not need casting once it is relocated

CORRECT ANSWER—D. *Rationales:* Casting of the wrist is done after relocation to immobilize the joint and prevent re-dislocation. Wrist dislocations commonly result from falling onto outstretched hands and frequently are associated with sporting events. Median nerve damage can result from wrist dislocations; therefore, neurovascular assessment distal to the area of injury should be done on all patients who present with an injured extremity.
Nursing process step: Analysis

19. Which surgical intervention is initially used to treat compartment syndrome?
A. Muscle flap
B. Fasciotomy
C. Incision and drainage
D. Amputation

CORRECT ANSWER—B. *Rationales:* Fasciotomy is a surgical intervention used to treat compartment syndrome. The surgeon makes longitudinal incisions along the affected extremity to relieve tissue pressure and limit compression damage. This procedure should be performed within 8 to 12 hours of the onset, before irreversible damage occurs. A muscle flap and incision and drainage are not interventions for compartment syndrome. Amputation is the surgical intervention of last resort.
Nursing process step: Intervention

20. Which of the following is the most common site of nerve entrapment syndrome?
   A. Arm
   B. Leg
   C. Thoracic vertebral column
   D. Lumbar vertebral column

CORRECT ANSWER—A. *Rationales:* Nerve entrapment syndrome occurs most often in the arm. The median nerve is involved in pronator syndrome (entrapment occurs at the forearm) and carpal tunnel syndrome (entrapment at the wrist). The ulnar nerve is involved in cubital entrapment syndrome (entrapment at the elbow). The leg, thoracic vertebral column, and lumbar vertebral column are not involved in nerve entrapment syndromes.
Nursing process step: Analysis

21. Ankle dislocations are commonly associated with which of the following conditions?
   A. Strain
   B. Sprain
   C. Fracture
   D. None of the above

CORRECT ANSWER—C. *Rationales:* Ankle dislocations are commonly associated with fractures. Ligament strains and tendon sprains do not lead to ankle dislocations.
Nursing process step: Assessment

22. Which of the following statements is appropriate when teaching a patient about a strained wrist?
   A. "You may resume normal activities on discharge."
   B. "Apply heat intermittently for the first 24 to 48 hours and then apply ice up to 72 hours."
   C. "Do not use a compression elastic bandage because it may cause compartment syndrome."
   D. "Elevate the injured wrist higher than the level of the heart for the first 24 hours to reduce swelling."

CORRECT ANSWER—D. *Rationales:* The patient should be instructed to rest the injured extremity for the first 24 to 48 hours and then gradually increase activity as tolerated. The appropriate intervention is to apply ice for the first 24 hours to reduce swelling and then apply heat. The use of a compression elastic bandage provides support and helps to decrease swelling; it does not cause compartment syndrome.
Nursing process step: Evaluation

23. Which of the following is a priority nursing diagnosis in a patient who is diagnosed with a nerve entrapment syndrome?
   A. Pain related to entrapment of nerves
   B. Anxiety related to symptoms and unknown prognosis
   C. Knowledge deficit related to therapeutic regimens
   D. Altered tissue perfusion related to nerve entrapment

CORRECT ANSWER—A. *Rationales:* Pain related to the entrapment of nerves is the priority nursing diagnosis for the patient with nerve entrapment syndrome. Therefore, pain management is an important aspect of the nursing care associated with this syndrome. Altered tissue perfusion does not occur with nerve entrapment syndromes. These syndromes are the result of nerve tissue compression, not vascular compression. Anxiety related to symptoms and unknown prognosis and knowledge deficit related to therapeutic regimens are appropriate for a patient with nerve entrapment syndrome; however, they are not considered high priority.
Nursing process step: Analysis/Nursing diagnosis

24. Which of the following structures is seldom dislocated?
A. Knee
B. Shoulder
C. Foot
D. Elbow

CORRECT ANSWER—**C.** *Rationales:* Dislocations of the foot are rare. Dislocations of the knee, shoulder, and elbow occur in greater frequency than the foot.
Nursing process step: Assessment

25. Which of the following interventions is a priority for a patient receiving conscious sedation for relocation of a dislocated shoulder?
A. Monitoring the patient's respiratory status
B. Assessing the patient to determine the need for additional sedation
C. Assessing the extremity's neurovascular status after the relocation is complete
D. Monitoring the patient until the level of consciousness returns to baseline

CORRECT ANSWER—**A.** *Rationales:* When administering conscious sedation, the priority intervention is to monitor the patient's respiratory status. Medications given for conscious sedation can cause respiratory depression that may lead to respiratory arrest. Therefore, resuscitation equipment should be readily available. Adequate sedation must be maintained to complete the procedure and provide maximal patient comfort. Once relocation is complete, the nurse needs to assure that the neurovascular status is intact. Patients undergoing conscious sedation should be observed until the level of consciousness has returned to baseline.
Nursing process step: Intervention

26. Which of the following is true about obtaining X-rays on a patient with an injured extremity?
A. Anterior, posterior, and lateral views are the only films needed
B. X-rays should include the joints immediately above and below the injury
C. X-rays are indicated only if there is an obvious deformity to the extremity
D. Open fractures usually do not need X-rays because the location and type of fracture are easily identified based on clinical assessment alone

CORRECT ANSWER—**B.** *Rationales:* X-rays of the injured extremity should include the joints immediately above and below the injured area. The views are necessary to determine if there are any fractures along the length of the bone or if there is any joint involvement. Anterior, posterior, and lateral views of an injured extremity do not always allow visualization of fractures, so an oblique view may be needed. All extremity injuries involving a suspected fracture must be evaluated by X-ray, regardless of the presence of deformities or degree of integumentary disruption; these indicators do not give insight to the location or severity of the fracture.
Nursing process step: Intervention

27. Which of the following injuries to bone is common in unrestrained front seat passengers involved in motor vehicle crashes?
A. Fractured foot
B. Ankle dislocation
C. Patella fracture
D. Hip dislocation

CORRECT ANSWER—B. *Rationales:* Unrestrained front seat passengers may suffer lower-extremity trauma as a result of striking the dashboard with their knees. These injuries include ankle dislocation, knee or patella dislocations, femur fractures, hip fractures or dislocations, and acetabular fractures as a result of the femoral head being pushed through the acetabulum. Patella, ankle, and foot fractures are not common occurrences in this group of patients.
Nursing process step: Assessment

28. Which of the following is a priority nursing diagnosis for a patient with a dislocation to the extremity?
A. Risk for altered tissue perfusion related to vessel compression
B. Pain related to soft tissue injury and pressure
C. Impaired physical mobility
D. Infection related to impaired skin integrity

CORRECT ANSWER—A. *Rationales:* The risk for altered tissue perfusion related to vessel compression is the priority nursing diagnosis for a patient with a dislocation. This is considered to be an orthopedic emergency. Dislocations can cause bone to compress blood vessels and nerves impeding circulation and causing neurovascular disruption. The dislocation results in pain as tissues are stretched and edema occurs. The patient will experience impaired physical mobility until healing and rehabilitation have occurred. Infection is not a common occurrence in dislocations that do not disrupt skin integrity.
Nursing process step: Analysis

29. Which of following is used for the initial splinting of a pelvic fracture?
A. Long spine board
B. Pneumatic antishock garment
C. Traction splint
D. Bilateral long leg splints

CORRECT ANSWER—A. *Rationales:* A long spine board is used for the initial splinting of a pelvic fracture. A pneumatic antishock garment may help stabilize a pelvic fracture and tamponade bleeding, but it is not considered the initial splinting device. Traction splints are indicated for femur and proximal tibial fractures only. Long leg splints are not indicated for pelvic fractures because they do not stabilize or immobilize the pelvis.
Nursing process step: Planning/Intervention

30. Which of the following is not a type of fracture?
A. Spiral fracture
B. Avulsion fracture
C. Torus fracture
D. Diagonal fracture

CORRECT ANSWER—D. *Rationales:* A diagonal fracture is not a type of fracture. A fracture break line does resemble a diagonal line, but it is not considered a diagonal fracture. An avulsion fracture refers to a bone injury in which a fragment of bone connected to a ligament breaks off from the rest of the bone. A torus fracture, which is a buckling of a bone's surface, is seen in children. A spiral fracture appears to twist with the surface of the affected bone.
Nursing process step: Assessment

31. Which of the following is not a typical mechanism of injury in the cause of pelvic fractures?
A. Penetrating trauma
B. Falls from a significant height
C. Motor vehicle ejections
D. Pedestrian struck by a motor vehicle

CORRECT ANSWER—A. *Rationales:* Pelvic fractures commonly result from a patient being hit by or thrown from a vehicle or from falling from a significant height. A pelvic fracture may result from penetrating trauma, but this is not a typical occurrence.
Nursing process step: Assessment

32. Compression fractures most commonly occur in which of the following?
A. Femur
B. Vertebrae
C. Humerus
D. Sternum

CORRECT ANSWER—B. *Rationales:* The bones of the vertebral column are susceptible to compression fractures. Axial loading forces result in compression of the bones along the vertebral column. The most common type of axial loading occurs with diving accidents and falls.
Nursing process step: Assessment

33. Which of the following factors increases the risk for increased blood loss after a fracture?
A. Blood disorders
B. Anemia
C. Alcohol abuse
D. All of the above

CORRECT ANSWER—D. *Rationales:* Blood disorders, anemia, and alcohol abuse can be contributing factors to increased blood loss after a fracture.
Nursing process step: Assessment

34. The following describes a fracture commonly associated with contact sports: The patient presents with the head tilted toward the injured area and the chin directed away from the side of the injury. What is the name of the injury?
   A. Shoulder fracture
   B. Clavicle fracture
   C. Scapular fracture
   D. Humerus fracture

CORRECT ANSWER—B. *Rationales:* The symptoms described are characteristic of a clavicle fracture. Additional symptoms include pain, point tenderness, swelling, crepitus, and deformity to the clavicle. In addition, the patient usually cannot raise the arm on the affected side. A shoulder fracture is actually a shoulder dislocation with an associated fracture of the proximal humerus. The patient complains of pain and the inability to move his shoulder. There may be a disruption of blood flow to the arm. Because of the location of the scapula, it may be fractured in many different areas; however, fractures of this bone are uncommon. Muscles and the ability of the scapula to move along the chest wall protect it from fractures. Great force is required to fracture the scapula.
Nursing process step: Assessment

35. Which of the following is not an expected outcome in a patient with fat embolism syndrome?
   A. The patient has normal vital signs and cardiac rhythm
   B. The patient has good skin color
   C. The patient is able to state interventions that might prevent recurrence of the syndrome
   D. The patient's arterial blood gas values are within normal limits

CORRECT ANSWER—C. *Rationales:* Fat embolism syndrome is an unpredictable complication of trauma to the skeleton, and there are no known self-care interventions that can prevent its occurrence. The expected outcome of treatment is the return of normal vital signs, cardiac rhythm, skin color, and arterial blood gas values.
Nursing process step: Evaluation

36. Elderly patients who fall are most at risk for which of the following injuries?
   A. Wrist fractures
   B. Humerus fractures
   C. Pelvic fractures
   D. Cervical spine fractures

CORRECT ANSWER—C. *Rationales:* Elderly patients who fall often sustain pelvic and lower-extremity fractures. These injuries are devastating because they can seriously alter an elderly patient's lifestyle and reduce functional independence. Wrist fractures usually occur with falls on an outstretched hand or from a direct blow. They are commonly found in young men. Humerus fractures and cervical spine fractures are not age-specific.
Nursing process step: Analysis

37. Which of the following forces does not play a role in causing fractures?
   A. Tension force
   B. Bending force
   C. Compression force
   D. Extension force

CORRECT ANSWER—D. *Rationales:* There is no such force as extension force relative to fractures. The forces that do result in fractures include tension (pulling), compression (longitudinal loading), bending, and torsion (twisting).
Nursing process step: Analysis

38. Which of the following injuries are commonly seen in adult pedestrians struck by motor vehicles?
A. Femur fractures
B. Humerus fractures
C. Wrist fractures
D. Forearm fractures

CORRECT ANSWER—A. *Rationales:* Many adult pedestrians who are struck by cars sustain leg fractures and dislocations. Fractures to the upper extremities are not typical in pedestrians hit by moving vehicles.
Nursing process step: Assessment

39. Which of the following laboratory studies is most relevant to treating a patient who has sustained a pelvic fracture?
A. Urine myoglobin
B. Urinalysis
C. Type and crossmatch
D. Serum ethanol

CORRECT ANSWER—C. *Rationales:* Because of the rich blood supply to the pelvis, fractures to this area can result in significant blood loss. Type and crossmatch is a priority laboratory test in preparing for fluid replacement. Urinalysis and serum ethanol, although part of the trauma workup, do not alter treatment of a pelvic fracture. Urine is not commonly analyzed for myoglobin with this injury unless the mechanism was a crush injury; even then, urinalysis is not as high a priority as type and crossmatch.
Nursing process step: Intervention

40. Which of the following is a potential complication of compartment syndrome?
A. Disseminated intravascular coagulation (DIC)
B. Anemia
C. Myoglobinuria
D. Osteomyelitis

CORRECT ANSWER—C. *Rationales:* Myoglobin may be present in the urine as a result of muscle breakdown. To prevent myoglobin from damaging the renal tubules, the kidneys must be thoroughly flushed. A minimum urine output of 75 to 100 ml/hour needs to be maintained. Sodium bicarbonate can be administered to alkalinize the urine and to decrease precipitation of myoglobin in the renal tubules. Myoglobin in the tubules can lead to renal failure. DIC and anemia are not complications of compartment syndrome. Osteomyelitis can occur if an infection is present, but it is not a complication of compartment syndrome.
Nursing process step: Assessment

41. Which of the following is an indication for splint application?
A. To prevent infection
B. To prevent dislocations
C. To prevent damage to blood vessels and nerves
D. To align bones

CORRECT ANSWER—C. *Rationales:* By immobilizing the injured extremity, the nurse is helping prevent potential damage to nerves and blood vessels. A splint does not prevent infections from occurring if the fracture is open. It is not indicated for dislocation prevention, and it is not used to align the bones of a comminuted fracture.
Nursing process step: Intervention

42. Which of the following necessitates removal of a cast before the fracture has healed?
A. If the patient complains of itching under the cast
B. If pain is still present the day after the injury
C. If it is believed that the patient is developing a pressure ulcer
D. If the patient can't seem to get used to crutches

CORRECT ANSWER—C. *Rationales:* If a pressure ulcer is developing, the cast should be removed and the extremity evaluated. Itching is a common complaint and occurs as the skin dries. The patient may experience pain during the first 24 hours after the injury. Pain medication and elevation of the injured extremity should help relieve the discomfort. Pain that continues beyond the first 24 hours should be evaluated by the patient's health care provider. If using crutches is a problem, the patient needs instruction. If inability to use crutches persists, alternate methods may be investigated, such as switching to a walking cast (if the type of fracture permits) or a wheelchair (usually an expensive alternative).
Nursing process step: Evaluation

43. Which of the following is not appropriate when teaching a patient who is using crutches for the first time?
A. Have the patient stand and balance on the crutches
B. Have the patient hold the crutches 4 inches to the side and 4 inches in front of the feet
C. Instruct the patient to place all the weight on the axilla when ambulating
D. Have the patient demonstrate a three-point gait.

CORRECT ANSWER—C. *Rationales:* By straightening the elbows, the patient should place all the weight on the hands. The patient should be instructed not to place any weight on the axilla, not even when resting. Weight on the axilla causes nerve compression and may lead to permanent nerve damage.
Nursing process step: Evaluation

44. Which of the following is an expected outcome for a patient with a contusion to the thigh?
A. The patient states that the pain has increased
B. Swelling continues to progress
C. The patient relates understanding of the signs and symptoms that require further evaluation
D. The patient verbalizes that follow-up care will be needed only if symptoms worsen

CORRECT ANSWER—C. *Rationales:* Contusion to the thigh is an injury to the soft tissue caused by blunt force. There is hemorrhage into the injured area of the thigh, pain, swelling, and ecchymosis. Treatment is aimed at controlling these symptoms. Swelling should begin to decrease if treatment interventions were effective. Interventions should include elevation and the use of cold packs. If the swelling continues, additional interventions will become necessary. Follow-up care is needed regardless of symptoms to assure resolution of the injury without complications.
Nursing process step: Evaluation

45. When treating a patient with a strained knee, RICE is recommended. Which of the following is not an appropriate component of the RICE mnemonic ?
   A. R-Rest the affected extremity
   B. I-Ice application
   C. C-Compression with elastic dressing
   D. E-Exercise of the affected extremity

CORRECT ANSWER—D. *Rationales:* The correct mnemonic intervention for the letter E is elevation, which reduces swelling and pain. Exercise should be avoided, and the patient should rest the affected extremity. Options A, B, and C are correct.
Nursing process step: Intervention

46. When does the onset of fat embolism syndrome usually occur?
   A. 1 to 2 hours after a traumatic event
   B. 4 to 6 hours after a traumatic event
   C. 6 to 10 hours after a traumatic event
   D. More than 12 hours after a traumatic event

CORRECT ANSWER—D. *Rationales:* Symptoms of fat embolism syndrome usually occur 12 to 72 hours after a traumatic event, but they may be seen up to 10 days later. All of the other options are incorrect.
Nursing process step: Assessment

47. Which of the following is a priority nursing diagnosis for the hypovolemic patient with a pelvic fracture?
   A. Fluid volume deficit
   B. Ineffective breathing pattern
   C. Impaired gas exchange
   D. Ineffective airway clearance

CORRECT ANSWER—A. *Rationales:* Because pelvic fractures are associated with a large amount of blood loss, the most appropriate diagnosis for this patient is fluid volume deficit. A patient with a pelvic fracture is at risk for developing fat emboli. If this syndrome does occur, the patient would show an ineffective breathing pattern and impaired gas exchange.
Nursing process step: Analysis

48. Which of the following is the most appropriate intervention to control hemorrhage associated with an extremity injury?
   A. Placing a tourniquet 3 to 4 inches above the site of hemorrhage
   B. Applying warm compresses to cause vasoconstriction
   C. Holding the extremity low and applying pressure
   D. Applying a pressure dressing to the site of bleeding

CORRECT ANSWER—D. *Rationales:* Applying a pressure dressing to the site of bleeding is the first-line intervention for hemorrhage associated with an extremity injury. Applying a tourniquet should be a last resort because it could cause tissue damage. Warmth causes vasodilation and increases bleeding. Holding the extremity below the level of the heart also increases bleeding.
Nursing process step: Intervention

49. Which of the following interventions is appropriate for a patient who has a traction splint in place on arrival at the emergency department?
A. Immediately remove the splint and assess the patient's distal neurovascular status.
B. Leave the splint in place and assess the patient's distal neurovascular status.
C. Change the traction splint to one that the hospital owns and give the other back to the ambulance crew.
D. Take the splint off if the patient's neurovascular status is normal.

CORRECT ANSWER—B. *Rationales:* If a patient arrives in the emergency department with a traction splint in place, the nurse should assure that neurovascular status distal to the injury is intact. Next, the nurse should elevate the affected limb. The splint should be left in place until radiographic studies are complete and a fracture is ruled out.
Nursing process step: Intervention

50. Which of the following is a common complication of a pelvic fracture?
A. Urethral injury
B. Muscle spasms
C. Neurovascular compromise
D. Rhabdomyolysis

CORRECT ANSWER—A. *Rationales:* Urethral injury is a complication of a pelvic fracture. Muscle spasms are common with femur fractures, and neurovascular compromise is seen in extremity trauma. Rhabdomyolysis is defined as the acute destruction of muscle. This is not a complication of a pelvic fracture.
Nursing process step: Evaluation

51. Which of the following indicates an understanding of discharge instructions given after long leg cast placement?
A. The patient calls the emergency department after noticing a foul odor from the cast
B. After 1 week, the patient comes to the emergency department to have the cast removed
C. The patient verbalizes the need to come to the emergency department weekly for cast replacement
D. The patient states that he can walk on the cast for short distances and to climb stairs

CORRECT ANSWER—A. *Rationales:* A foul-smelling odor coming from the cast may indicate an infection, and the patient should return to a heath care professional or the emergency department. The cast will not be removed after 1 week, nor will it require weekly removal if cared for properly. The patient should not ambulate on a long leg cast; doing so stresses the cast and causes damage to the cast and possibly the broken leg.
Nursing process step: Evaluation

52. Which of the following type of splint is used to immobilize a fractured upper extremity?
A. Traction splint
B. Soft splint
C. Long spine board
D. Cervical collar

CORRECT ANSWER—B. *Rationales:* Four basic types of splints are available for immobilizing extremity fractures: soft splints, such as a pillow; hard splints, which have a firm surface; air splints, which are inflatable and provide support; and traction splints, which provide support and traction. Long spine boards and cervical collars are used to immobilize the spine and are not indicated for upper-extremity splinting.
Nursing process step: Intervention

53. Uric acid crystals that collect in the synovial fluid of joints can lead to erythema, warmth, and extreme pain. What is this condition called?
A. Bursitis
B. Rheumatoid arthritis
C. Uremia
D. Gout

CORRECT ANSWER—**D.** *Rationales:* Urate crystals that collect in the synovial fluid of joints cause rapid inflammation, often in just a few hours. The pain is severe. Bursitis is the inflammation of the synovial cavities that surround joints. It commonly occurs in the knee or elbow. Rheumatoid arthritis includes joint pain that is often accompanied by deformity. Uremia is associated with renal insufficiency and is caused by retention of a nitrogenous substance that is normally excreted by the kidneys.
Nursing process step: Assessment

54. In which of the following is replantation unlikely to be successful?
A. Multiple digits
B. The thumb
C. Pediatric extremity amputations
D. Injuries at multiple levels on the same extremity

CORRECT ANSWER—**D.** *Rationales:* Injuries at multiple levels on the same extremity make it unlikely that replantation will be successful. Replantation should be considered under the following circumstances. Loss of several digits: Hand function would be seriously compromised without them. Loss of the thumb: It constitutes 40% to 50% of the functional value of the hand because of its role in opposition and grasp, and replantation has a high success rate. In children: Their transected nerves regenerate well, and they readily adapt to using a replanted part.
Nursing process step: Evaluation

MENTAL HEALTH EMERGENCIES

CHAPTER 12

Mental Health Emergencies

Questions 1 through 3 refer to the following information:
After being struck by a car, a 3-year-old child is brought to the emergency department by paramedics. The parents arrive shortly afterward and are informed by the doctor that their child is dead. The mother becomes hysterical, throws herself on the floor, and begins screaming.

1. Which of the following interventions would be most appropriate for the mother at this time?
A. Support and encourage the mother's expression of grief and provide her with privacy.
B. Tell her to get off the floor. Her behavior is inappropriate.
C. Obtain a doctor's order and administer 5 mg of diazepam (Valium) by mouth.
D. Provide the family with accurate information regarding the incident.

CORRECT ANSWER—A. *Rationales:* Families need to be encouraged to express grief in whatever way they desire, as long as they do not harm themselves or others. Nursing's role is to help families focus on the grief, not to alleviate it. Families need accurate information to deal with the death of a loved one. However, they must be able to listen at the time the information is given. Diazepam may cloud or even delay the grieving process.
Nursing process step: Intervention

2. When communicating with a grieving family, the emergency nurse should do which of the following?
A. Use words such as dead, died, or death.
B. Tell the family, "Everything will be all right."
C. Tell the family, "It was for the best."
D. Tell the family that the patient did not suffer.

CORRECT ANSWER—A. *Rationales:* Using words such as dead, died, or death reinforces reality, prevents denial, and supports the grief process. Telling the family that "everything will be all right" or that "it was for the best" only minimizes their feelings. Telling the family that the patient did not suffer is helpful but should be stated only if it is true.
Nursing process step: Intervention

3. What would be a realistic short-term goal for the mother?
  A. Making funeral arrangements
  B. Sharing her feelings with the nurse
  C. Cleaning out the child's closet
  D. Leaving the emergency department just after learning about the death

CORRECT ANSWER—**B.** *Rationales:* By being able to share her feelings, the mother is acknowledging the death and beginning the work of grief. This step should begin in the emergency department. Making funeral arrangements and cleaning out the child's closet take more time. They are not short-term goals and are not realistic in the initial stages of grief. It is not desirable for the mother to leave the emergency department until she has had time to process and accept the information.
Nursing process step: Evaluation

4. Which of the following is the priority when assessing the suicidal patient who has ingested a handful of unknown pills?
  A. Determine if the patient was trying to harm himself or herself
  B. Determine if the patient has a support system
  C. Determine if the patient's physical condition is life-threatening
  D. Determine if the patient has a history of suicide attempts

CORRECT ANSWER—**C.** *Rationales:* If the patient's physical condition is life-threatening, the priority is to treat the medical condition. Any compromise in the patient's airway, breathing, or circulation must be addressed immediately. It is also imperative to determine the time of ingestion because this may determine treatment. The psychiatric evaluation, which includes intent to harm oneself, adequate support system, and history, can be done once the patient is medically stable.
Nursing process step: Assessment

5. Which is the most appropriate nursing diagnosis for a grieving family?
  A. Altered family process
  B. Powerlessness
  C. Grieving from experienced loss
  D. Ineffective coping

CORRECT ANSWER—**C.** *Rationales:* Grieving related to experienced loss most accurately describes the problem; therefore, nursing care in the emergency department should be based on this diagnosis. Families may not have altered family processes or suffer from ineffective coping. Although the family may feel powerless, this is not the most accurate diagnosis.
Nursing process step: Analysis

6. Initial interventions for the patient with acute anxiety include all except which of the following?
  A. Providing the patient with a safe, quiet, and private place
  B. Encouraging the patient to verbalize feelings and concerns
  C. Approaching the patient in a calm, confident manner
  D. Touching the patient in an attempt to comfort

CORRECT ANSWER—**D.** *Rationales:* The emergency nurse must establish rapport and trust with the anxious patient before using therapeutic touch. Touching an anxious patient may actually increase anxiety. Trust can be established by approaching the patient in a calm and confident manner; providing a place that is quiet, safe, and private; and encouraging the patient to verbalize feelings and concerns.
Nursing process step: Intervention

Questions 7 through 9 refer to the following information:

A 25-year-old man on a psychiatric hold is brought to the emergency department by police. He is in four-point restraints. The patient was reportedly observed running through the street naked, smashing windows, and screaming. He is now calm, nonverbal, and diaphoretic and has both vertical and horizontal nystagmus. He is noted to have a 2-inch laceration to his right arm.

7. What is the priority when assessing this patient?

A. To evaluate his mental status and obtain a full set of vital signs

B. To perform a primary assessment quickly and rule out other signs of trauma

C. To determine if the patient can cooperate so that the restraints can be removed

D. To send a urine specimen for toxicology screening

CORRECT ANSWER—B. *Rationales:* A quick primary assessment is indicated on all patients in the emergency department. This patient is a danger to himself and may have sustained other life-threatening injuries not noted by the police. The mental status exam and vital signs need to be done but are not the priority. Removing the restraints before fully examining the patient may place both the patient and the emergency department staff at great risk. Obtaining a urine specimen for toxicology screening takes time and should not determine the initial care.

Nursing process step: Assessment

8. What is the most appropriate immediate intervention for this patient?

A. Suturing his arm laceration

B. Obtaining an order and administering haloperidol (Haldol) 5 mg I.M. or I.V.

C. Leaving him in restraints because he is potentially violent and a danger to himself and others

D. Obtaining a psychiatric consult

CORRECT ANSWER—C. *Rationales:* Assuring the safety of the patient and staff is a top priority. Patients with a history of violence in the prehospital setting are at risk for violence in the emergency department. They should be fully evaluated before restraints are removed. Suturing can be done later, and a psychiatric consult is not indicated until the patient is medically stable. Haloperidol may be ordered after an evaluation by the doctor.

Nursing process step: Intervention

9. Which of the following is important when restraining a violent patient?

A. Have three staff members present: one for each side of the body and one for the head.

B. Always tie restraints to side rails.

C. Have an organized, efficient team approach once the decision is made to restrain the patient.

D. Secure restraints to the gurney with knots to prevent escape.

CORRECT ANSWER—C. *Rationales:* Emergency department personnel should use an organized, team approach when restraining violent patients so that no one is injured in the process. The leader, located at the patient's head, should take charge; four staff members are required to hold and restrain the limbs. For safety reasons, restraints should be fastened to the bed frame instead of the side rails. For quick release, loops should be used instead of knots.

Nursing process step: Intervention

10. Which of the following medications would the nurse expect to order to reverse a dystonic reaction?
A. Prochlorperazine (Compazine)
B. Diphenhydramine (Benadryl)
C. Haloperidol (Haldol)
D. Midazolam (Versed)

CORRECT ANSWER—B. *Rationales:* Diphenhydramine, 25 to 50 mg I.M. or I.V., would quickly reverse this condition. Prochlorperazine and haloperidol are both capable of causing dystonia, not reversing it. Midazolam would make this patient drowsy.
Nursing process step: Intervention

11. Which is the most appropriate nursing diagnosis for a violent patient in the emergency department?
A. Ineffective individual coping related to inadequate coping skills
B. Powerlessness related to lack of control over the event or situation
C. Risk for injury related to violent behavior
D. All of the above

CORRECT ANSWER—D. *Rationales:* All the answers are correct. A violent patient is unable to cope with the event or situation, feels powerless, and uses violent behavior to attempt to gain control. The patient and emergency department staff are at risk for injury from this reckless behavior. Nursing interventions should be focused on these diagnoses.
Nursing process step: Analysis

12. The emergency nurse determines that a suicidal patient is a danger to himself. Appropriate nursing interventions include all except which of the following?
A. Communicating with the family regarding the plan of care
B. Ensuring that a psychiatric consult is obtained
C. Ensuring that a psychiatric hold is written and placed on the medical record
D. Allowing the patient to ambulate around the emergency department to work off his nervous energy

CORRECT ANSWER—D. *Rationales:* It is the nurse's responsibility to protect the suicidal patient by providing a safe environment. Thus, suicidal patients must remain under close observation at all times. It is not appropriate for suicidal patients to wander around the emergency department alone. The emergency nurse must ensure that a psychiatric consultation is obtained so that the patient can be placed on a psychiatric hold and detained for further psychiatric evaluation. Communicating with the family regarding the plan of care is also essential.
Nursing process step: Intervention

13. Victims of domestic violence should be assessed for what important information while they are in the emergency department?
A. The reasons they stay in abusive relationships (for example, lack of financial autonomy and isolation)
B. Readiness to leave the perpetrator and knowledge of resources
C. The use of drugs or alcohol
D. A history of previous victimization

CORRECT ANSWER—B. *Rationales:* Victims of domestic violence must be assessed for their readiness to leave the perpetrator and their knowledge of the resources available to them. Nurses can then provide the victims with information and options to enable them to leave when they are ready. The reasons they stay in the relationship are complex and can be explored at a later time. The use of drugs or alcohol is irrelevant. There is no evidence to suggest that previous victimization results in a person's seeking or causing abusive relationships.
Nursing process step: Assessment

14. Which of the following nursing diagnoses is appropriate for a patient with a dystonic reaction?
A. Pain
B. Body image disturbance
C. Fear
D. All of the above

CORRECT ANSWER—**D.** *Rationales:* All the listed nursing diagnoses apply to a patient with a dystonic reaction. The patient can experience contractions of neck muscles, protruding or retracting of the tongue, and facial grimacing. The symptoms can be frightening and uncomfortable and can alter the patient's physical appearance.
Nursing process step: Analysis

15. Which of the following nursing diagnoses would not apply to a victim of domestic violence?
A. Ineffective individual coping
B. Risk of injury or trauma
C. Knowledge deficit regarding resources
D. Social isolation and powerlessness

CORRECT ANSWER—**A.** *Rationales:* The situation is not the victim's fault, and it is not due to ineffective coping mechanisms. It is the perpetrator who is not able to cope and who uses violence and aggression. The victim of domestic violence is at risk for injury or trauma from the perpetrator. Additionally, the victim may not be aware of the resources available. Gradually, the victim becomes isolated from friends and family because the perpetrator refuses to allow the victim to remain in contact with them.
Nursing process step: Analysis

16. In a toddler, which of the following injuries is probably the result of child abuse?
A. A hematoma on the occipital region of the head
B. A 1-inch forehead laceration
C. Several small, dime-sized circular burns on the child's back
D. A small isolated bruise on the right lower extremity

CORRECT ANSWER—**C.** *Rationales:* Small circular burns on a child's back are no accident and may be from cigarettes. Toddlers are injury prone because of their developmental stage, and falls are frequent because of their unsteady gait. Therefore, head injuries are not uncommon. A small area of ecchymosis is not suspicious in this age-group.
Nursing process step: Assessment

17. Which of the following statements would be most appropriate or therapeutic when the emergency department nurse suspects domestic violence?
A. Ask directly, "Is someone hurting you at home?" Let the patient know that she is not alone and that there is help when she is ready to leave.
B. Comment, "This doesn't look like you fell. Is there something else you want to tell me?"
C. Tell her, "You should leave him. You do not deserve this!" Call the police and encourage her to press charges.
D. State, "Wow, you're really injury prone."

CORRECT ANSWER—**A.** *Rationales:* Victims of domestic violence want to be asked directly. It is important to let them know that help is available when they are ready and that they are not alone. They should be given the resources to leave when it is safe for them to do so. The statements in Options B and D are indirect and imply that the emergency department nurse really doesn't want to know. The statement in Option C is judgmental.
Nursing process step: Intervention

18. Which intervention would not be appropriate for a suspected rape victim?
  A. Emphasize that you are there to help and that she is safe now.
  B. Encourage the patient to verbalize what happened.
  C. Provide the patient with privacy (by leaving her alone) until she is ready to talk.
  D. Offer to call friends or family for her when she is ready.

CORRECT ANSWER—C. *Rationales:* Never leave a rape victim alone. This increases feelings of isolation, fear, and anxiety. Emphasizing that you are there to help and that she is safe establishes rapport and trust. Encouraging a patient to talk helps her sort through her thoughts and feelings and lowers her anxiety level. Friends and family can provide a feeling of safety when the patient is ready.
Nursing process step: Intervention

19. Which of the following groups of characteristics would the emergency department nurse expect to see in the schizophrenic patient?
  A. Disheveled appearance, flight of ideas, grandiose delusions, and auditory hallucinations
  B. Periods of hyperactivity and irritability alternating with depression
  C. Delusions of jealousy and persecution, paranoia, and mistrust
  D. Sadness, apathy, feelings of worthlessness, anorexia, and weight loss

CORRECT ANSWER—A. *Rationales:* A disheveled appearance, flight of ideas, grandiose delusions, and auditory hallucinations are all characteristic of the classic schizophrenic patient. These patients are not able to care for their physical appearance. They frequently hear voices telling them to do something either to themselves or to others. Additionally, they verbally ramble from one topic to the next. Periods of hyperactivity and irritability alternating with depression is characteristic of bipolar or manic disease. Delusions of jealousy and persecution, paranoia, and mistrust are characteristics of paranoid disorders. Sadness, apathy, feelings of worthlessness, anorexia, and weight loss are characteristics of depression.
Nursing process step: Assessment

20. Which of the following is not a true statement about child abuse?
  A. Nurses are required by law to report only actual cases of child abuse, not cases of suspected abuse.
  B. Nurses should be direct and nonjudgmental when communicating with parents who are suspected of abusing their children.
  C. It should be documented on the medical record that a report was made to the Child Protective Agency.
  D. Whenever possible, photographs should be taken to provide evidence of visible injuries.

CORRECT ANSWER—A. *Rationales:* Nurses are required by law to report both actual and suspected cases of child abuse. Nurses should be direct and nonjudgmental when communicating with parents who are suspected of abusing their children. The medical record should show documentation that the Child Protective Agency was notified of the case. Whenever possible, photographs should be taken to provide evidence of visible injuries.
Nursing process step: Intervention

21. What medication would probably be ordered for the schizophrenic patient?
A. Chlorpromazine (Thorazine)
B. Haloperidol (Haldol)
C. Lithium carbonate (Lithonate)
D. Amitriptyline (Elavil)

CORRECT ANSWER—**B.** *Rationales:* Haloperidol administered I.M. or I.V. is the drug of choice for acute psychotic behavior. Chlorpromazine is also an antipsychotic drug; however, it causes more pronounced sedation than haloperidol. Lithium carbonate is useful in bipolar or manic disorder, and amitriptyline is used for depression.
Nursing process step: Intervention

22. Sudden infant death syndrome (SIDS) is one of the most common causes of death in infants. At what age is the diagnosis of SIDS most likely?
A. At 1 to 2 years of age
B. At 1 week to 1 year of age, peaking at 2 to 4 months
C. At 6 months to 1 year of age, peaking at 10 months
D. At 6 to 8 weeks of age

CORRECT ANSWER—**B.** *Rationales:* SIDS can occur any time between 1 week and 1 year of age; the incidence peaks at 2 to 4 months of age.
Nursing process step: Assessment

23. When interviewing the parents of an injured child, which of the following is the strongest indicator that child abuse may be a problem?
A. The injury is not consistent with the history or the child's age.
B. The mother and father tell different stories regarding what happened.
C. The family is poor.
D. The parents are argumentative and demanding with emergency department personnel.

CORRECT ANSWER—**A.** *Rationales:* When the child's injuries are inconsistent with the history given or impossible because of the child's age and developmental stage, the emergency department nurse should be suspicious that child abuse is occurring. The parents may tell different stories because their perception may be different regarding what happened. If they change their story when different health care workers ask the same question, this is a clue that child abuse may be a problem. Child abuse occurs in all socioeconomic groups. Parents may argue and be demanding because of the stress of having an injured child.
Nursing process step: Assessment

24. When communicating with the grieving family after a sudden infant death syndrome (SIDS) death, it is most important that the emergency department nurse do which of the following?
A. Stress that the death is not the parents' fault, that is was unpreventable and unpredictable
B. Stress that an autopsy must be done to confirm the diagnosis
C. Stress that the parents are still young and can have more children
D. Instruct the parents to place other infants on their backs to sleep

CORRECT ANSWER—**A.** *Rationales:* The cause of SIDS is unclear. These deaths are unexpected and sudden. It is most important that the parents do not believe that the death is their fault or that they could have prevented it. Although it is important to inform the parents that an autopsy needs to be performed, it is secondary. Stressing that they are still young and can have more children minimizes their feelings of grief. Instructing the parents to place other infants on their backs to sleep implies that the parents did something to cause the death.
Nursing process step: Intervention

25. When discharging a patient after treatment for a dystonic reaction, it is most important that the emergency department nurse ensure that the patient understands which of the following?
A. Results of treatment are rapid and dramatic but may not last
B. Although uncomfortable, this reaction is not serious
C. The patient should not buy drugs on the street again
D. The patient must continue to take diphenhydramine (Benadryl) for the next 2 to 3 days to prevent a return of symptoms

CORRECT ANSWER—**D.** *Rationales:* Phenothiazines have a half life of 24 hours; therefore, oral diphenhydramine must be continued for the next 2 days to prevent the return of symptoms. Results of treatment are rapid and dramatic and will last if the patient receives and understands appropriate discharge instructions. Dystonic reactions can be life-threatening when airway patency is compromised. Lecturing the patient about buying drugs on the street is not appropriate.
Nursing process step: Evaluation

26. Which of the following histories is most consistent with the diagnosis of sudden infant death syndrome (SIDS)?
A. The child had been physically abused and is usually found in the evening
B. The infant was considered ill and had many medical problems
C. The infant was healthy and was found dead shortly after being put down to sleep
D. The child is usually described as lethargic, irritable, and feeding poorly

CORRECT ANSWER—**C.** *Rationales:* Children who are diagnosed with SIDS are typically healthy with no previous medical problems. They are usually found dead sometime after being put down to sleep. Depending on how long the infant has been dead, a SIDS baby may have a mottled complexion with extreme cyanosis of the lips and fingertips, or pooling of blood in the legs and feet that may be mistaken for bruises.
Nursing process step: Assessment

Questions 27 and 28 refer to the following information:
A middle-aged woman brings her mother to the emergency department. The mother has multiple bruises and skin breakdown. The woman states that her mother has lived with her for the past 5 years and that the mother is confused and falls all the time. The daughter states: "You know, she has Parkinson's disease and can't even dress herself." On examination, the patient is fully oriented but unable to ambulate alone.

27. When eliciting a history from the daughter, it is most important that the emergency nurse do which of the following?
A. Agree with the daughter that older people do fall all the time and that it is impossible to prevent them from getting skin breakdown from immobility
B. Ask specifically if the daughter is experiencing great stress and frustration caring for her mother at home, whether she has multiple demands, and if she has any resources available to her
C. Determine if there is a history of family violence, including domestic violence and child abuse
D. Inquire about a history of alcoholism

CORRECT ANSWER—B. *Rationales:* Elder abuse is often rooted in frustration and stress on the part of the abuser. The family member caring for the parent may feel overburdened and exhausted and may need support. Asking the family member about the stress and frustration associated with caring for a parent demonstrates concern and appreciation for the situation. Emergency department nurses can then help families mobilize community resources. That older people fall a lot is a misconception that contributes to the underdetection of elder abuse. Determining if there is a history of family violence or alcoholism is important. Patients and their families may not offer this information freely, and it is not as important as determining the caretaker's stressors.
Nursing process step: Assessment

28. What is the best approach for the nurse to take when an elderly patient does not acknowledge the abuse and wants to stay in the home?
A. Provide the patient and family with appropriate resources and report the abuse as required by state law
B. Call the police and have the patient removed from the home
C. Arrange for a visiting nurse to make home visits
D. Insist that the patient confront the situation so that a crisis intervention plan can be initiated

CORRECT ANSWER—A. *Rationales:* When the patient is alert and oriented, the patient should be provided with choices and the nurse should respect whatever decision the patient makes. Nurses must report elder abuse as required by their state law. Forcefully removing a patient from the home is not advisable. Patients have the right to stay in the abusive relationship if they choose to do so. A visiting nurse is only one resource available to family members, and they should be provided with several options. Insisting that the patient confront the situation is not appropriate. The patient may not have the required coping mechanisms and may not be ready to confront the situation at this time.
Nursing process step: Intervention

29. A 40-year-old executive who was laid off from work unexpectedly 2 days earlier presents to the emergency department. He is complaining of fatigue and inability to cope. He admits drinking excessively over the past 48 hours. This is an example of which of the following conditions?
  A. Alcoholism
  B. A manic episode
  C. Situational crisis
  D. Depression

CORRECT ANSWER—C. *Rationales:* A situational crisis results from a specific event in a person's life. The person is overwhelmed by the situation and reacts emotionally. Fatigue, insomnia, and inability to make a decision are common. The situational crisis may precipitate behavior that in turn causes a crisis (alcohol or drug abuse). There is not enough information to label this patient an alcoholic. A manic episode is characterized by euphoria and labile affect. Symptoms of depression are usually present for 2 or more weeks.
Nursing process step: Assessment

30. Victims of sexual assault can experience post-traumatic stress reactions after the attack. Which of the following statements does this include?
  A. Denial of the event
  B. Anger, guilt, and humiliation
  C. Fatigue and self-blame
  D. Flashbacks, recurring dreams, and numbness

CORRECT ANSWER—D. *Rationales:* Posttraumatic stress involves recurring dreams about the event or flashbacks to the event. The victims feel a general sense of numbness and estrangement from others. Emotional reactions such as denial of the event, anger, guilt, humiliation, fatigue, and self-blame are all normal feelings after rape but are not consistent with posttraumatic stress.
Nursing process step: Assessment

31. What is an expected outcome for the violent patient in the emergency department?
  A. The patient and staff are not injured
  B. The patient verbalizes feelings of frustration
  C. The patient does not demonstrate any further signs of aggressive behavior
  D. All of the above

CORRECT ANSWER—D. *Rationales:* Avoiding injury to the staff and patient, allowing the patient to verbalize feelings of frustration, and avoiding further demonstrations of aggressive behavior are all expected outcome for the violent patient in the emergency department.
Nursing process step: Evaluation

32. Which of the following is not true about sudden cardiac death syndrome survivors?
  A. Their usual coping behaviors may be inadequate
  B. The event represents a threat to their survival
  C. The person is physiologically stable on arrival at the emergency department.
  D. Loss and grief reactions may occur

CORRECT ANSWER—C. *Rationales:* The survivor of sudden cardiac death is physiologically unstable either before arrival or on arrival at the emergency department. These people have survived resuscitation and experienced a close brush with death. Their usual coping mechanisms may not be adequate, and both loss and grief reactions may occur.
Nursing process step: Assessment

33. Which of the following is the most important nursing diagnosis for the manic patient while in the emergency department?
A. Altered thought process related to mental disorder
B. Noncompliance with medication related to poor impulse control
C. Risk for injury related to grandiose delusions and impaired judgment
D. Altered health maintenance related to inability to make decisions

CORRECT ANSWER—C. *Rationales:* Patients in the manic phase of their bipolar disorder are at high risk for injuring themselves and others because of their reckless behavior. Therefore, nursing interventions should be aimed at preventing injury. Although the other diagnoses are applicable, they are not the priority in the emergency department setting.
Nursing process step: Analysis

34. A patient presents to the emergency department with signs of ineffective coping. What is the most realistic nursing goal for this patient while in the emergency department?
A. To help the patient improve coping skills
B. To help the patient develop a plan for better communication
C. To help the patient identify the precipitating event and select realistic options
D. To help the patient develop a plan to deal with stress more effectively

CORRECT ANSWER—C. *Rationales:* In the emergency department, it is realistic for the nurse to help the patient identify the precipitating event and possible options. It is not realistic to strive for improvement in coping skills, better communication, or dealing with stress more effectively. These goals require long-term planning that cannot be done in the emergency department.
Nursing process step: Evaluation

35. Which are appropriate nursing interventions for the patient with bipolar disorder?
A. Obtaining a lithium level and urine toxicology screen for drugs
B. Orienting the patient to current reality (person, place, and time) if delusional
C. Restraining the patient as needed for safety
D. All of the above

CORRECT ANSWER—D. *Rationales:* All answer options are appropriate interventions. Lithium carbonate (Lithonate) is the drug of choice for bipolar disorder, and drug levels should be measured. A toxicology screen is important to rule out substance toxicity, which can mimic psychiatric illness. Delusional patients should be reoriented to reality. If mania is not controlled, patients are at risk of harming themselves and others. Restraints may be necessary.
Nursing process step: Intervention

36. What is the most appropriate nursing diagnosis for the survivor of sudden cardiac death?
A. Grieving related to anticipated loss
B. Anxiety related to actual threat of death
C. Powerlessness related to fear of nonsurvival (death)
D. All of the above

CORRECT ANSWER—D. *Rationales:* All the nursing diagnoses listed are appropriate for the survivor of sudden cardiac death. It is common for the survivor to experience grief and feelings of loss as well as anxiety and powerlessness.
Nursing process step: Analysis

37. For which of the following reasons are antidepressants not usually prescribed for depressed patients being discharged from the emergency department?

A. Therapeutic responses take several weeks to months

B. Overdoses are lethal

C. Patients need to return for appropriate psychiatric follow-up, and they might not comply if they are given the medication

D. All of the above

CORRECT ANSWER—D. *Rationales*: Patients who are depressed need to receive psychiatric follow-up and not simply be given antidepressants. Patients on antidepressants need to be followed carefully because therapeutic response may not be seen for several weeks to months and overdoses of the drugs can be lethal.

Nursing process step: Intervention

38. A patient presents to the emergency department after being attacked and sexually assaulted. What is the most accurate nursing diagnosis for this patient?

A. Rape-trauma syndrome

B. Fear

C. Anxiety

D. Helplessness

CORRECT ANSWER—A. *Rationales*: The nursing diagnosis rape-trauma syndrome refers to both the acute and the long-term phases experienced by the victim of sexual assault. Specific nursing interventions can be planned based on this diagnosis. The rape victim may also experience fear, anxiety, and helplessness; however, these diagnoses are not specific.

Nursing processes step: Analysis/Nursing diagnosis

39. A dystonic reaction can be caused by which of the following medications?

A. Diazepam (Valium)

B. Haloperidol (Haldol)

C. Amitriptyline (Elavil)

D. Clonazepam (Klonopin)

CORRECT ANSWER—B. *Rationales*: Haloperidol is a phenothiazine and is capable of causing dystonic reactions. Diazepam and clonazepam are benzodiazepines, and amitriptyline is a tricyclic antidepressant. Benzodiazepines and tricyclic antidepressants do not cause dystonic reactions. Benzodiazepines can cause drowsiness, lethargy, and hypotension. Tricyclics can cause a decreased level of consciousness, tachycardia, dry mouth, and dilated pupils.

Nursing process step: Intervention

PATIENT CARE MANAGEMENT

CHAPTER 13

Patient Care Management

1. A patient presenting to the emergency department has ventricular tachycardia at a rate of 170 beats/minute, and blood pressure is 90/60 mm Hg. The patient is awake and oriented and has substernal chest pain. During synchronized cardioversion, the patient becomes unconscious and her cardiac rhythm changes to ventricular fibrillation. Which of the following is the priority of the emergency nurse?
A. Administer amiodarone (Cordarone) by I.V. bolus
B. Administer bretylium tosylate (Bretylol) by I.V. bolus
C. Administer synchronized countershock at 300 joules
D. Defibrillate at 200 joules

CORRECT ANSWER—D. *Rationales:* According to the standards of the American Heart Association, the patient should be defibrillated and then given epinephrine. Patients in ventricular fibrillation cannot be cardioverted using the synchronization mode. Although amiodarone and bretylium may be used in the treatment of ventricular fibrillation, they are not considered first-line pharmacologic agents.
Nursing process step: Intervention

2. Which physiologic abnormalities can occur as a result of multiple packed red blood cell transfusions?
A. Hypocalcemia and hypothermia
B. Hyperchloremic acidosis, hypothermia, and vasodilation
C. Hyponatremia
D. Hypercalcemia

CORRECT ANSWER—D. *Rationales:* Hypercalcemia can occur after massive blood transfusion because of the presence of the preservative EDTA. Hypothermia, hypernatremia, and hyperchloremic acidosis can also occur.
Nursing process step: Assessment

3. Why should topical nitroglycerin agents be removed from the chest before defibrillation?
A. Massive drug administration
B. Deactivation of the drug
C. Electrical arcing
D. Reflex tachycardia

CORRECT ANSWER—C. *Rationales:* Electrical arcing can occur when topical medications are present. These agents should be removed or wiped off before defibrillation. Defibrillation has no effect on administration or deactivation of topical nitroglycerin. Nitroglycerin in combination with defibrillation does not cause reflex tachycardia.
Nursing process step: Intervention

4. Which agent is used in the treatment of organo-
phosphate poisoning?
  A. Naloxone (Narcan)
  B. Atropine sulfate
  C. Activated charcoal
  D. Flumazenil (Romazicon)

CORRECT ANSWER—**B.** *Rationales:* Organophosphate insecticides (cholinesterase inhibitors)
bind to prevent the breakdown of acetylcholine, resulting in pulmonary edema. Atropine
sulfate (an anticholinergic agent) promotes
drying of pulmonary secretions and is considered an end point in treatment. Flumazenil is
used in the treatment of barbiturate overdose;
naloxone is used in the treatment of opioid toxicity; and activated charcoal is used to facilitate
binding of the ingested toxic substance and to
promote excretion of the substance through
the GI tract.
Nursing process step: Intervention

5. When administering agents by way of an endotracheal tube, the nurse should do which of the
following?
  A. Stop cardiopulmonary resuscitation, administer the agent, and then hyperventilate the patient
  B. Continue cardiopulmonary resuscitation, administer the agent, and then resume normal
ventilations
  C. Continue cardiopulmonary resuscitation, administer the agent, and then flush with sterile
water
  D. Place the syringe needle deep into the endotracheal tube and vigorously instill the agent

CORRECT ANSWER—**A.** *Rationales:* Medication
administration by way of an endotracheal tube
requires momentary cessation of cardiopulmonary resuscitation, followed by hyperventilation to nebulize the medication. Needles
should never be placed in the endotracheal
tube. Resuming normal ventilations does not
propel the drug into the lungs or clear the tube
of any remaining drug. Flushing the tube with
sterile water places excess fluid in the lungs,
further compromising the patient's oxygenation.
Nursing process step: Intervention

6. In which of the following is cardioversion con-
traindicated?
  A. Methemoglobinemia
  B. Cyanide toxicity
  C. Hypermagnesemia
  D. Digoxin toxicity

CORRECT ANSWER—**D.** *Rationales:* Elective cardioversion should be avoided in the presence
of digoxin toxicity because there is a likelihood
of arrhythmogenesis. Cardioversion can be
safely used with methemoglobinemia, cyanide
toxicity, and hypermagnesemia.
Nursing process step: Analysis

7. What is the criterion for the determination of
death in the United States?
  A. Irreversible cessation of circulatory functions
  B. Irreversible cessation of respiratory functions
  C. Irreversible cessation of all functions of the
entire brain, including the brain stem
  D. All of the above

CORRECT ANSWER—**D.** *Rationales:* According
to the Uniform Determination of Death Act,
death can be pronounced in the United States
when there is irreversible cessation of circulatory and respiratory functions *or* irreversible cessation of all functions of the entire brain, including the brain stem. Death must be
pronounced according to accepted medical
standards.
Nursing process step: Assessment

8. A patient presenting to the emergency department has a narrow complex tachycardia at a rate of 160 beats/minute and is unresponsive. Blood pressure is 70/50 mm Hg. Which is the highest treatment priority?
  A. Administer synchronized cardioversion
  B. Administer oxygen at 100% by way of a non-rebreather mask
  C. Administer verapamil (Calan) 5 mg by I.V. bolus
  D. Administer asynchronized cardioversion

CORRECT ANSWER—**A.** *Rationales:* The treatment of choice in patients with symptomatic narrow complex tachycardia is synchronized cardioversion. Asynchronized cardioversion is indicated in pulseless ventricular tachycardia or ventricular fibrillation. This patient, although unstable, has a pulse (blood pressure of 70/50 mm Hg), so synchronized cardioversion is the treatment choice. Oxygen and verapamil are secondary options.
Nursing process step: Intervention

9. Metastatic disease is an absolute contraindication for all except which of the following?
  A. Heart valve donation
  B. Eye (cornea) donation
  C. Saphenous vein donation
  D. Bone donation

CORRECT ANSWER—**B.** *Rationales:* Transmissibility of malignant cells is possible with heart valve, saphenous vein, and bone donation because of the vascularity of these tissues. The cornea is not vascular, thus eliminating the possibility of disease transmission.
Nursing process step: Analysis

10. Which drug is used to treat symptomatic bradycardia in a patient who has had a heart transplant?
  A. Epinephrine (Adrenalin)
  B. Atropine sulfate
  C. Isoproterenol (Isuprel)
  D. Adenosine (Adenocard)

CORRECT ANSWER—**C.** *Rationales:* Isoproterenol is the drug of choice in the treatment of symptomatic bradycardia after heart transplantation because of its potent beta-adrenergic effect in patients with intact vagal innervation. Adenosine slows electrical conduction through the atrioventricular node and is used to treat symptomatic supraventricular tachycardia. Atropine is an anticholinergic agent used in the treatment of symptomatic bradycardia in patients with intact vagal innervation. Epinephrine is a potent sympathomimetic agent that mimics the sympathetic nervous system.
Nursing process step: Intervention

11. What is a normal systolic blood pressure for a 3-year-old child?
  A. 100 mm Hg
  B. 86 mm Hg
  C. 120 mm Hg
  D. 60 mm Hg

CORRECT ANSWER—**B.** *Rationales:* Using the formula systolic blood pressure = 80 + age in years × 2, the estimated blood pressure for a 3-year-old child is 80 + (3 × 2) = 86.
Nursing process step: Assessment

12. Which is the most common cause of trauma deaths in infants?
A. Homicide
B. Drowning
C. Motor vehicle crashes
D. Fires and burn injuries

CORRECT ANSWER—C. *Rationales:* According to the Centers for Disease Control and Prevention, motor vehicle crashes are the number one cause of pediatric deaths, followed by homicide, suicide, drowning, pedestrian injuries, fires, and burns.
Nursing process step: Evaluation

13. To decrease the likelihood of bradyarrhythmias in children during endotracheal intubation, succinylcholine (Anectine) is used with which of the following agents?
A. Epinephrine (Adrenalin)
B. Isoproterenol (Isuprel)
C. Atropine sulfate
D. Lidocaine hydrochloride (Xylocaine)

CORRECT ANSWER—C. *Rationales:* Succinylcholine is an ultra-short-acting depolarizing agent used for rapid-sequence intubation. Bradycardia can occur, especially in children. Atropine is the drug of choice in treating succinylcholine-induced bradycardia. Lidocaine is used in adults only. Epinephrine bolus and isoproterenol are not used in rapid-sequence intubation because of their profound cardiac effects.
Nursing process step: Intervention

14. Which of the following agents cannot be administered by way of intraosseus infusion?
A. Sodium bicarbonate
B. Dopamine (Intropin)
C. Calcium chloride
D. Isoproterenol (Isuprel)

CORRECT ANSWER—D. *Rationales:* The following agents can be safely administered by way of intraosseus infusion: sodium bicarbonate, calcium, bretylium, glucose, crystalloids, colloids, blood, dopamine, epinephrine, and dobutamine. Isoproterenol, which does not fall into any of the above categories, cannot be administered by the intraosseus route.
Nursing process step: Intervention

15. What is the circulating blood volume in a 20-kg child?
A. 1,500 ml
B. 1,600 ml
C. 1,700 ml
D. 1,800 ml

CORRECT ANSWER—B. *Rationales:* Children have a circulating blood volume of 80 ml/kg. Therefore, a 20-kg child has a circulating blood volume of 1,600 ml.
Nursing process step: Analysis

16. When assessing an elderly patient with upper GI bleeding, the nurse should determine that which of the following is not a risk factor?
A. Nonsteroidal anti-inflammatory drug use
B. Gender
C. *Heliobacter pylori* infection
D. Smoking

CORRECT ANSWER—B. *Rationales:* Gender has not been identified as a risk factor in upper GI bleeding. Cigarette smoking, nonsteroidal anti-inflammatory drugs, and *Heliobacter pylori* infection have been implicated as major risk factors.
Nursing process step: Assessment

17. Which of the following is not seen in a brain dead person?
A. Neurogenic pulmonary edema
B. Neurogenic hyperthermia
C. Neurogenic diabetes insipidus
D. Neurogenic shock

CORRECT ANSWER—**B.** *Rationales:* After permanent interruption of cerebral circulation (brain death), the patient frequently experiences pulmonary edema, diabetes insipidus, or neurogenic shock. Loss of thermoregulatory mechanisms result in hypothermia.
Nursing process step: Assessment

18. A medical examiner's case may include all except which of the following?
A. Homicide or suspicion of homicide
B. Unwitnessed cardiac arrest
C. Traumatic death
D. Poisoning

CORRECT ANSWER—**B.** *Rationales:* Forensic examination of patients after their death is common when the cause of death is suspected of being unnatural. Homicide or suspected homicide, death after traumatic injury, and poisoning may be attributed to malicious acts or product failure involving others. Further investigation is required in these cases. Unwitnessed cardiac arrest is not considered unnatural.
Nursing process step: Analysis

19. Management of the potential organ donor includes which of the following steps?
A. Maintaining urine output above 100 ml/hour
B. Maintaining hematocrit above 30%
C. Manipulating the ventilatory settings to maintain a PCO_2 of 60 mm Hg
D. Maintaining central venous pressure less than 2 mm Hg

CORRECT ANSWER—**A.** *Rationales:* Maintaining urine output above 100 ml/hour in a potential organ donor ensures adequate perfusion of the renal glomeruli. Systolic blood pressure should be maintained above 100 mm Hg. Central venous pressure should be maintained within normal limits to prevent neurogenic pulmonary edema. Hematocrit should be maintained above 30% to ensure adequate intravascular fluid volume. Oxygen and carbon dioxide levels are maintained within normal limits to ensure organ and tissue oxygenation.
Nursing process step: Intervention

20. Which site is the most reliable in assessing the pulse of a hemodynamically unstable adult?
A. Radial
B. Popliteal
C. Carotid
D. Dorsalis pedis

CORRECT ANSWER—**C.** *Rationales:* Because of sympathetic nervous system influences resulting in peripheral vasoconstriction, the central carotid pulse is the most reliable site in assessing pulse quality in the hemodynamically unstable adult. Radial, dorsalis pedis, and popliteal pulses are generally palpable in patients with a systolic pressure greater than 80 mm Hg. Femoral pulses are palpable in patients with a systolic pressure greater than 70 mm Hg, and carotid pulses are palpable in patients with a systolic pressure greater than 60 mm Hg.
Nursing process step: Assessment

21. Why might diabetic patients with myocardial ischemia not have classic chest pain?
   A. Aspartame (Nutra-Sweet) use
   B. Insulin use
   C. Sulfonylurea agent use
   D. Chronic neuropathy

CORRECT ANSWER—**D.** *Rationales:* Chronic neuropathy, commonly seen in patients with diabetes mellitus, interferes with the transmission of pain impulses. Diabetics with myocardial ischemia may be pain free. Careful history combined with subjective findings should be used in diagnosing cardiac emergencies in diabetic patients. The use of aspartame, sulfonylurea agents, or insulin does not interfere with pain impulse transmission to the brain.
Nursing process step: Assessment

22. The nurse would expect to see respiratory acidosis as a result of which of the following?
   A. Salicylate toxicity
   B. Aldosteronism
   C. Severe scoliosis
   D. High altitudes

CORRECT ANSWER—**C.** *Rationales:* Scoliosis prevents the thoracic cage from expanding and, therefore, decreases tidal volumes. Respiratory acidosis occurs in severe cases of scoliosis. High altitudes, aldosteronism, and salicylate toxicity produce respiratory alkalosis.
Nursing process step: Assessment

23. Encouraging fantasy, play, and participation in their care is a useful developmental approach for which pediatric age-group?
   A. Preschool age (3 to 5 years)
   B. Adolescence (10 to 19 years)
   C. School age (5 to 10 years)
   D. Toddler (1 to 3 years)

CORRECT ANSWER—**A.** *Rationales:* Children in the preschool age-group have a rich fantasy life and think about magic. Combined with their strong concept of self, fantasy play and participation in care can minimize the trauma of being in the emergency department. Adolescents should be allowed choices and control. School-age children are modest and need to have their privacy respected. Procedures should be explained to them. Toddlers should be examined in the presence of their parents because they fear separation. Allow choices when possible.
Nursing process step: Intervention

24. After any type of traumatic injury, a child may experience which of the following?
   A. Bradycardia
   B. Aerophagia
   C. Hypothermia
   D. Cushing's phenomenon

CORRECT ANSWER—**B.** *Rationales:* Swallowing of air (aerophagia) occurs in children, causing gastric dilatation that impedes diaphragmatic expansion. Cushing's phenomenon is bradycardia in the presence of increasing blood pressure; it is associated with an increase in intracranial pressure. Hypothermia is seen when the child's clothing is removed and the child is exposed to the ambient environment.
Nursing process step: Assessment

25. Which of the following is an ominous sign of cardiac arrest in children?
A. Tachycardia
B. Increased peripheral vascular resistance
C. Tachypnea
D. Bradycardia

CORRECT ANSWER—D. *Rationales:* Bradycardia is an ominous sign of cardiac arrest in children and should be considered the result of hypoxia until proven otherwise. Tachypnea is indicative of respiratory distress or anxiety; tachycardia is seen with febrile illness. Increased peripheral resistance is not a common finding in children and is associated with ingestion of pharmacologic agents.
Nursing process step: Assessment

26. Which is a late sign of hypovolemic shock in a child?
A. Absence of bilateral breath sounds
B. Presence of hypotension
C. Presence of flushing of the skin
D. Presence of tachycardia

CORRECT ANSWER—B. *Rationales:* Because children are able to compensate for blood loss by increasing their intrinsic heart rate and their peripheral vascular resistance, up to 33% of blood volume may be lost before a change in blood pressure. Capillary refill is a sensitive indicator of perfusion in the pediatric patient. Absence of breath sounds is commonly seen in patients with pneumothorax. Tachycardia is commonly seen with anxiety or febrile illness. Flushing of the skin is seen with toxic ingestion.
Nursing process step: Assessment

27. Which of the following medications cannot be administered by way of an endotracheal tube?
A. Naloxone (Narcan)
B. Bretylium (Bretylol)
C. Epinephrine (Adrenalin)
D. Atropine

CORRECT ANSWER—B. *Rationales:* Naloxone, atropine, diazepam, epinephrine, and lidocaine are the five agents that can be administered by way of an endotracheal tube.
Nursing process step: Intervention

28. Verbalization of which of the following by the nurse demonstrates successful teaching about adenosine (Adenocard) administration?
A. Adenosine should be given by I.V. push over 1 to 3 minutes.
B. Adenosine should be given by continuous I.V. infusion over 20 to 30 minutes.
C. Adenosine should be given by deep I.M. injection.
D. Adenosine should be given by I.V. push over 1 to 3 seconds, followed by a 10-ml flush with normal saline.

CORRECT ANSWER—D. *Rationales:* The half-life of adenosine is 10 seconds; thereby, it requires rapid I.V. push administration, followed by a 10-ml infusion with normal saline.
Nursing process step: Evaluation

29. A patient is chosen as a match for a donor heart based on which of the following?
  A. Blood type only
  B. Blood type and donor-recipient weight compatibility
  C. HLA crossmatch compatibility only
  D. Donor-recipient age compatibility

CORRECT ANSWER—B. *Rationales:* A patient is compatible with a donor heart if ABO type and body weight are compatible. HLA-antigen typing may be used for high-risk patients. Age, HLA crossmatch compatibility, and ABO type are not used in determining allocation independent of one another.
Nursing process step: Assessment

30. Anencephalics cannot become organ donors for which reason?
  A. They do not fully meet the criteria for brain death.
  B. They have multiple congenital anomalies, which preclude transplantation.
  C. They are medical examiner cases that require autopsy.
  D. It is recommended that families not be approached about donation after the loss of an anencephalic infant.

CORRECT ANSWER—A. *Rationales:* Organ donation in the United States occurs after the determination of death using neurologic criteria (brain death). The Uniform Determination of Death Act states that death is determined when there is irreversible damage to the entire brain. Because anencephalics are born without a cerebrum, they cannot fulfill this criterion. Anencephalics commonly have multiple congenital anomalies, although these are not what exclude them from donation. Organ donation can occur in medical examiner cases. Federal law requires that all families be approached with the option of organ or tissue donation after the loss of a loved one, unless prior documentation indicates that this is not their wish.
Nursing process step: Analysis

31. What is critical incident stress?
  A. Defined by each individual
  B. Seen frequently throughout the career of emergency providers
  C. Seen as occupation-related stress
  D. Seen only in the direct caregiver

CORRECT ANSWER—A. *Rationales:* There is no exact definition for critical incident stress; it is a personally defined term. What one person determines as critical incident stress may have no significant impact on another person. Therefore, all individuals should be evaluated based on their perception versus that of the examiner. Comparisons between involved individuals may obscure the diagnosis. Critical incident stress does not happen frequently, and it may or may not be occupation-related stress. It can involve on-scene and off-scene personnel.
Nursing process step: Analysis

32. Dopamine hydrochloride (Intropin) is ordered for administration to a patient with hypotension. Which agent is used to counteract soft tissue necrosis after extravasation?
  A. Sodium bicarbonate
  B. Phentolamine (Regitine)
  C. Naloxone (Narcan)
  D. Ranitidine (Zantac)

CORRECT ANSWER—B. *Rationales:* Phentolamine is used both prophylactically and in the treatment of dopamine extravasation to prevent tissue sloughing and necrosis. Sodium bicarbonate promotes further tissue damage. Naloxone is used to reverse the effects of narcotic analgesics. Ranitidine is used as a prophylactic H$_2$-blocking agent.
Nursing process step: Intervention

33. A transplant recipient verbalizes an understanding of discharge teaching when stating which of the following?
  A. "I should take acetaminophen (Tylenol) if I have a fever."
  B. "I should have flank pain for a few weeks postoperatively."
  C. "I should notify the doctor immediately if I develop flank pain, fever, or weakness."
  D. "I can stop taking my immunosuppressant drugs when I begin to feel better."

CORRECT ANSWER—C. *Rationales:* Successful discharge teaching should show evidence that the patient can identify signs and symptoms of rejection. They include fever, malaise, flank pain or tenderness, and a decrease in urine output. Once these symptoms are identified, the patient should understand the importance of reporting them to the doctor immediately so that immunosuppressive therapy can be increased. The patient should also understand that immunosuppressive therapy must continue for life.
Nursing process step: Evaluation

34. Dopamine (Intropin) is inappropriate for a patient with which of the following conditions?
  A. Hypotension secondary to tachyarrhythmias
  B. Euvolemic hypotension
  C. Continued hypovolemic hypotension after fluid resuscitation
  D. Concomitant dobutamine infusion

CORRECT ANSWER—A. *Rationales:* Dopamine is a potent alpha, beta, and dopaminergic receptor-stimulating agent that is used in the treatment of hypotension after correction of hypovolemia. Tachycardia is a common side effect of dopamine at high doses; therefore, it is contraindicated in the treatment of tachyarrhythmia-induced hypotension. Dopamine is indicated for treating euvolemic hypotension and continued hypovolemic hypotension after fluid resuscitation combined with surgical intervention. It is also used concomitantly with dobutamine to increase systemic blood pressure and cardiac output.
Nursing process step: Evaluation

35. Which of the following cadaveric tissues cannot be banked for future transplantation?
  A. Heart valves
  B. Bone marrow
  C. Meniscus and cartilage
  D. Saphenous veins

CORRECT ANSWER—B. *Rationales:* Bone marrow cannot be stored and must be transplanted shortly after procurement. Heart valves, saphenous veins, and meniscus and cartilage can be cryopreserved for later transplantation.
Nursing process step: Analysis

36. The doctor orders a continuous infusion of lidocaine (Xylocaine) at 3 mg/minute for the treatment of premature ventricular complexes after a lidocaine bolus administration. Lidocaine is mixed in a concentration of 1 g in 250 ml of D$_5$W by way of an infusion pump. What is the infusion rate in milliliters per hour (assuming the use of microdrip 60 gtt/ml tubing)?
  A. 15 ml/hour
  B. 75 ml/hour
  C. 45 ml/hour
  D. 30 ml/hour

CORRECT ANSWER—C. *Rationales:* First, determine the concentration of the lidocaine by changing 1 g to 1,000 mg. Then, divide 1,000 mg by 250 ml, which is 4 mg/ml. So, the concentration of the lidocaine is 4 mg/ml. Then, use the following formula: dosage in milligrams per minute multiplied by 60 minutes divided by the concentration in milligrams per milliliter equals the pump setting in milliliters per hour.
3 mg/minute × 60 = (180) divided by 4 = 45 ml/hour
Nursing process step: Intervention

37. Which is the most commonly reported emotional change resulting from critical incident stress?
  A. Panic
  B. Euphoria
  C. Hebephrenia
  D. Depression

CORRECT ANSWER—A. *Rationales:* Panic is the most commonly reported emotional change. Euphoria, hebephrenia, and depression are not seen after critical incident stress and are attributed to other mental illnesses.
Nursing process step: Assessment

38. Which test would best detect signs of rejection in a patient who has received a liver transplant?
  A. Blood culture
  B. White blood cell count
  C. Liver biopsy
  D. Decreased activated partial thromboplastin time (APTT)

CORRECT ANSWER—C. *Rationales:* After liver transplantation, a liver biopsy is primarily used to monitor patients for rejection. Positive blood cultures in the liver transplant patient would indicate infection. The patient's white blood cell count would probably not be elevated because of the immunosuppressive therapy used to prevent rejection. The patient's APTT would probably be increased because the liver is not functioning properly.
Nursing process step: Evaluation

39. The doctor orders a continuous infusion of dopamine (Intropin) 400 mg in 250 ml of D$_5$W at 10 mcg/kg/minute by way of an infusion pump in a 70-kg patient. What is the infusion rate in milliliters per hour (assuming the use of microdrip 60 gtt/ml tubing).

  A. 26 ml/hour
  B. 30 ml/hour
  C. 36 ml/hour
  D. 40 ml/hour

CORRECT ANSWER—A. *Rationales:* The concentration of dopamine is 1,600 mcg/ml (change 400 mg to 400,000 mcg and then 400,000 mcg divided by 250 ml = 1,600 mcg/ml). To infuse 10 mcg/kg/minute, the nurse should infuse 26 ml/hour. Use the following formula: Dosage in microgram per kilogram per minute multiplied by the patient's weight in kilograms, multiplied by 60 minutes, divided by the drug concentration in micrograms per milliliter.
10 mcg/kg/minute × 70 kg = (700) × 60 minutes = (42,000) divided by 1,600 mcg/ml = 26 ml/hour
Nursing process step: Intervention

40. Which is the most appropriate nursing diagnosis for the kidney transplant patient who is not following treatment protocols?

  A. Anxiety
  B. Fear
  C. Defensive coping
  D. Ineffective management of therapeutic regimen

CORRECT ANSWER—D. *Rationales:* The transplant recipient may suffer from anxiety, fear, and defensive coping, but the most appropriate diagnosis is ineffective management of therapeutic regimen. Transplant patients initially are excited to receive a second chance through transplantation, but the lifelong drug therapy, expense, and risk of infection or rejection can lead to noncompliance with the treatment regimen.
Nursing process step: Analysis/Nursing diagnosis

41. Nitroglycerin (Tridil) is ordered to be administered at 50 mcg/minute by way of an infusion pump. The infusion is prepared as nitroglycerin 100 mg in 250 ml of D$_5$W. What is the infusion rate in milliliters per hour (assuming the use of microdrip 60 gtt/ml tubing)?

  A. 10 ml/hour
  B. 6 ml/hour
  C. 8 ml/hour
  D. 12 ml/hour

CORRECT ANSWER—C. *Rationales:* The concentration of nitroglycerin is 0.04 mg/ml or 400 mcg/ml (100 mg divided by 250 ml = 0.04 mg/ml). To infuse 20 mcg/minute, the nurse should infuse 8 ml/hour. Use the following formula: Dosage in micrograms per minute multiplied by 60 minutes, divided by the concentration of drug = pump setting.
50 mcg/minute × 60 minutes = (3,000) divided by 400 mcg/ml = 7.5 or 8 ml/hour
Nursing process step: Intervention

42. Dobutamine (Dobutrex) is ordered to be administered at 6 mcg/kg/minute by way of an infusion pump in a 75-kg patient. The concentration is 500 mg in 250 ml of D$_5$W. What is the infusion rate in milliliters per hour (assuming the use of 60 gtt/ml tubing)?
   A. 12 ml/hour
   B. 11 ml/hour
   C. 14 ml/hour
   D. 15 ml/hour

CORRECT ANSWER—C. *Rationales:* The concentration of dobutamine is 2 mg/ml or 2,000 mcg/ml (500 mg divided by 250 ml = 2 mg/ml). To infuse 6 mcg/kg/minute, the nurse should infuse 14 ml/hour. Use the following formula: Dosage in micrograms per kilogram per minute multiplied by the patient's weight in kilograms, multiplied by 60 minutes, divided by the concentration of drug in micrograms per milliliter.
6 mcg/kg/minute × 75 kg = (450) x 60 minutes = (27,000) divided by 2,000 mcg/ml = 13.5 or 14 ml/hour
Nursing process step: Intervention

43. Which of the following nursing diagnoses is a priority for the kidney transplant recipient?
   A. Fluid volume excess
   B. Pain
   C. Altered sexuality patterns
   D. Risk for infection

CORRECT ANSWER—D. *Rationales:* The highest priority nursing diagnosis in the kidney transplant recipient is risk for infection because of the immunosuppressive therapy. The recipient should have a normal fluid balance if the kidney is functioning properly, so fluid volume excess should not be a problem. The patient will have normal postoperative pain and altered sexuality patterns because of the risk for infection; however, these diagnoses do not take priority over the need to prevent infection.
Nursing process step: Analysis/Nursing diagnosis

44. Which of the following statements is true about administering nitrous oxide–oxygen 50:50 mixture (Nitronox)?
   A. It is safe for use in the first and second trimesters of pregnancy
   B. The patient self-administers the drug until pain is relieved
   C. Prolonged use may produce tachypnea
   D. It may be beneficial in relieving pain from pneumothorax or abdominal obstruction

CORRECT ANSWER—B. *Rationales:* Nitronox is self-administered by the patient until adequate analgesia is obtained. Nitrous oxide use is safe only in the third trimester of pregnancy, and it may worsen pneumothorax or intestinal obstruction. Prolonged use of nitrous oxide does not result in tachypnea.
Nursing process step: Evaluation

45. Which of the following is a necessary coenzyme in the metabolism of glucose?
A. Thiamine (vitamin B$_1$)
B. Protamine
C. Aspartame
D. Levothyroxine (Synthroid)

CORRECT ANSWER—A. *Rationales:* Thiamine is a water-soluble vitamin that is a necessary coenzyme in most human metabolic processes, especially carbohydrate (glucose) metabolism. Protamine is used to reverse the effects of heparin sodium. Aspartame is an artificial sweetener that has no medicinal value. Levothyroxine is used for treating hypothyroidism.
Nursing process step: Analysis

46. Which of the following best defines magnesium sulfate?
A. Stimulates the central nervous system
B. Depresses the central nervous system
C. Is used in the treatment of atrioventricular block
D. Is used to promote diuresis in patients with renal disease

CORRECT ANSWER—B. *Rationales:* Magnesium sulfate depresses smooth, cardiac, and skeletal muscle in addition to depressing the central nervous system. It is commonly used to treat ventricular arrhythmia, torsades de pointes, and hypomagnesemia. It is also used in the postpartum management of preeclampsia and eclampsia. Magnesium sulfate is contraindicated in patients with preexisting renal disease and atrioventricular block.
Nursing process step: Analysis

47. A patient will receive a kidney-pancreas transplant based on which of the following?
A. Blood type only
B. Blood type and donor-recipient weight compatibility
C. Blood type and HLA compatibility
D. HLA compatibility only

CORRECT ANSWER—C. *Rationales:* Allocation of a combined cadaver kidney-pancreas for transplantation is based on donor-recipient ABO type and HLA compatibility. ABO type, donor-recipient weight compatibility, and HLA compatibility are not used independent of one another in determining pancreas allocation.
Nursing process step: Assessment

48. While assessing a patient in triage, the nurse notices that the patient is dyspneic and short of breath. These signs and symptoms are usually associated with which of the following?
A. Bradycardia
B. Eupnea
C. Tachycardia
D. Bradypnea

CORRECT ANSWER—C. *Rationales:* Dyspnea and shortness of breath stimulate the sympathetic nervous system, causing catecholamine release, and result in tachycardia. Bradycardia is seen with vagal stimulation. Eupnea is a normal finding. When patients are short of breath, their respiratory rate increases, thereby eliminating bradypnea as a possible choice.
Nursing process step: Assessment

49. Increased cardiac responsiveness to catecholamines is the desired effect of which of the following?
  A. Bretylium (Bretylol)
  B. Dopamine (Intropin)
  C. Sodium bicarbonate
  D. Atropine

CORRECT ANSWER—C. *Rationales:* Sodium bicarbonate stabilizes ion balance and potentiates the effects of sympathomimetic (catecholamine) agents such as dopamine. Bretylol is used in the treatment of ventricular arrhythmias; atropine is used in the treatment of bradyarrhythmias.
Nursing process step: Evaluation

50. When communicating with someone whose primary language is not English, it is best to do which of the following?
  A. Use slang or jargon instead of actual terms
  B. Avoid use of the word not
  C. Use the passive voice instead of the active voice
  D. Repeat misunderstood statements using the same words

CORRECT ANSWER—B. *Rationales:* The nurse should avoid using the word not; it can become lost in a sentence and create the opposite meaning. Likewise, active voice should be used in communication. Jargon and slang are not readily translatable across languages or dialects. When statements are misunderstood, they should be repeated using different words.
Nursing process step: Intervention

51. Which of the following indicates that the nurse has observed the appropriate procedure for administering a continuous I.V. infusion of nitroglycerin (Tridil)?
  A. The I.V. bag is wrapped in aluminum foil to prevent exposure to light
  B. Filtered I.V. tubing is used
  C. Polyvinylchloride tubing is used
  D. The infusion is diluted in D5W in a glass bottle

CORRECT ANSWER—D. *Rationales:* Nitroglycerin must be mixed in D5W in a glass bottle and administered by way of nonfiltered, nonpolyvinylchloride (plastic) tubing. A plastic container or tubing will absorb up to 80% of diluted nitroglycerin. Aluminum foil is wrapped around the I.V. bag when administering nitroprusside (Nipride).
Nursing process step: Evaluation

52. Teaching is effective when the patient receiving monoamine oxidase (MAO) inhibitor agents verbalizes which of the following?
  A. "I should avoid using antihistamines."
  B. "I can no longer eat bread."
  C. "I must avoid decaffeinated cola."
  D. "I must refrain from eating ham and pork."

CORRECT ANSWER—A. *Rationales:* When taking an MAO inhibitor, the patient must avoid using antihistamines, which can potentiate the MAO inhibitor's effects and result in acute hypertensive crisis. The patient should also avoid foods that contain tryptophan or tyramine. If the patient requires elective surgery with general anesthesia or cocaine or a local anesthetic that contains sympathomimetic vasoconstrictors, the MAO inhibitor should be discontinued within 10 days of the surgery.
Nursing process step: Evaluation

53. Anticholinergic crisis (toxicity) after antihistamine overdose is treated with which of the following?
A. Pralidoxime (2-PAM chloride)
B. Naloxone (Narcan)
C. Dopamine (Intropin)
D. Dobutamine (Dobutrex)

CORRECT ANSWER—A. *Rationales:* Anticholinergic crisis may be caused by various medications and plant alkaloids. It produces hypertension, tachycardia, mydriasis, decreased bowel sounds, urine retention, and dry skin. The treatment is administration of atropine and pralidoxime. Naloxone is used to reverse the effects of narcotic analgesics. Dopamine and dobutamine are used to increase systemic blood pressure and cardiac output.
Nursing process step: Intervention

54. Continuous I.V. nitroglycerin (Tridil) infusion in a patient with acute myocardial infarction is effective when which of the following happens?
A. Pain and ventricular preload are reduced
B. Pain and ventricular afterload are reduced
C. Pain is reduced and ventricular afterload is increased
D. Pain is reduced and ventricular preload is increased

CORRECT ANSWER—A. *Rationales:* Nitroglycerin is a potent preload reducer. It is used after an acute myocardial infarction to relieve pain and to decrease atrial and ventricular preload to minimize myocardial oxygen consumption and ischemia.
Nursing process step: Evaluation

55. The emergency department triage nurse should give highest priority to which of the following patients?
A. The patient with crushing chest pain
B. The patient with seizures
C. The patient with severe abdominal pain
D. The patient with congestive heart failure

CORRECT ANSWER—A. *Rationales:* The patient with crushing chest pain is probably presenting with an acute myocardial infarction and should be seen immediately. The patient with seizures, who is not in status epilepticus, can be seen within 30 to 60 minutes of arrival at the emergency department. The patient with abdominal pain, who does not present with signs of shock, and the patient with congestive heart failure, who is not in acute distress, can also be seen within 30 to 60 minutes of arrival.
Nursing process step: Assessment

56. A multiple-trauma patient with a hemothorax arrives in the emergency department. A chest tube is placed. Initially 500 ml of blood drains from the tube. The patient's vital signs are blood pressure 146/74 mm Hg and heart rate 138 beats/minute. Respirations are controlled by mechanical ventilation at a rate of 16 breaths/minute. Which assessment parameter should be closely monitored over the next hour?

A. Vital signs
B. Central venous pressure
C. Chest tube drainage
D. Urine output

CORRECT ANSWER—**C.** *Rationales*: The initial drainage from the chest tube was 500 ml, so the chest tube drainage should be monitored closely. If the patient continues to lose blood at a rate of 200 ml/hour or more, the patient may require surgical intervention to identify and repair the source of bleeding. Monitoring vital signs, central venous pressure, and urine output are all important in assessing fluid status, but monitoring the chest drainage is highest priority.
Nursing process step: Assessment

57. A child with a history of varicella and aspirin intake is brought to the emergency department. The nurse suspects Reye's syndrome. Which assessment findings are consistent with this syndrome?

A. Fever, decreased level of consciousness, and impaired liver function
B. Joint inflammation, red macular rash with a clear center, low-grade fever
C. Peripheral edema, fever for 5 or more days, "strawberry tongue"
D. Red, raised "bull's eye"-shaped rash; malaise; joint pain

CORRECT ANSWER—**A.** *Rationales:* Reye's syndrome occurs in children with a history of a viral infection, varicella, or influenza. It is often associated with the administration of aspirin. The child presents with fever and decreased level of consciousness, which can lead to coma and death. As the disease progresses, the child also develops impaired liver function. A child with joint pain, a red macular rash with a clear center, and a low-grade fever probably has rheumatic fever. The child presenting with peripheral edema, fever for more than 5 days, and a "strawberry tongue" probably has Kawasaki syndrome. The child with a red, raised bull's eye rash; malaise; and joint pain should be tested for Lyme disease.
Nursing process step: Assessment

RESPIRATORY EMERGENCIES

CHAPTER 14

Respiratory Emergencies

Questions 1 through 3 refer to the following information:
An unrestrained passenger is thrown 20 feet from a car that hit an embankment. On admittance, the patient is conscious, and vital signs are pulse 130 beats/minute, respirations 26 breaths/minute and shallow, blood pressure 90/60 mm Hg, and weak radial pulses. The patient's skin is pale and cool, and capillary refill is delayed. The patient is confused and restless; the lungs are clear bilaterally with diminished breath sounds on the right. Paradoxical chest movement is noted on the right side. Arterial blood gas analysis shows increased pH, decreased $PaCO_2$, and diminished PaO_2. A chest film shows a right pneumothorax and multiple rib fractures on the right (4th to 7th).

1. Which is the most likely diagnosis for this patient?
  A. Tension pneumothorax
  B. Flail chest
  C. Ruptured diaphragm
  D. Massive hemothorax

CORRECT ANSWER—B. *Rationales:* This patient's multiple rib fractures caused a flail chest. Signs include bruised skin, extreme pain, paradoxical chest movements, rapid and shallow respirations, tachycardia, hypotension, respiratory acidosis, and cyanosis. Flail chest also can cause tension pneumothorax, a condition in which air enters the chest but can't be ejected during exhalation. Classic signs are tracheal deviation (away from the affected side), cyanosis, severe dyspnea, absent breath sounds on the affected side, distended jugular veins, and shock. The patient with a ruptured diaphragm presents with hyperresonance on percussion, hypotension, dyspnea, dysphagia, shifted heart sounds, and bowel sounds in the lower to middle chest. A patient with massive hemothorax shows signs of shock (tachycardia, hypotension), dullness on percussion on the injured side, decreased breath sounds on the injured side, respiratory distress and, possibly, mediastinal shift.
Nursing process step: Assessment

2. What is the definition of flail chest?

   A. An unstable segment of the chest wall that moves paradoxically with respirations

   B. A compressed rib cage with open chest wound

   C. A fracture of two adjacent ribs, bilaterally

   D. A fracture of two or more ribs in two or more places

CORRECT ANSWER—D. *Rationales:* The definition of flail chest is a fracture of two or more ribs in two or more places. The result is a free-floating segment of the chest wall. Paradoxical chest movement is often a sign of flail chest; however, until the chest muscles relax or pain relief is achieved, paradoxical movements are unlikely to be seen. Flail chest usually is a closed injury. Bilateral injury is not required. If bilateral injury is present, the mortality increases drastically.

Nursing process step: Assessment

3. An appropriate nursing diagnosis for a patient with flail chest is which of the following?

   A. Decreased cardiac output related to hypovolemia

   B. Impaired gas exchange related to pain

   C. Potential for infection related to altered skin integrity

   D. Ineffective airway clearance related to pain

CORRECT ANSWER—B. *Rationales:* The correct response is impaired gas exchange related to pain. The pain associated with flail chest limits chest expansion and potentiates impaired gas exchange. Adequate pain control is a priority therapy for a patient with flail chest. The patient's blood pressure is borderline (90/60 mm Hg). The most probable explanation is the presence of a right pneumothorax and increased intrathoracic pressure. Because the patient has a closed chest wound, risk for infection related to altered skin integrity is inappropriate. Ineffective airway clearance could occur in a patient with flail chest if the pain is not adequately controlled.

Nursing process step: Analysis/Nursing diagnosis

4. The most likely laboratory finding in a patient with acute respiratory distress syndrome (ARDS) is which of the following?

   A. Elevated carboxyhemoglobin level

   B. Decreased PaO_2

   C. Elevated $PaCO_2$

   D. Decreased HCO_3-

CORRECT ANSWER—B. *Rationales:* Hypoxemia is a universal finding in ARDS. The $PaCO_2$ is low early in the disease because of hyperventilation, and it rises later in the disease because of fatigue and worsening clinical status. The bicarbonate level may be low in ARDS and is related to reduced oxygenation to tissue. Reduced oxygenation leads to anaerobic metabolism and accumulating lactate. The bicarbonate in the serum combines with the lactate, reducing circulating bicarbonate levels. The carboxyhemoglobin level is increased in a patient with an inhalation injury, which commonly progresses to ARDS. This is not a common cause of ARDS.

Nursing process step: Assessment

5. The most appropriate intervention for a patient with chronic obstructive pulmonary disease (COPD) is which of the following?
A. Administer 100% oxygen by way of a nonrebreather mask
B. Obtain and monitor arterial blood gas levels
C. Restrict fluids
D. Place the patient in a supine position

CORRECT ANSWER—B. *Rationales:* The patient with COPD presenting to the emergency department has abnormal arterial blood gas levels, which may predispose the patient to respiratory distress. The patient is hypoxemic with hypercapnia. Oxygen should be administered at low concentrations to maintain hypoxic drive. If the PaO_2 remains inadequate at low dose, the nurse should increase the oxygen while continuously monitoring the patient's respiratory status. Patients with COPD usually benefit from adequate hydration to liquefy secretions. Allow the patient to assume a position that facilitates ventilation. This usually is high Fowler's and leaning forward.
Nursing process step: Intervention

6. An appropriate nursing diagnosis for a patient with acute respiratory distress syndrome (ARDS) is which of the following?
A. Impaired gas exchange related to noncompliant lungs and impaired pulmonary capillary permeability
B. Fluid volume deficit related to underhydration
C. Ineffective airway clearance related to bronchoconstriction
D. Decreased cardiac output related to poor cardiac contractility

CORRECT ANSWER—A. *Rationales:* The hallmark of ARDS is impaired gas exchange. This is because noncompliant lungs and increased capillary permeability lead to pulmonary edema. A patient with ARDS would be likely to have fluid volume excess related to overhydration. Ineffective airway clearance could occur owing to possible injury and increased secretions. Decreased cardiac output related to high positive end-expiratory pressure could occur in ARDS management.
Nursing process step: Analysis/Nursing diagnosis

7. The patient with chronic obstructive pulmonary disease (COPD) is given discharge instructions regarding nutritional support. Which of the following statements identifies the need for further teaching?
A. "I should eat five or six small meals each day."
B. "I will limit my fluid intake at mealtime."
C. "I should select most of my foods from the carbohydrate group."
D. "I should rest for 30 minutes before each meal."

CORRECT ANSWER—C. *Rationales:* The patient with COPD should rest for 30 minutes before each meal to conserve energy and decrease dyspnea. The patient should also avoid exercise and breathing treatments for at least 1 hour before and after eating. The patient with emphysema has a markedly increased need for protein and calories to maintain an adequate nutritional status. The patient's diet, high in both protein and calories, should be divided into five or six small meals a day, and fluid intake should be maintained at 3 L/day unless contraindicated. Fluids should be taken between meals to reduce gastric distention and pressure on the diaphragm.
Nursing process step: Evaluation

8. A consequence of pulmonary emboli can be the development of right-sided heart failure. Which of the following findings is consistent with this development?
A. Physiologic S_2 split heart sound
B. Peaked P wave on ECG
C. Expiratory wheeze
D. Pericardial friction rub

CORRECT ANSWER—B. *Rationales:* Elevated pulmonary pressures resulting from pulmonary emboli can lead to dysfunction of the right heart. This can lead to an increase in right atrial volume, showing an altered P wave on the ECG. The lead to monitor for this finding is lead II. In lead II, the P wave is taller and more peaked than a normal P wave. A physiologic S_2 split is normal. When pulmonary pressures become severely elevated, the split becomes pathologic. Breath sounds are generally clear in a patient with pulmonary emboli. In extreme cases, there may be crackles in the bases. A pleural friction rub may be heard in patients with pulmonary emboli and must be differentiated from a pericardial friction rub.
Nursing process step: Assessment

9. The primary nursing diagnosis for a patient with asthma is which of the following?
A. Ineffective airway clearance related to bronchospasm
B. Decreased cardiac output related to tachycardia
C. Knowledge deficit related to therapeutic regimen
D. Altered tissue perfusion related to hypoxemia

CORRECT ANSWER—A. *Rationales:* A definitive finding in asthma is bronchospasm that causes ineffective airway clearance. The heart rate in the asthmatic patient increases as a compensatory mechanism to improve cardiac output. An acute exacerbation does not necessarily mean that the patient does not understand the therapeutic regimen. Specific questions would need to be asked to determine if a knowledge deficit is present. Even in an acute episode, the patient may not have severe hypoxemia resulting in decreased tissue perfusion.
Nursing process step: Analysis/Nursing diagnosis

10. The diagnostic study that most accurately identifies the presence of a pulmonary embolus is which of the following?
A. Bronchoscopy
B. Chest X-ray
C. Ventilation/perfusion (V/Q) scan
D. Pulmonary angiography

CORRECT ANSWER—D. *Rationales:* A chest X-ray is usually done to rule out other pulmonary problems, such as pneumonia and atelectasis. A V/Q scan is used to locate the inadequately perfused area; however, results are often not definitive. Although riskier than a V/Q scan, pulmonary angiography confirms the presence of pulmonary emboli. Bronchoscopy is often used to differentially diagnose pneumonia.
Nursing process step: Assessment

11. Which of the following drugs may be given safely to the patient with asthma?
A. Beta-adrenergic blocking agents
B. Beta₂-agonists
C. Aspirin
D. Nonsteroidal anti-inflammatory drugs

CORRECT ANSWER—B. *Rationales:* Beta₂-agonists are the first-line drugs of choice for the asthma patient. They relax bronchial smooth muscle and enhance mucociliary clearance. Beta-adrenergic blocking agents, aspirin, and nonsteroidal anti-inflammatory drugs all worsen asthma.
Nursing process step: Intervention

12. In a patient with a hemothorax, a sign or symptom consistent with blood loss greater than 1,500 ml is which of the following?
A. Mediastinal shift
B. Blood pressure less than 80 mm Hg systolic
C. Capillary refill greater than 4 seconds
D. All of the above

CORRECT ANSWER—D. *Rationales:* A mediastinal shift, systolic blood pressure less than 80 mm Hg, and a capillary refill greater than 4 seconds can all be associated with a hemothorax greater than 1,500 ml. The patient with a massive hemothorax has mediastinal shift, blood pressure depicting decompensation, diminished peripheral blood flow, decreased urine output, and respiratory distress.
Nursing process step: Assessment

13. After teaching the patient with asthma about inhalers, which of the following statements indicates the need for further instruction?
A. "I should hold the inhaler upright and shake it well."
B. "I should hold my breath for 5 to 10 seconds after each puff."
C. "I should hold the inhaler 1 to 2 inches from my mouth."
D. "I should hold my head back and forcefully exhale."

CORRECT ANSWER—D. *Rationales:* If the patient states "I should hold my head back and forcefully exhale," further teaching is necessary. The correct technique for using an inhaler is as follows: The inhaler must be mixed thoroughly before administration. The patient's breath should be held for 5 to 10 seconds to allow the medication to reach as far as possible into the lungs. If the patient has difficulty with this technique, a spacer device may be added to the inhaler. A forced exhalation isn't recommended because coughing, small-airway closure, and air trapping may result.
Nursing process step: Evaluation

14. The initial treatment for a patient with pulmonary emboli should include which of the following?
A. Correcting the hypoxia with oxygen by way of a mask
B. Administering heparin (Calciparine) at 1,000 to 3,000 units/hour
C. Considering thrombolytic therapy
D. Administering morphine to treat pain

CORRECT ANSWER—A. *Rationales:* The priority is always airway, breathing, and circulation. Provide oxygen by face mask. If hypocapnia is present on admission, arterial blood gas analysis should be repeated within 15 to 20 minutes. Worsening hypercapnia with progressive obtundation is an indication for emergency intubation. A loading dose of heparin should be administered, followed by a continuous drip. The heparin should be titrated to an activated partial thromboplastin time 1.5 to 2 times the control. Heparin therapy is sufficient treatment for most patients with pulmonary emboli. For patients who present with significant hemodynamic compromise, streptokinase (Streptase), urokinase (Abbokinase), and tissue plasminogen activator (Activase) have been approved for use in pulmonary emboli. Pain increases oxygen demand and anxiety, and it should be treated with morphine or meperidine (Demerol). The nurse should monitor arterial blood gas levels carefully to prevent carbon dioxide retention.
Nursing process step: Intervention

15. The goals of successful asthma management include measurement of lung function. This can be accomplished with peak expiratory flow rate (PEFR). What is the optimal PEFR?
A. PEFR greater than 80% of predicted or personal best
B. PEFR variability 20% to 30%
C. PEFR less than 50% of predicted or personal best
D. PEFR variability less than 30%

CORRECT ANSWER—A. *Rationales:* The optimal PEFR is greater than 80% of predicted or personal best with a variability of less than 20%. Monitoring PEFR helps assess the severity of obstruction. The nurse should evaluate the patient's response to treatment and detect changes in airflow. If PEFR is increasing and subjective symptoms are decreasing, there is no need to change medication or dosage. If PEFR is decreasing and symptoms are increasing, the patient can better judge his status and adjust medications appropriately.
Nursing process step: Evaluation

16. Which is the most likely finding on a lateral neck X-ray in a child with epiglottitis?
    A. Supraglottic narrowing
    B. Steeple sign
    C. Thickened mass
    D. Subglottic narrowing

CORRECT ANSWER—C. *Rationales:* X-ray assessment of the lateral neck assists in diagnosing common respiratory emergencies in children. The lateral neck X-ray of a child with epiglottitis shows a thickened mass. The steeple sign is found in the patient with viral croup syndrome. Subglottic narrowing with membranous tracheal exudate is found in bacterial tracheitis. Supraglottic narrowing is not a diagnostic indicator.
Nursing process step: Assessment

17. Which of the following interventions would be least effective for a patient who is breathing deeply and coughing productively?
    A. Incentive spirometry every 2 hours
    B. Sitting in a chair at the bedside three times each day
    C. Splinting the abdomen when coughing
    D. Suctioning the patient every 2 hours and when necessary

CORRECT ANSWER—D. *Rationales:* If the patient is effectively removing secretions, suctioning can be harmful. Suctioning can cause mucosal trauma, hypoxemia, and even pulmonary infection. Incentive spirometry every 2 hours, sitting in a chair at bedside three times each day, and splinting the abdomen to facilitate coughing all are measures to prevent pneumonia.
Nursing process step: Intervention

18. Diagnostic tests that might be helpful in supporting a diagnosis of pneumonia include which of the following?
    A. Complete blood count, chest X-ray, and cold agglutinins
    B. Complete blood count, chest X-ray, and lumbar puncture
    C. Chest X-ray and sedimentation rate
    D. Complete blood count with differential and electrolytes

CORRECT ANSWER—A. *Rationales:* A complete blood count is helpful in determining the presence of infection and identifying the microbial (viral, bacterial, fungal) agent. A chest film can identify the location of the pneumonia. Cold hemagglutination is useful in identifying a mycoplasmic infection. Sedimentation rate, electrolytes, and lumbar puncture do not assist in the differential diagnosis of pneumonia.
Nursing process step: Assessment

19. Which of the following is the priority intervention for a child with epiglottitis?
A. Administering oxygen by face mask
B. Administering parenteral antibiotics
C. Assisting with intubation
D. Monitoring the ECG for arrhythmias

CORRECT ANSWER—C. *Rationales:* The most important intervention for a child with epiglottitis is airway management. Children are at high risk for developing abrupt airway obstruction. Intubation should be performed as soon as possible in a controlled environment. Children need supplemental oxygen, but most are so anxious that they will never allow a mask to stay in place. Provide humidified "blow-by" oxygen administered by the parent, if possible. The child needs parenteral antibiotics; however, the priority is airway management. The most common rhythm in this patient is sinus tachycardia related to compensation.
Nursing process step: Intervention

Questions 20 through 22 refer to the following information:
A patient was admitted to the emergency department after being involved in a single-car accident. Symptoms include dyspnea, respirations shallow at a rate of 40 breaths/minute, restlessness, confusion, apprehension, cyanosis, and pleuritic chest pain. On inspection, the nurse finds tachypnea, bulging of the intercostal spaces on the left side, labored breathing with accessory muscle use, and distended neck veins. On percussion, there is hyperresonance on the left side. Auscultation reveals absent breath sounds on the left. Arterial blood gas levels are pH, 7.2; $PaCO_2$, 50 mm Hg; and PaO_2, 69 mm Hg. A bag-valve-mask device is in place, but it is difficult to ventilate the patient.

20. Which is the most likely diagnosis, based on the findings above?
A. Tension pneumothorax
B. Flail chest
C. Ruptured diaphragm
D. Massive hemothorax

CORRECT ANSWER—A. *Rationales:* Tension pneumothorax presents with severe respiratory distress, hypotension, diminished breath sounds over the affected area, hyperresonance, distended neck veins and, eventually, tracheal shift. A finding of multiple rib fractures in a patient with respiratory distress verifies a diagnosis of flail chest. A patient with a ruptured diaphragm presents with hyperresonance on percussion, hypotension, dyspnea, dysphagia, shifted heart sounds, and bowel sounds in the lower to middle chest. A patient with massive hemothorax shows signs of shock (tachycardia, hypotension), dullness on percussion on the injured side, decreased breath sounds on the injured side, respiratory distress and, possibly, mediastinal shift.
Nursing process step: Assessment

21. Which is the most common cause of traumatic pneumothorax?
A. Broken ribs
B. Gunshot wound
C. Barotrauma
D. Central line insertion

CORRECT ANSWER—A. *Rationales:* The most common cause of traumatic pneumothorax is broken ribs. Other common causes include penetrating trauma (gunshot or knife wound), insertion of a central venous pressure catheter, barotrauma in mechanically ventilated patients, and closed pleural biopsy.
Nursing process step: Assessment

22. Which finding indicates that a chest tube is not effective in the management of a pneumothorax?
A. Patient resting quietly, respirations 12 breaths/minute
B. Breath sounds equal bilaterally, equal chest excursion
C. Patient anxious, respirations 36 breaths/minute, with cyanosis
D. Trachea midline, neck veins not distended

CORRECT ANSWER—C. *Rationales:* After chest tube insertion, the patient should be calm. A patient who is anxious with cyanosis and rapid respirations is showing signs of respiratory distress. If the chest tube is effective, respirations should be within normal limits for the age of the patient. Breath sounds should be heard in all lobes bilaterally with equal excursion of chest. The trachea should be midline without jugular venous distention.
Nursing process step: Evaluation

23. What is the primary goal in the treatment of a patient with acute respiratory distress syndrome (ARDS)?
A. Identifying and treating the underlying condition
B. Maintaining nutritional requirements
C. Maintaining adequate tissue oxygenation
D. Preventing secondary infection

CORRECT ANSWER—A. *Rationales:* Identifying and treating the underlying condition is the primary goal. If the condition causing ARDS is not treated, injury to the lung continues, preventing adequate tissue oxygenation and predisposing the patient to secondary infection. The nurse should also provide adequate nutritional support in the form of increased protein and calories and limit carbohydrate intake.
Nursing process step: Intervention

24. Which of the following is a nursing diagnosis for a patient with a massive hemothorax?
A. Impaired gas exchange related to paradoxical chest motion
B. Ineffective airway clearance related to increased mucus production
C. Fluid volume deficit related to blood loss
D. Risk for infection related to increased pulmonary secretions

CORRECT ANSWER—C. *Rationales:* Bleeding and accumulation of blood in the pleural space can result from chest wall injury, great vessel disruption, or lung injury. A massive hemothorax produces signs and symptoms consistent with hypovolemic shock. Impaired gas exchange can occur when blood accumulates in the pleural space, leading to mediastinal shift and lung compression. There is no increased mucus production in the patient with a massive hemothorax; therefore, ineffective airway clearance and risk for infection related to increased secretions are inappropriate diagnoses for this patient.
Nursing process step: Analysis/Nursing diagnosis

25. The bronchodilator most appropriate for a patient who is taking a nonselective beta-adrenergic blocker is which of the following?
A. Ephedrine (Efedron)
B. Epinephrine (Adrenalin)
C. Metaproterenol (Alupent)
D. Theophylline (Theo-Dur)

CORRECT ANSWER—C. *Rationales:* The use of a beta$_2$-agonist bronchodilator, such as metaproterenol or terbutaline (Brethaire), would be most effective. Nonselective beta-adrenergic blockers interfere with the bronchodilating effects of ephedrine, theophylline, and epinephrine. The beta-adrenergic effects of epinephrine remain unblocked, increasing systemic vasoconstriction.
Nursing process step: Intervention

26. What is the definitive therapy for a patient with a massive hemothorax?
A. Emergency thoracotomy
B. Chest tube insertion
C. Fluid resuscitation
D. Supplemental oxygenation

CORRECT ANSWER—A. *Rationales:* The definitive treatment for a patient with massive hemothorax is emergency thoracotomy. It is imperative to identify and repair the source of bleeding. Temporary measures to stabilize the patient include chest tube insertion and, possibly, autotransfusion, fluid resuscitation (crystalloids and colloids), and supplemental oxygenation.
Nursing process step: Intervention

27. Which is the most serious injury associated with a fracture of the first or second rib?
A. Cervical spine injury
B. Aortic rupture
C. Tracheal tear
D. Clavicular fracture

CORRECT ANSWER—B. *Rationales:* Although a cervical spine injury, tracheal tear, or clavicular fracture can be associated with a fracture of the first or second rib, the most serious injury is aortic rupture. An aortic rupture often results in immediate death from severe hemodynamic compromise. The injury commonly is caused by rapid deceleration. Such injuries occur in high-speed motor vehicle collisions and falls from great heights. Suspect an aortic rupture in a trauma patient with motor, sensory, or pulse deficits in the lower extremities. Such deficits usually result from disruption of blood flow to the spinal cord. Other symptoms include unexplained hypotension and chest or back pain. A cervical spine injury can also be serious, especially if it involves a C-3, C-4, or higher lesion, which can result in respiratory depression. Tracheal tears lead to pneumomediastinum and have the potential for tension pneumothorax if undetected. Clavicular fractures cause great pain; however, they seldom cause more severe consequences.
Nursing process step: Assessment

28. Which is the most important treatment for the patient with tension pneumothorax?
A. Position the patient with the head of the bed elevated
B. Administer 100% oxygen by way of a non-rebreather mask
C. Infuse normal saline solution at a keep-vein-open rate
D. Assist with needle decompression

CORRECT ANSWER—D. *Rationales:* All the options listed are important in the treatment of tension pneumothorax, but the most definitive is needle decompression. A 14-gauge needle is inserted into the second intercostal space at the midclavicular line on the affected side. A chest tube insertion should follow needle decompression.
Nursing process step: Intervention

29. Which is the most appropriate position to facilitate oxygen exchange in the patient with acute respiratory distress syndrome (ARDS)?
A. Side-lying position with the right lung down
B. Side-lying position with the left lung down
C. Prone position slightly on the right side
D. Semi-Fowler position lying on the left side

CORRECT ANSWER—C. *Rationales:* Research has shown that improved oxygenation parameters are seen when a patient with ARDS is placed in the prone position. In ARDS, neither lung is functioning properly; therefore, the good lung down doesn't help determine positioning. Changing the patient's position at least every 2 hours is important. The right lung down usually produces the next best oxygenation parameters. This lung has three lobes and is not compressed by the heart. The nurse should allow 15 minutes after each turn for stabilization of parameters. If they do not improve, the patient should be turned to a more functional position.
Nursing process step: Intervention

30. Which finding is often associated with a poor outcome in a patient with a pulmonary contusion?
A. Temperature of 100.4° F (38° C)
B. Crackles in the bases
C. Hemoptysis
D. White blood cell count of 30,000 mm^3

CORRECT ANSWER—B. *Rationales:* Fluid overload, as evidenced by crackles in the bases, is consistently associated with a poor outcome in these patients. A pulmonary contusion causes an inflammatory response that results in an increase in temperature and white blood cells; however, the levels are not elevated as high as those seen in options A and D. The patient with pulmonary contusion is expected to have hemoptysis. The blood may be expectorated or suctioned from the endotracheal tube, if the patient is intubated. Restriction of fluids, meticulous monitoring of intake and output, and monitoring of central venous pressure are appropriate interventions.
Nursing process step: Assessment

31. Which is the most appropriate intervention for a patient with a pulmonary contusion?
A. Restrict fluid administration if there are no signs of shock
B. Provide supplemental humidified oxygen
C. Position the patient to facilitate breathing
D. Assist with removal of secretions

CORRECT ANSWER—A. *Rationales:* The intervention identified with the best outcome for a patient with a pulmonary contusion is restricted fluid administration during initial care. If the patient is not exhibiting signs and symptoms of hypovolemic shock, fluids should be kept at a keep-vein-open rate. Providing supplemental oxygen, positioning the patient to facilitate breathing, and assisting with removal of secretions are all treatments for pulmonary contusion.
Nursing process step: Intervention

32. Effective treatment for a patient with pulmonary contusion is best identified by which of the following?
A. Diminished breath sounds in right lower lobe
B. Increased respiratory rate and effort
C. Decreased complaints of pain
D. Respiratory acidosis with hypoxemia

CORRECT ANSWER—C. *Rationales:* Effective treatment of a patient with pulmonary contusion is evidenced by equal bilateral breath sounds; improved respiratory rate, rhythm, depth, and effort; vital signs within normal limits; arterial blood gases within acceptable limits; decreased complaints of pain; and improved skin and mucous membrane color.
Nursing process step: Evaluation

33. Treatment of a patient with a rib fracture includes which of the following?
A. Placing the patient in the supine position
B. Taping the chest circumferentially to relieve pain
C. Controlling pain to assist with breathing
D. Forcing fluids to prevent dehydration

CORRECT ANSWER—C. *Rationales:* Pain control for a patient with rib fractures is a priority to ensure adequate expansion of lung tissue and to facilitate turning, coughing, and deep breathing. The patient should be placed in high Fowler's position to facilitate gas exchange and breathing. Avoid circumferential taping of the chest because it predisposes the patient to atelectasis. The lung directly below the fractured rib is often bruised (pulmonary contusion). Fluids should be monitored closely to decrease the risk of pulmonary edema.
Nursing process step: Intervention

Questions 34 through 36 refer to the following information:
A patient presents with a history of mild respiratory infection and a dry cough for the past week. The patient has recently developed a loose, productive cough. The patient is afebrile, appears nontoxic, and has had no difficulty eating or drinking. There is no history of allergies.

---

34. Which is the most likely diagnosis for this patient?
   A. Acute asthma
   B. Acute bronchitis
   C. Pneumonia
   D. Chronic obstructive pulmonary disease (COPD)

CORRECT ANSWER—B. *Rationales:* Patients with acute bronchitis initially have dry coughs that become more productive; they usually appear nontoxic. Most patients with asthma have exposure to allergens as an important history finding. A patient with pneumonia usually has an elevated temperature, productive cough, and coarse crackles. A patient with COPD has a chronic productive cough, exercise intolerance, and increased anteroposterior diameter of the chest. Infection is the most common cause of acute respiratory arrest in asthma patients who appear toxic on admission.
Nursing process step: Assessment

35. Which is the most appropriate treatment for a patient with bronchitis?
   A. Antibiotic therapy for 7 to 10 days
   B. Supportive care, including increased fluids, rest, and humidity
   C. Expectorants every 4 to 6 hours during the day and cough suppressants at night
   D. Beta$_2$-agonist inhaler (two puffs every 6 hours)

CORRECT ANSWER—B. *Rationales:* Therapy for a patient with acute bronchitis includes humidified air, increased fluids, and rest. The most likely medications are bronchodilators, corticosteroids, and antianxiety drugs. These patients need a calm environment and benefit from postural drainage. Cough suppressants may help at night.
Nursing process step: Intervention

36. Which of the following statements indicates successful education of a patient with acute bronchitis?
   A. "As long as I limit my fluid intake, I should not have further symptoms."
   B. "I can continue smoking as long as I don't smoke in a closed area."
   C. "I should wear a mask when around people with a cold."
   D. "I should use my bronchodilators to reduce symptoms."

CORRECT ANSWER—D. *Rationales:* The medications prescribed for acute bronchitis may include bronchodilators, corticosteroids, expectorants, and antianxiety drugs. The patient must increase fluid intake to liquefy secretions. Bronchitis is an inflammation resulting from irritation of the bronchial mucosa by pollen, smoking, or inhalation of irritating substances. The environmental irritant must be removed. A cold does not cause acute bronchitis.
Nursing process step: Evaluation

37. The patient with acute bronchitis requires careful monitoring when receiving which of the following treatments?
   A. Oxygen therapy
   B. Fluid resuscitation
   C. Humidified air
   D. Postural drainage

CORRECT ANSWER—A. *Rationales:* The patient should be given low-flow oxygen to decrease chances of depressing the respiratory drive. Increasing fluids to liquefy secretions, humidifying the air, and performing postural drainage are also important therapy for a patient with acute bronchitis.
Nursing process step: Intervention

38. Which is the most common cause of chest trauma–related deaths?
A. Falls
B. Assaults
C. Firearms
D. Motor vehicle accidents

CORRECT ANSWER—**D.** *Rationales:* Motor vehicle accidents account for two thirds of all chest trauma–related deaths. Other causes of thoracic injuries are falls, assaults, firearms, stabbings, crush injuries, and motor vehicle–pedestrian accidents.
Nursing process step: Assessment

39. Which respiratory sound is most often associated with laryngotracheobronchitis (croup)?
A. Crackles
B. Barky cough
C. Rales
D. Wheezing

CORRECT ANSWER—**B.** *Rationales:* A barky cough occurs most often with croup; coughing frequency increases at night. Crackles, or rales, are popping noises heard most often during inspiration. They indicate that fluid, pus, or mucus is in the smaller airways. When heard, the nurse should instruct the patient to cough and breathe deeply; the nurse should then auscultate again. The sounds may have cleared. Wheezing is a high-pitched musical sound. It can be heard during inspiration and expiration and usually accompanies an asthma attack or bronchospasm.
Nursing process step: Assessment

40. High levels of oxygen in a patient with chronic obstructive pulmonary disease (COPD) can result in which of the following conditions?
A. Increased ventilatory drive
B. Diminished ventilatory drive
C. A mismatch between ventilation and perfusion
D. Profound decrease in P_{CO_2}

CORRECT ANSWER—**B.** *Rationales:* A patient with COPD has had an elevated carbon dioxide level for a prolonged time and no longer depends on carbon dioxide level changes to regulate ventilations. The patient depends on hypoxia or lower PaO_2 level changes to regulate ventilations. If high levels of oxygen are administered, the patient will lose the hypoxic respiratory drive and respirations will decrease or even stop. As respirations decrease, P_{CO_2} levels rise, not decrease. COPD leads to a ventilation/perfusion mismatch. The alveoli enlarge and overdistend, thereby decreasing the surface area of alveoli to capillary. Increasing the oxygen level does not increase the ventilation/perfusion mismatch.
Nursing process step: Intervention

41. Which is the most appropriate nursing diagnosis for a child with croup?
A. Risk for altered nutrition, less than body requirements
B. Risk for infection
C. Risk for altered parent/child attachment
D. Risk for ineffective airway clearance

CORRECT ANSWER—D. *Rationales:* A child with croup has difficulty eating; however, with proper therapy, the child will show decreased symptoms and improved feeding. Croup is usually preceded by an upper respiratory tract infection. There is a risk for altered parent/child attachment. The caregiver should be instructed to remain calm and to stay with the child at all times. The most significant complication of croup is ineffective airway clearance, which often leads to hospitalization.
Nursing process step: Analysis/Nursing diagnosis

42. Which finding is consistent with a diagnosis of hyperventilation?
A. Increased mental acuity
B. Respiratory acidosis
C. Left arm pain
D. Carpopedal spasms

CORRECT ANSWER—D. *Rationales:* Patients with hyperventilation exhibit carpopedal spasms, anxiety, jaw pain, tachypnea, diffuse chest pain, confusion, diaphoresis, and headache. They exhibit respiratory alkalosis, not acidosis.
Nursing process step: Assessment

43. A life-threatening condition that occurs with penetrating chest wounds and results in impaired gas exchange and risk for fluid volume deficit is which of the following?
A. Pneumothorax
B. Cardiac contusion
C. Open pneumothorax
D. Ruptured esophagus

CORRECT ANSWER—C. *Rationales:* An open pneumothorax, which causes equalization of atmospheric and intrathoracic pressures, leads to lung collapse and impaired gas exchange. A hemothorax is commonly associated with an open pneumothorax and results in a risk for fluid volume deficit. Cardiac contusion usually results from blunt trauma. A ruptured esophagus does have the risk for fluid volume deficit; however, the most serious complications are from infection.
Nursing process step: Assessment

44. Which is the most appropriate nursing diagnosis for a child with epiglottitis?
 A. Anxiety related to separation from parent
 B. Decreased cardiac output related to bradycardia
 C. Ineffective airway clearance related to laryngospasm
 D. Impaired gas exchange related to non-compliant lungs

CORRECT ANSWER—C. *Rationales:* Epiglottitis is an immediate threat to life because complete upper airway obstruction may occur suddenly and be precipitated by improper examination or intervention. The upper airway obstruction is the result of laryngospasm and edema. The patient is anxious because of respiratory distress. The nurse should allow a parent to stay with the child and should encourage the parent to hold and reassure the child. The child has impaired gas exchange from impeded air flow, not from a noncompliant lung. The child will probably be tachycardic until respiratory failure ensues.
Nursing process step: Analysis/Nursing diagnosis

45. Which is the most appropriate treatment for a patient with a stable open pneumothorax?
 A. Chest tube insertion
 B. Emergency thoracotomy
 C. Autotransfusion
 D. I.V. infusion of D₅W

CORRECT ANSWER—A. *Rationales:* If the patient's vital signs are stable with no signs of shock, the most appropriate intervention is chest tube insertion for reexpansion of the lung. If the patient is unstable, an emergency thoracotomy is the definitive therapy. Autotransfusion may be used to stabilize the patient until transportation to surgery. Lactated Ringer's solution and normal saline are the only crystalloids that are acceptable in traumatic emergencies.
Nursing process step: Intervention

46. A patient with an open pneumothorax is admitted to the emergency department. A nonporous dressing was placed in the field. Which finding suggests worsening of the patient's condition?
 A. Respiratory rate within normal limits
 B. Decreased breath sounds on the affected side
 C. Tracheal shift with distended neck veins
 D. Blood pressure 120/80 mm Hg

CORRECT ANSWER—C. *Rationales:* The finding that suggests a worsening of the patient's condition is a tracheal shift with distended neck veins, indicating tension pneumothorax. The respiratory rate within normal limits and blood pressure 120/80 mm Hg are acceptable outcomes. The patient will have decreased breath sounds until reexpansion of the lung has been achieved.
Nursing process step: Evaluation

47. Which is the definitive diagnostic study for a patient with suspected esophageal disruption?
A. Chest X-ray
B. Complete blood count with differential
C. Esophagography
D. Esophagoscopy

CORRECT ANSWER—D. *Rationales:* The most definitive study is esophagoscopy. It is used in a patient who has a negative esophagogram but is suspected of having esophageal disruption. Chest films often show mediastinal widening, which occurs in aortic and tracheobronchial ruptures. A complete blood count with differential will not assist with the differential diagnosis of an esophageal rupture.
Nursing process step: Assessment

48. Which is the treatment of choice for a patient with a pneumothorax?
A. Chest tube insertion
B. Emergency thoracotomy
C. Needle thoracostomy
D. Emergent intubation

CORRECT ANSWER—A. *Rationales:* A pneumothorax is treated with the insertion of a chest tube that is connected to an underwater seal until reexpansion of the lung has been achieved. An emergency thoracotomy is reserved for a hemodynamically unstable patient. Needle thoracostomy is used in the treatment of tension pneumothorax. Most patients with pneumothorax do not require emergent intubation.
Nursing process step: Intervention

49. Which is the most likely intervention for a patient with a suspected diaphragmatic rupture?
A. Needle thoracostomy
B. Rapid infusion of I.V. fluids
C. Preparation for surgical intervention
D. Transfer to unit for observation

CORRECT ANSWER—C. *Rationales:* Preparing a patient for surgical intervention is the most important intervention. Needle thoracostomy is contraindicated in this patient because of the risk of puncturing the bowel and releasing its contents into the chest cavity. The potential for serious complications would deter from transfer for observation. I.V. fluids may be necessary if the bowel compresses large vessels, causing a decrease in preload. A gastric tube should also be inserted.
Nursing process step: Intervention

50. A patient who has sustained chest trauma and is suspected of having rib involvement will be hospitalized if which of the following conditions exists?
A. The patient is elderly or has chronic pulmonary disease
B. There is a fracture of more than three ribs
C. Rib one or two has been fractured
D. All of the above

CORRECT ANSWER—D. *Rationales:* Admission to the hospital for patients with rib fractures is based on the number of fractures (more than three ribs), location of the fracture (first or second rib), severity of the fracture (displaced or comminuted rib fractures) and preexisting factors (elderly or patients with chronic pulmonary disease).
Nursing process step: Intervention

51. Which is the initial treatment for a patient with a tracheobronchial injury?
A. Suctioning to maintain airway patency
B. Preparing for chest tube insertion
C. Intubating and providing mechanical ventilation
D. Preparing for surgical intervention

CORRECT ANSWER—A. *Rationales:* The priority intervention is to maintain airway patency, which is accomplished by suctioning. Chest tube insertion and surgical intervention will be necessary after the patient is stabilized. If the patient is intubated, the end of the endotracheal tube must be positioned distal to the injury. It is also advisable to monitor for possible pneumothorax.
Nursing process step: Intervention

52. Which is the most likely nursing diagnosis for a patient with chronic obstructive pulmonary disease (COPD)?
A. Impaired gas exchange related to increased mucus production
B. Risk for infection related to retained secretions
C. Ineffective airway clearance related to structural damage
D. Ineffective airway clearance related to thick secretions

CORRECT ANSWER—C. *Rationales:* The correct response is ineffective airway clearance related to structural damage to the alveoli. Impaired gas exchange in the patient with COPD results from hypoxemia and hypercarbia, not increased mucus production. The patient with COPD does not have a problem with retained secretions. Thick secretions are more often found in a patient with bronchitis, not COPD.
Nursing process step: Analysis/Nursing diagnosis

53. Which finding indicates effective treatment of a tracheobronchial injury?
A. Respiratory rate of 36 breaths/minute
B. Tracheal shift
C. Distended neck veins
D. Improved arterial blood gas levels

CORRECT ANSWER—D. *Rationales:* Findings consistent with improved status after tracheobronchial injury include vital signs within normal limits, decreased air leak, improved arterial blood gas levels, improved tissue perfusion, and no increase in subcutaneous emphysema. Tachypnea and tracheal shift with distended neck veins suggest tension pneumothorax, a possible complication of tracheobronchial injury.
Nursing process step: Evaluation

54. Which is the most appropriate nursing diagnosis for a patient with pneumonia?
A. Fluid volume deficit
B. Decreased cardiac output
C. Impaired gas exchange
D. Risk for infection

CORRECT ANSWER—C. *Rationales:* Impaired gas exchange is the most appropriate diagnosis for a patient with pneumonia. The patient is prone to fluid volume excess. Decreased cardiac output is unlikely in a patient with pneumonia. A patient with pneumonia already has an infection.
Nursing process step: Analysis/Nursing diagnosis

55. Which is the most appropriate nursing diagnosis for a patient with a pulmonary embolus?

A. Ineffective airway clearance related to increased secretions

B. Risk for infection related to interventions

C. Impaired gas exchange related to impeded air flow

D. Altered tissue perfusion related to occlusion of vessel

CORRECT ANSWER—**D.** *Rationales:* Pulmonary emboli occurs when a thrombus lodges in a branch of the pulmonary artery and causes total or partial occlusion. The lung is adequately ventilated but not perfused. There is no increase in secretions. Most of the interventions for pulmonary emboli are noninvasive and do not increase the risk for infection.

Nursing process step: Analysis/Nursing diagnosis

56. Which is the most appropriate nursing diagnosis for a patient who is hyperventilating?

A. Anxiety related to a precipitating event

B. Pain related to oxygen supply or demand imbalances

C. Fluid volume deficit related to osmotic diuresis

D. Impaired gas exchange related to abnormal neurologic function

CORRECT ANSWER—**A.** *Rationales:* The most common medical causes of hyperventilation are myocardial infarction (MI), intracerebral bleeding, ketoacidosis, and salicylate overdose. These causes must be ruled out before treatment. Pain related to oxygen supply or demand imbalances is a viable diagnosis for the MI patient who is hyperventilating. A patient with diabetic ketoacidosis hyperventilates as a compensatory mechanism to correct acidosis and exhibits diuresis as well. A patient with intracerebral bleeding may have neurogenic hyperventilation, which impairs gas exchange.

Nursing process step: Analysis/Nursing diagnosis

SHOCK AND MULTISYSTEM TRAUMA EMERGENCIES

CHAPTER 15

Shock and Multisystem Trauma Emergencies

1. What is the initial rate at which a patient in hemorrhagic hypovolemic shock should have I.V. crystalloid fluid replaced?
A. 20 to 40 ml/kg
B. 5 to 10 ml/kg
C. 80 to 90 ml/kg
D. 200 to 300 ml/kg

CORRECT ANSWER—**A.** *Rationales:* The standard therapy for a hemodynamically unstable patient in hemorrhagic hypovolemic shock is rapid infusion of crystalloid fluid at 20 to 40 ml/kg. The minimal rate of fluid replacement, 5 to 10 ml/kg, may not be sufficient to raise the circulating volume. A rate of 80 to 300 ml/kg may result in dilution of the remaining red blood cell mass, platelets, and coagulation factor. Clot formation in the injured vessels may be disrupted, and homeostasis of the injured site will not be maintained.
Nursing process step: Intervention

Questions 2 through 4 refer to the following information:
A patient who was involved in a motor vehicle accident is brought to the emergency department by a local emergency medical service unit. The patient was an unrestrained driver of a compact automobile that had an impact on the driver's side. The patient sustained severe abdominal injuries, bilateral fractured femurs, and a 4-cm laceration to the right arm. On arrival at the emergency department, the patient was pale, diaphoretic, and talking incoherently. Vital signs on arrival were blood pressure, 50/40 mm Hg; heart rate, 130 beats/minute; respiratory rate, 36 breaths/minute; and tympanic temperature, 98.2° F (36.8° C).

2. Which of the following is the priority for assessing a patient with multisystem trauma?

A. Airway with cervical spine stabilization, breathing, level of consciousness and pupillary response, and circulation

B. Level of consciousness and pupillary response, airway with cervical spine stabilization, breathing, and circulation

C. Breathing, airway with cervical spine stabilization, circulation, and level of consciousness and pupillary response

D. Airway with cervical spine stabilization, breathing, circulation, and level of consciousness and pupillary response

CORRECT ANSWER—D. *Rationales:* The initial assessment of a patient in shock must be rapid and begins with the primary survey. The airway, if not patent, must be opened while maintaining cervical spine stabilization. Breathing effectiveness needs to be assessed, and supplemental oxygen should be administered in the most appropriate route based on the patient's condition. Assessment of circulation should be done by noting the patient's skin temperature, moisture, and color. Capillary refill time in an adult (normal, 2 to 3 seconds; delayed, more than 3 seconds) is of questionable value but may still be included during the assessment as a baseline parameter. The patient's level of consciousness must be evaluated next because cerebral perfusion may be affected by low-perfusion blood flow. If circulation is compromised, two I.V. lines with 14G to 16G catheters should be started with warmed lactated Ringer's solution or normal saline. Pupillary response assessment is performed to determine the equality of pupil size and response to light stimulation. The assessment is organized to identify and correct the most life-threatening conditions first.

Nursing process step: Assessment

3. This patient has which type of shock?
A. Cardiogenic
B. Septic
C. Hypovolemic
D. Neurogenic

CORRECT ANSWER—C. *Rationales:* The patient is hypotensive with a narrow pulse pressure, tachycardia, and altered level of consciousness. These signs and symptoms indicate that the patient is in a compensatory phase of a hypovolemic shock condition. The mechanism of injury (unrestrained driver in a motor vehicle accident) suggests blunt trauma to the abdomen. The most common form of shock in trauma patients is hypovolemic shock. Cardiogenic shock is typically caused by myocardial infarction. Septic shock is most frequently caused by gram-negative and gram-positive bacteria. Neurogenic shock results from a severe brain stem injury at the level of the medulla, an injury to the spinal cord, or spinal anesthesia. A patient with neurogenic shock has a different presentation than one with hypovolemic shock. Signs and symptoms of neurogenic shock include peripheral vasodilation and severe hypotension from loss of sympathetic tone. On assessment, the patient is hypotensive with warm, flushed skin.
Nursing process step: Assessment

4. Which is the most appropriate nursing diagnosis for this patient?
A. Altered cerebral tissue perfusion related to shock state
B. Posttrauma response related to the motor vehicle accident
C. Hypothermia related to prolonged exposure to cold
D. Impaired skin integrity related to skin lacerations

CORRECT ANSWER—A. *Rationales:* During low cerebral blood flow, the body strives to maintain blood flow to the vital centers in the brain stem. Agitation, irritability, and anxiety may be caused by pain, but they may also be early signs of decreased cerebral perfusion. The patient may later develop psychological effects from the accident, but currently cerebral perfusion and cognitive ability are decreased. Hypothermia is not appropriate at this time, but the patient may become hypothermic if measures to prevent body heat loss are not implemented. Impaired skin integrity related to skin lacerations is not a priority nursing diagnosis during initial stabilization unless bleeding is uncontrolled.
Nursing process step: Analysis/Nursing diagnosis

5. Which nursing diagnosis best describes a trauma patient with a central venous pressure (CVP) reading of 3 cm H$_2$O?

A. Fluid volume deficit

B. Impaired gas exchange

C. Risk for fluid volume deficit

D. Fluid volume excess

CORRECT ANSWER—A. *Rationales:* Normal CVP readings range from 4 to 10 cm H$_2$O. A reading above 10 cm H$_2$O indicates volume overload; readings below 4 cm H$_2$O identify fluid volume deficit. Impaired gas exchange is not an appropriate diagnosis for a decreased CVP reading; it would be more appropriate with an alteration in pulmonary function. Risk for fluid volume deficit is incorrect because the patient is beyond that risk; the patient is experiencing actual fluid volume deficit, evidenced by the CVP reading of 3 cm H$_2$O.

Nursing process step: Intervention

6. Which is the most common form of shock in trauma patients?

A. Hypovolemic

B. Cardiogenic

C. NeurogenicRD.Anaphylactic

CORRECT ANSWER—A. *Rationales:* Hypovolemic shock is the most common form of shock in trauma patients. It occurs as a result of inadequate intravascular volume from the loss or redistribution of whole blood, plasma, or other body fluids. Hypovolemic shock is commonly caused by the loss of whole blood (hemorrhage). Additional causes are dehydration from body fluid loss and displaced fluid, as seen in thermal injuries. Cardiogenic shock is caused by myocardial infarction. Neurogenic shock is caused by loss of sympathetic tone brought on by spinal anesthesia or injury to the spinal cord. Anaphylactic shock is most commonly caused by parenterally administered penicillin and insect stings.

Nursing process step: Assessment

7. What should be the initial bolus of crystalloid fluid replacement for a pediatric patient in shock?

A. 20 ml/kg

B. 10 ml/kg

C. 30 ml/kg

D. 15 ml/kg

CORRECT ANSWER—A. *Rationales:* Fluid volume replacement must be calculated to the child's weight to avoid overhydration. Initial fluid bolus is administered at 20 ml/kg, followed by another 20 ml/kg bolus if there is no improvement in volume status. All other options are incorrect.

Nursing process step: Intervention

8. In which of the following conditions is the pneumatic antishock garment (PASG) contra-indicated?
A. Bilateral femur fractures
B. Anaphylactic shock
C. Pelvic fracture
D. Right-sided tension pneumothorax

CORRECT ANSWER—D. *Rationales:* Prehospital providers routinely use the PASG to control hemorrhage and support blood pressure. Inflation of the device causes tamponade of soft tissue hemorrhage and raises blood pressure by increasing systemic vascular resistance. The PASG is contraindicated with a right-sided tension pneumothorax because it further elevates venous pressure associated with the tension pneumothorax. The PASG is also useful for unstable pelvic and femur fractures. In these cases, the garment stabilizes the fractures and tamponades retroperitoneal hemorrhage. Patients in anaphylactic shock may benefit from the PASG because it increases preload and enhances cardiac output.
Nursing process step: Intervention

9. What effect does alpha-adrenergic receptor stimulation have on the peripheral and central circulation vessels?
A. Vasodilation
B. No effect, vascular circulation
C. Vasoconstriction
D. Vasodilatation, then vasoconstriction

CORRECT ANSWER—C. *Rationales:* Alpha-adrenergic receptor stimulation results in vasoconstriction of the vascular beds. This occurs as a compensatory mechanism to enhance the central circulation by increasing diastolic blood pressure and maintaining systolic blood pressure. Beta-adrenergic receptor stimulation results in bronchodilation and postcapillary vasodilation. Options B and D are incorrect.
Nursing process step: Assessment

10. Which patient has the lowest probability of developing septic shock?
A. A geriatric patient with pneumonia
B. A patient who has sustained second degree burns to 30% of body surface area
C. A patient with cancer who is receiving chemotherapy
D. A patient with a 3-cm laceration to the hand sustained while washing dishes

CORRECT ANSWER—D. *Rationales:* The most common organism responsible for septic shock is gram-negative bacteria, which releases endotoxins that activate various hormone and chemical mediators. Other causative organisms of septic shock are gram-positive bacteria, fungi, viruses, and rickettsiae. The patient who received a 3-cm laceration on the hand while washing dishes has the lowest probability of developing septic shock because the injury occurred in a clean environment. Populations at risk for developing septic shock are the very young, the very old, multiple-injury patients, debilitated individuals, and immunosuppressed patients.
Nursing process step: Assessment

11. In addition to whole blood or packed red blood cells, what clotting component should be replaced in a patient with hemorrhagic shock?
  A. Albumin
  B. Dextran
  C. Fresh frozen plasma or platelets
  D. Washed red blood cells

CORRECT ANSWER—C. *Rationales:* In addition to whole blood or packed red blood cells, fresh frozen plasma or platelets should be replaced in a patient with hemorrhagic shock. Red blood cells have minimal clotting factors and platelets available. To decrease the probability of a patient's developing coagulopathy deficits, 1 to 2 units of fresh frozen plasma or platelets are often administered after the infusion of 5 units of blood. Albumin is administered to expand the plasma volume rapidly and may not be necessary as long as blood has been replaced. Dextran and washed red blood cells are not clotting components.
Nursing process step: Intervention

12. A patient with a 7.5-cm laceration on the right arm is admitted to the emergency department. The wound is bleeding profusely. Which nursing intervention should be performed immediately to control the bleeding?
  A. Inject epinephrine into the wound
  B. Apply a tourniquet above the injury site
  C. Apply direct pressure to the wound
  D. Suture the wound

CORRECT ANSWER—C. *Rationales:* Direct pressure applied to the laceration is the most immediate nursing intervention to control bleeding. Applying a tourniquet above the injury may result in permanent damage to the circulatory and nervous pathways in the arm. Injecting epinephrine into the arm and suturing the wound are usually done by the medical staff and require some preparation.
Nursing process step: Intervention

13. Cardiogenic shock results from all except which of the following conditions?
  A. Myocardial infarction
  B. Myocardial contusion
  C. Cardiac failure
  D. Intestinal obstruction

CORRECT ANSWER—D. *Rationales:* Intestinal obstruction results in hypovolemic shock because of fluid that's trapped in the interstitial spaces of the intestinal lumen. Cardiogenic shock is caused by inadequate contractility of the cardiac muscle and results in reduced cardiac output. Myocardial infarction, myocardial contusion, and cardiac failure are causes of cardiogenic shock.
Nursing process step: Assessment

14. Distributive shock is caused by all except which of the following conditions?
   A. Neurogenic shock
   B. Anaphylactic shock
   C. Septic shock
   D. Hypovolemic shock

CORRECT ANSWER—D. *Rationales:* Hypovolemic shock results from inadequate circulating volume and produces changes in the systemic vascular compartments. Distributive shock results from inadequate blood flow and is caused by neurogenic, anaphylactic, and septic shock. Peripheral vasodilatation occurs and leads to inadequate venous return. Neurogenic shock is caused by an injury to the spinal cord above the level of T-6. Because the autonomic sympathetic nervous system is unable to initiate reflux vasoconstriction, systemic vasodilation occurs. Septic shock occurs as a result of a widespread systemic response to an organism. Endotoxins are released into the circulation and create a complex series of events in the cellular, humoral, and immunologic systems. During the hyperdynamic phase, systemic vascular resistance is decreased and peripheral pooling occurs. During the hypodynamic phase, systemic vascular resistance is increased.
Nursing process step: Assessment

15. A patient in septic shock has received a rapid infusion of 3 liters of lactated Ringer's solution and now has a urine output of 35 ml/hour. Based on this finding, which action is required next?
   A. Infuse another 2 liters of lactated Ringer's solution
   B. Change I.V. fluid to normal saline
   C. Infuse lactated Ringer's solution at 125 ml/hour and continue to monitor urine output
   D. Infuse rapidly 1 liter of lactated Ringer's solution

CORRECT ANSWER—C. *Rationales:* The patient's urine output is within the normal range (equal to or greater than 30 ml/hour). Based on this, the patient is experiencing adequate renal perfusion, so the I.V. fluids should be decreased. The nurse should continue to monitor the urine output to determine whether or not the patient is perfusing the viscera. It is not necessary to infuse another 2 liters of lactated Ringer's solution because the patient has adequate urine output. It is not necessary to change the I.V. fluid to normal saline unless the patient is hyponatremic.
Nursing process step: Evaluation

Questions 16 through 18 refer to the following information:
A patient who has fallen from a second-story balcony is admitted to the emergency department. On arrival, the patient is unconscious with a Glasgow coma scale score of 8. Admission vital signs were blood pressure, 70/50 mm Hg; pulse, 64 beats/minute; respiratory rate, 8 breaths/minute; and tympanic temperature, 98° F (36.6° C). The patient has been immobilized on a backboard and has a rigid cervical collar in place. Respirations are being assisted with a bag-valve-mask device on 100% oxygen.

---

16. What is the priority of assessment for this patient?

A. Airway with cervical spine stabilization, breathing, circulation, disability, vital signs, and head-to-toe exam

B. Vital signs, airway with cervical spine stabilization, breathing, circulation, disability, and head-to-toe exam

C. Head-to-toe exam, vital signs, airway with cervical spine stabilization, breathing, circulation, and disability

D. Airway with cervical spine stabilization, breathing, circulation, disability, vital signs, history, and head-to-toe exam

CORRECT ANSWER—D. *Rationales:* Initial assessment of a trauma patient begins with patency of the airway with simultaneous cervical spine stabilization, effectiveness of breathing, adequacy of circulation, and disability (level of consciousness and pupillary response). After all life-threatening conditions have been addressed, the nurse should remove all of the patient's clothing while keeping him warm with heated blankets or radiant heaters. Next, the nurse should get a complete set of vital signs, record present injuries and past medical conditions (if information is available from a significant other or medical records), and logroll the patient to inspect the posterior surface for injuries.

Nursing process step: Assessment

17. Which diagnosis best fits this patient's clinical presentation?

A. Hypovolemic shock

B. Neurogenic shock

C. Cardiogenic shock

D. Septic shock

CORRECT ANSWER—B. *Rationales:* Injury to the cervical spinal cord affects the autonomic nervous system. Below the injury, there is a blocking of sympathetic vasomotor regulation, resulting in extreme vasodilation and maldistribution of the circulating volume. Neurogenic shock occurs as a result of peripheral vasodilation with decreased venous return. The patient's skin is warm, dry, and flushed. The patient is hypotensive and bradycardic. Options A, C, and D do not represent the patient's assessment findings.

Nursing process step: Assessment

18. Which nursing diagnosis reflects respiratory function for this patient?
   A. Risk for injury
   B. Pain
   C. Altered cerebral tissue perfusion
   D. Ineffective breathing pattern

CORRECT ANSWER—D. *Rationales:* The patient's respirations are being assisted with a bag-valve-mask device on high-flow oxygen. Current spontaneous respiratory rate is inadequate for maintaining normal gas exchange. Patients with cervical spine injury may be unable to sustain spontaneous ventilations. Therefore, ineffective breathing pattern is the only diagnosis that reflects the respiratory function for this patient. The other diagnoses are also appropriate for this patient. The patient is at high risk for injury because of the decreased level of consciousness. The patient has decreased cerebral tissue perfusion because the mean arterial pressure is low. Pain cannot be adequately assessed, but most patients who suffer multiple trauma have pain.
Nursing process step: Analysis/Nursing diagnosis

19. A patient with blunt trauma to the chest is admitted to the emergency department. The patient has no breath sounds on the right side of the chest, neck veins are distended, and the trachea is shifted to the left. Admission vital signs are blood pressure 88/56 mm Hg, pulse rate 128 beats/minute, respiratory rate 32 breaths/minute, and a tympanic temperature of 98.4° F (36.9° C). The patient's skin is pale, cool, and clammy. Which type of shock does this patient have?
   A. Hypovolemic
   B. Obstructive
   C. Septic
   D. TNeurogenic

CORRECT ANSWER—B. *Rationales:* The patient has a right-sided tension pneumothorax. It is creating an obstruction from the increased intrathoracic pressure that displaces the inferior vena cava and obstructs venous return to the right atrium. Preload is decreased, and the patient's vital signs exhibit a sympathetic response. Hypovolemic shock results in flat neck veins from the low-volume state and the trachea is not affected. Patients with septic shock do not typically have alterations in the trachea, and neck veins are not generally distended. Neurogenic shock results in bradycardia from the depressed sympathetic nervous system innervation.
Nursing process step: Assessment

20. Early shock class I is characterized by which of the following conditions?

A. Normal or falling systolic pressure and rising diastolic pressure

B. Rising systolic pressure and falling diastolic pressure

C. Falling systolic and diastolic pressures

D. Increased systolic and diastolic pressures

CORRECT ANSWER—**A.** *Rationales:* Early shock (class I) is characterized by normal or falling systolic blood pressure and rising diastolic pressure. Sympathetic stimulation occurs as specialized cells in the carotid and aorta sense a decrease in oxygen and an increase in carbon dioxide in the circulating blood. Catecholamines are released to produce peripheral vasoconstriction and an increase in total peripheral resistance. This action results in an increase in diastolic pressure as a means of increasing preload and cardiac output. All other options are incorrect.

Nursing process step: Assessment

21. Rapid I.V. infusion of lactated Ringer's solution to a patient in shock can best be accomplished by using which of the following?

A. Large-bore long catheter

B. Long I.V. tubing

C. Short I.V. pole

D. Large-bore short catheter

CORRECT ANSWER—**D.** *Rationales:* Rapid I.V. infusion of a crystalloid can best be accomplished by using a large-bore short catheter. A large-bore long catheter and long I.V. tubing or extension sets increase the infusion time. A short I.V. pole does not allow I.V. fluids to flow rapidly because of the decreased gravitational pull.

Nursing process step: Intervention

22. Blood products should be infused only through an I.V. line containing which crystalloid solution?

A. Lactated Ringer's solution

B. D_5W

C. Normal saline

D. Dextran

CORRECT ANSWER—**C.** *Rationales:* Blood should be infused through an I.V. line with normal saline. Lactated Ringer's solution contains enough ionized calcium (3 mEq/L) to overcome the anticoagulant effect of CPDA-1 and allow the development of small clots, which may precipitate in the I.V. line. Dextran and D_5W contain glucose, which causes clumping of the red cells in the tubing and results in swelling and hemolysis of the red blood cells. The blood should be administered through a filter. Although filters come in mesh and microaggregate types, the latter is preferred, especially when transfusing multiple units of blood.

Nursing process step: Intervention

23. Which clinical manifestation of shock in a pediatric patient indicates the late stage of shock?
A. Cyanosis
B. Delayed capillary refill
C. Cool, clammy skin
D. Hypotension

CORRECT ANSWER—**D.** *Rationales:* Hypotension is a late sign of shock in a pediatric patient. A child's cardiovascular system is relatively healthy and may be capable of sustaining cardiac output for a period of time. During the early phase of shock, compensatory mechanisms are implemented to augment circulating volume and venous return. Cyanosis, delayed capillary refill, and cool, cold skin result from sympathetic nervous system innervation, which occurs in the early phase of shock.
Nursing process step: Evaluation

24. The abdominal section of the pneumatic anti-shock garment (PASG) should not be inflated in the patient with which condition?
A. Pelvic fractures
B. Pregnancy
C. Bilateral femur fractures
D. Blunt trauma to the abdomen

CORRECT ANSWER—**B.** *Rationales:* The abdominal section of the PASG should not be inflated in pregnant trauma patients because of potential injury to the fetus. Use of the PASG to augment circulating volume is controversial, but it can assist circulation by decreasing the volume loss from abdominal and extremity injuries.
Nursing process step: Intervention

25. A pediatric patient with a history of vomiting and diarrhea for 2 days is admitted to the emergency department. Which assessment finding indicates that the child is in the late stages of shock?
A. Tachycardia
B. Bradycardia
C. Irritability
D. Urine output 1 to 2 ml/kg/hour

CORRECT ANSWER—**B.** *Rationales:* Bradycardia is a sign of late shock in a pediatric patient. Cardiovascular dysfunction and impairment of cellular function lead to lowered perfusion pressures, increased precapillary arteriolar resistance, and venous capacitance. Decreased cardiac output occurs in late shock if the lost circulating volume is not replaced. Sympathetic nervous innervation has limited compensatory mechanisms if the volume is not replaced. Tachycardia and irritability occur during the early phase of shock as compensatory mechanisms are implemented to increase cardiac output. Normal urine output for a pediatric patient is 1 to 2 ml/kg/hour; volumes less than this would indicate a decrease in renal perfusion and activation of the renin-angiotensin-aldosterone system to decrease water and sodium excretion.
Nursing process step: Evaluation

26. Which procedure should be completed before initiating antibiotic therapy on a patient diagnosed with septic shock?

A. Urine culture, complete blood count, and one set of blood cultures

B. Lumbar puncture, urine culture, urinalysis, and complete blood count

C. Complete blood count, urinalysis, serum electrolyte levels, prothrombin time, and partial thromboplastin time

D. Two separate sets of blood cultures from different venipuncture sites and a urine culture

CORRECT ANSWER—D. *Rationales:* Before administering antibiotic therapy, the nurse should obtain cultures of blood and urine to identify the bacteria responsible for the septic condition. Blood cultures should be obtained from two separate venipuncture sites to avoid false results from skin contamination. Lumbar puncture should be done if a patient has a clinical sign, such as nuchal rigidity, that indicates central nervous system infection. Complete blood count, urinalysis, serum electrolyte levels, prothrombin time, and partial thromboplastin time are laboratory tests that should be done as part of the basic examination and do not need to be completed before initiating antibiotic therapy.

Nursing process step: Intervention

27. Which is the major pulmonary cause of septic shock?

A. Tuberculosis

B. Bronchitis

C. Pulmonary embolus

D. Acute bacterial pneumonia

CORRECT ANSWER—D. *Rationales:* The major pulmonary cause of septic shock is acute bacterial pneumonia. The most common causative organisms are *Streptococcus pneumoniae* and *Staphylococcus aureus.* Tuberculosis differs from other bacterial pulmonary diseases in that it is a chronic condition. Once the organism has spread to the regional lymph nodes and disseminated hepatogenously, cell-mediated immunity occurs and halts further bacterial growth. Bronchitis is an inflammatory response of the bronchi caused by pollen, smoking, pollution, or inhalation of irritating substances. It is characterized by increased mucus production. Pulmonary embolus is caused by a clot lodging in the pulmonary artery (or one the smaller branches) and obstructing blood flow distally.

Nursing process step: Assessment

28. Which nursing diagnosis is most appropriate for an infant with irritability, poor dietary intake, sunken fontanels, and poor skin turgor?
A. Fluid volume deficit related to inadequate fluid intake
B. Ineffective airway clearance related to retained secretions
C. Impaired gas exchange related to exudate accumulation
D. Activity intolerance related to irritability

CORRECT ANSWER—A. *Rationales:* The most appropriate nursing diagnosis for this infant is fluid volume deficit related to inadequate fluid intake. Irritability, sunken fontanels, and poor skin turgor are all clinical signs of dehydration. Ineffective airway clearance and impaired gas exchange will occur if the volume deficit is not corrected. Activity intolerance related to irritability is a result of fluid volume deficit; decreased perfusion to the central nervous system produces impaired mentation; and the patient may exhibit irritability, agitation, confusion, lethargy, or coma.
Nursing process step: Analysis/Nursing diagnosis

29. Which of the following represents the estimated blood loss in a trauma patient with bilateral femur fractures and a fractured pelvis?
A. 2 units of blood
B. 4 units of blood
C. 1 unit of blood
D. More than 5 units of blood

CORRECT ANSWER—D. *Rationales:* This patient's blood loss is estimated to be more than 5 units. A closed femur fracture can result in up to 2 units of blood loss, and fractures of the pelvis can result in a blood loss of 2 to 20 units. Pelvic fractures frequently disrupt adjacent blood vessels. The blood loss for pelvic fractures is gauged as 1 unit for each fracture of the pelvis. All other options are incorrect.
Nursing process step: Assessment

30. Which nursing diagnosis best describes small petechial hemorrhages on the face and chest?
A. Impaired skin integrity
B. Impaired tissue integrity
C. Risk for impaired skin integrity
D. Risk for infection

CORRECT ANSWER—B. *Rationales:* The nursing diagnosis that best fits this patient is impaired tissue integrity related to altered clotting mechanisms that result in disseminated intravascular coagulation (DIC). In septic shock, microorganisms enter the body and release endotoxins. These endotoxins inhibit platelet function and injure the endothelium while activating the intrinsic clotting factors that result in DIC. Impaired skin integrity may result from the patient's immobility.
Nursing process step: Analysis/Nursing diagnosis

31. The administration of dopamine hydrochloride (Intropin) would be least beneficial in which shock state?

A. Hypovolemic
B. Septic
C. Cardiogenic
D.TNeurogenic

CORRECT ANSWER—A. *Rationales:* The administration of dopamine hydrochloride is least beneficial for a patient in hypovolemic shock. Studies have shown that raising the blood pressure with vasopressors increases the mortality potential. Blood pressure in patients in hypovolemic shock should be raised by replacing red blood cells and circulating volume. Vasopressors are effective in raising blood pressure in all forms of shock in which peripheral vasodilation has occurred.
Nursing process step: Intervention

Questions 32 through 34 refer to the following information:
A patient with increased urination and hunger and elevated temperature for 4 days is admitted to the emergency department. Admission vital signs are blood pressure, 82/52 mm Hg; pulse rate, 132 beats/minute; respirations, 28 breaths/minute and shallow; and oral temperature, 102° F (38.9° C). Laboratory studies reveal a blood glucose of 880 mg/dl, serum potassium of 2.8 mEq/L, serum sodium of 128 mEq/L, serum osmolality of 368 mOsm/kg, and absence of ketoacidosis.

---

32. Which is the most appropriate nursing diagnosis for this patient?

A. Risk for fluid volume deficit
B. Impaired gas exchange
C. Fluid volume excess
D. Fluid volume deficit

CORRECT ANSWER—D. *Rationales:* This patient is suffering from hyperosmolar hyperglycemic nonketotic syndrome (HNKS). HNKS is characterized by a serum osmolality greater than 350 mOsm/kg, blood glucose greater than 600 mg/dl, and the absence of ketoacidosis in a patient with an altered level of consciousness. The priority nursing diagnosis for this patient is fluid volume deficit from the hyperosmolar condition that results in osmotic diuresis. Hyperglycemia causes water to be drawn from the intracellular space to the extracellular space as well as a fall in the serum sodium concentration. This patient is beyond risk for fluid volume deficit. Impaired gas exchange is not the priority currently, but if the fluid volume deficit is not corrected, it will become a priority. Fluid volume excess is inappropriate for this diagnosis.
Nursing process step: Analysis/Nursing diagnosis

33. Which intervention is most important for this patient?

A. Insertion of an orogastric tube
B. Insertion of an indwelling urinary catheter
C. Initiation of an I.V. line
D. Collection of blood sample for culturing

CORRECT ANSWER—C. *Rationales:* The most important intervention for this patient is the initiation of an I.V. line for fluid replacement. Patients can lose up to 25% of their total body water with hyperosmolar hypoglycemic non-ketotic syndrome; elderly patients can lose up to 50%. One half of the estimated water deficit should be replaced during the first 12 hours and the remainder during the next 24 hours. Insertion of an orogastric tube is not necessary at this time. Insertion of an indwelling urinary catheter can be completed to monitor urine output but is not a priority before the replacement of circulating volume. The patient's elevated temperature is probably caused by dehydration and does not require the collection of blood samples.
Nursing process step: Intervention

34. During the initial phase of fluid resuscitation, which I.V. solution should be infused?

A. Normal saline solution
B. Lactated Ringer's solution
C. Dextran 40
D. Plasma-lyte A

CORRECT ANSWER—A. *Rationales:* Initial fluid resuscitation should consist of normal saline solution. In patients who are hypertensive and have significant hypernatremia, a hypotonic saline solution (0.45% sodium chloride) should be used. Normal saline corrects the extracellular volume deficit, increases blood pressure, and maintains adequate urine output. Once these physiologic conditions have been corrected, hypotonic saline can be administered to provide free water for correction of intracellular volume deficits. Dextran 40 is a glucose polysaccharide and worsens dehydration. Plasma-lyte A contains glucagon and increases blood glucose levels.
Nursing process step: Intervention

35. A pregnant trauma patient in hemorrhagic shock can lose up to what percentage of her circulating volume before exhibiting hypotension?

A. 15%
B. 20%
C. 30%
D. 50%

CORRECT ANSWER—C. *Rationales:* A pregnant patient becomes hypervolemic during pregnancy, and blood volume increases 45% to 50% above normal by term. Because the increase in plasma is more than that of red blood cells, the patient manifests a relative anemia. The increase in plasma volume allows the patient to lose up to 30% of the circulating volume before vital signs change to reflect a hypovolemic state. All other options are incorrect.
Nursing process step: Assessment

36. Which statement best describes neurogenic shock?
  A. Decrease in respiratory function
  B. Loss of sympathetic vasomotor regulation
  C. Inadequate cellular perfusion
  D. Loss of parasympathetic vasomotor regulation

CORRECT ANSWER—B. *Rationales:* Neurogenic shock follows compression or transection of the spinal cord above the 6th thoracic vertebrae and affects the autonomic nervous system. Other causes of neurogenic shock are the administration of anesthetic agents and the ingestion of drugs (barbiturates or tranquilizers). All causes block the sympathetic vasomotor regulation below the level of the injury. Parasympathetic stimulation is unopposed, resulting in venous dilation, decreased venous return, decreased cardiac output, and decreased tissue perfusion. A decrease in respiratory function may occur, depending on the level of injury. Venous vasodilation affects inadequate tissue perfusion because of decreases in cardiac output.
Nursing process step: Assessment

37. Which is the best early clinical indicator of hypovolemic shock in children?
  A. Blood pressure
  B. Respiratory rate
  C. Pulse rate and skin temperature and color
  D. Urine output

CORRECT ANSWER—C. *Rationales:* The best early indicators of hypovolemic shock in children are pulse rate and skin temperature and color. Low-volume receptors (baroreceptors) located in the aortic arch and carotid bodies sense a decrease in circulating volume and increase sympathetic nervous system stimulation. The sympathetic nervous system increases catecholamine release, which increases the heart rate. Peripheral vasoconstriction occurs in an effort to increase cardiac output. The peripheral vasoconstriction causes the skin temperature to become cool. If the low flow is not corrected, the skin color will become cyanotic. Capillary refill may be longer than 3 seconds. During low-flow states, initial compensatory mechanisms maintain near normal blood pressure because the child has a relatively healthy cardiovascular system. Hypotension occurs late in a shock state. Respiratory rate may be unaffected in the initial low-flow state. Normal urine output may be affected in the initial low-flow state as a result of decreased perfusion to the kidneys. Urinary output must be monitored to identify alterations in renal perfusion.
Nursing process step: Assessment

Questions 38 through 40 refer to the following information:
An infant with an upper respiratory tract infection and irritability for 4 days is admitted to the emergency department. On admission, vital signs are blood pressure, 48/30 mm Hg; pulse rate, 160 beats/minute; respiratory rate, 60 breaths/minute; and tympanic temperature, 96.5° F (35.8° C). The infant is lethargic, extremities are cool and cyanotic, and capillary refill is delayed (longer than 3 seconds). There is a petechial rash on the abdomen.

38. The clinical manifestations describe which type of shock condition?
  A. Hypovolemia
  B. Anaphylactic
  C. Septic
  D. Cardiogenic

CORRECT ANSWER—C. *Rationales:* The clinical manifestations describe septic shock that probably is caused by a gram-negative organism. Endotoxin causes a decrease in intravascular volume from increased venous capacitance. Cardiac output falls as the compensatory mechanisms fail to support circulation with the initial increased sympathetic stimulation. Endotoxins injure the endothelium and alter platelet function, causing the activation of intrinsic clotting factors, which leads to the development of disseminated intravascular coagulation. This is evidenced by the petechial rash on the abdomen. Petechiae on the abdomen may be a sign of meningococcemia, and the patient should be immediately isolated.
Nursing process step: Assessment

39. Which is the priority intervention for this patient?
  A. Initiate an I.V. line
  B. Obtain blood cultures
  C. Give oxygen therapy with the device best tolerated by the patient
  D. Insert an indwelling urinary catheter to determine urine output

CORRECT ANSWER—C. *Rationales:* The priority intervention for this patient is to support respirations with supplemental oxygen therapy. The nurse should use the device best tolerated by the child; fighting an oxygen device may use up the child's oxygen reserves. In septic shock, the child's respiratory efforts may quickly lead to fatigue, so the child requires close monitoring for signs of respiratory failure. Oxygen saturation can be monitored with pulse oximetry. Intubation and mechanical ventilation equipment should be readily accessible. Septic shock creates a hypovolemic state; therefore, fluid replacement should be started as soon as possible after the airway is secure. To isolate the causative organism, blood cultures and urine cultures should be done before antibiotics are administered. The nurse should insert an indwelling urinary catheter after stabilizing airway, breathing, and circulation.
Nursing process step: Intervention

40. Medication therapy should include all except which of the following?
   A. Ceftriaxone sodium (Rocephin)
   B. D$_{25}$W
   C. Dopamine hydrochloride (Intropin)
   D. Atropine sulfate

CORRECT ANSWER—D. *Rationales:* Atropine sulfate is not indicated at this time. It is an anticholinergic drug that blocks parasympathetic action on the sinoatrial node. It thereby improves conduction through the atrioventricular node and results in an increased heart rate. Antibiotics are recommended after obtaining at least one blood culture. Ceftriaxone sodium is a third-generation cephalosporin used in the treatment of septic shock. Glycogen stores are limited in infants and rapidly depleted during periods of stress; therefore, D$_{25}$W (2 to 4 ml/kg) is used to treat the hypoglycemic state. Dopamine hydrochloride is recommended in low doses of 2 to 5 mcg/kg/minute to increase renal and mesenteric blood flow; doses of 5 to 20 mcg/kg/minute increase heart rate and contractility of the myocardium and thereby raise cardiac output. Doses greater than 20 mcg/kg/minute cause systemic vasoconstriction.
Nursing process step: Intervention

41. Which statement best describes anaphylactic shock?
   A. Loss of sympathetic vasomotor function
   B. Systemic antigen-antibody response
   C. Endothelial surface damage from endotoxin
   D. Decreased catecholamine release

CORRECT ANSWER—B. *Rationales:* Anaphylactic shock occurs from a systemic antigen-antibody response in which massive quantities of chemical mediators are released from the mast cells and basophils throughout the body. For anaphylaxis to occur, there must be previous sensitization to a foreign substance. On reexposure to the substance, the foreign antigen binds to immunoglobulin E (IgE), which was made during the initial exposure. Once the IgE bonds to the mast cells and basophils, chemical mediators (histamine, kallikrein, leukotrienes, heparin, prostaglandins, protease, and platelet-activating factor) are released. Loss of sympathetic vasomotor function occurs in neurogenic shock. Endothelial surface damage from endotoxin occurs in septic shock. Catecholamines are released during the stress response and result in tachycardia. Histamine, prostaglandins, and kallikrein lead to peripheral vasodilation regardless of the vasoconstrictive efforts of the catecholamines.
Nursing process step: Assessment

42. Adequate fluid resuscitation in pediatric patients is best characterized by which of the following urine outputs?
A. 0.5 ml/kg/hour
B. 10 to 15 ml/kg/hour
C. 3 to 4 ml/kg/hour
D. 1 to 2 ml/kg/hour

CORRECT ANSWER—D. *Rationales:* Adequate renal perfusion is best characterized by a urine output of 1 to 2 ml/kg/hour. During fluid resuscitation, urine output must be monitored to assess the effectiveness of renal function. All other options are incorrect.
Nursing process step: Evaluation

43. Which of the following is the priority when implementing initial treatment of patients in anaphylactic shock?
A. Administering antihistamines
B. Maintaining airway patency
C. Establishing I.V. access
D. Infusing a bolus of 200 ml of lactated Ringer's solution

CORRECT ANSWER—B. *Rationales:* The priority in the initial treatment of patients in anaphylactic shock is maintaining airway patency. Anaphylactic shock is associated with the sudden onset of severe respiratory distress. Bronchospasm and laryngeal edema may lead to airway obstruction. I.V. access should be initiated to administer antihistamines and other drugs. Infusing a bolus of crystalloids is not necessary because the hypotension in this type of shock is caused by vasodilation, not hypovolemia. Therefore, the patient's blood pressure would remain low even after the fluid bolus.
Nursing process step: Intervention

44. In the treatment of shock, when peripheral cannulation is unsuccessful, intraosseous cannulation is usually recommended in which age-group?
A. No age limit
B. Younger than 2 years
C. Younger than 6 years
D. Younger than 13 years

CORRECT ANSWER—C. *Rationales:* Intraosseous cannulation is most frequently used with children less than 6 years of age, although it can be used with a child of any age. Intraosseous cannulation allows rapid access for fluid or drug resuscitation. The procedure is usually done after three attempts at peripheral I.V. insertion have been made. An intraosseous infusion is started by inserting a rigid needle into the medullary cavity of a long bone (tibia). When initiating intraosseous access, only one attempt should be made in each bone. Drugs, fluids, and blood may be infused by way of this access.
Nursing process step: Intervention

45. A patient who was stung by 30 hornets was brought to the emergency department. Which is the most critical nursing diagnosis for this patient?
A. Fluid volume deficit
B. Ineffective airway clearance
C. Pain
D. Altered cerebral tissue perfusion

CORRECT ANSWER—B. *Rationales:* The most critical nursing diagnosis for this patient is ineffective airway clearance related to the allergic response from the hornet stings. Respiratory distress may occur from the angioedema of the upper airways, and laryngeal and bronchial spasms may create an airway obstruction. Fluid volume deficit is related to peripheral vasodilation that occurs as a result of the release of mediators from the mast cells and basophils. These mediators are responsible for the increased vascular permeability and vasodilation. Fluid resuscitation measures may be refractory because of the generalized vasodilation. Pain is not a priority at this time. The patient will develop altered cerebral tissue perfusion if the anaphylaxis is not corrected.
Nursing process step: Analysis/Nursing diagnosis

46. During a shock state, the renin-angiotensin-aldosterone system has which of the following expected outcomes on renal function?
A. Decreased urine output, increased reabsorption of sodium and water
B. Decreased urine output, decreased reabsorption of sodium and water
C. Increased urine output, increased reabsorption of sodium and water
D. Increased urine output, decreased reabsorption of sodium and water

CORRECT ANSWER—A. *Rationales:* The renin-angiotensin-aldosterone system alters renal function by decreasing urine output and increasing reabsorption of sodium and water. Reduced renal perfusion stimulates the renin-angiotensin-aldosterone system in an effort to conserve circulating volume.
Nursing process step: Evaluation

47. A trauma patient with a fractured femur and a fractured pelvis has been transfused with 2 units of packed red blood cells. Which measurements indicate that this patient has received adequate replacement of circulating volume?
A. pH 7.22, $PaCO_2$ 45, PaO_2 88, HCO_3- 15
B. SaO_2 76%
C. Blood pressure 88/76 mm Hg, pulse 120 beats/minute
D. pH 7.35, $PaCO_2$ 40, PaO_2 95, HCO_3- 22

CORRECT ANSWER—D. *Rationales:* These blood gas values reflect a normal acid-base state, indicating that the patient has received adequate blood replacement. All other assessments indicate a hypovolemic state that has not been corrected.
Nursing process step: Evaluation

48. An indwelling urinary catheter has been inserted in an adult patient who was dehydrated from vomiting. Which urine output indicates that the patient has received adequate fluid replacement?
A. 15 ml/hour
B. 25 ml/hour
C. 30 ml/hour
D. 5 ml/hour

CORRECT ANSWER—C. *Rationales:* A urine output of 30 ml/hour or more indicates that the patient has received adequate volume replacement and that renal perfusion is normal. All other options indicate the need for more fluids.
Nursing process step: Evaluation

49 Which of the following is the expected outcome of administering pharmacologic agents in the treatment of cardiogenic shock?
A. Decrease preload, increase contractility, increase peripheral resistance
B. Increase contractility, decrease peripheral resistance and afterload, increase cardiac output
C. Increase preload, increase peripheral resistance, increase afterload
D. Decrease cardiac output, decrease cardiac contractility, decrease peripheral resistance

CORRECT ANSWER—B. *Rationales:* Administering dopamine hydrochloride (Intropin), dobutamine hydrochloride (Dobutrex), nitroprusside sodium (Nipride), and nitroglycerine (Nitro-Bid)) to treat cardiogenic shock should result in decreased peripheral resistance and afterload, increased contractility, and increased cardiac output. All other options are incorrect.
Nursing process step: Evaluation

50. Administering dopamine hydrochloride (Intropin) at 2 mcg/kg/minute results in which of the following?
A. Decreased renal perfusion
B. Decreased reabsorption of sodium and water
C. Increased renal perfusion
D. Increased reabsorption of sodium and water

CORRECT ANSWER—C. *Rationales:* Dopamine hydrochloride, when administered at low doses of 0.5 to 3 mcg/kg/minute, produces primarily alpha-adrenergic effects and increases renal perfusion. Doses over 10 mcg/kg/minute result in renal vasoconstriction. Dopamine does not directly affect the reabsorption of sodium and water other than to dilate renal arterioles.
Nursing process step: Evaluation

51. A patient with a fractured pelvis and retroperitoneal hemorrhage has received 10 units of packed red blood cells. The nurse notices that blood is oozing from abrasions and puncture sites. Which is the most appropriate intervention for this patient?
A. Administer blood without warming it
B. Administer fresh frozen plasma and platelets
C. Discontinue further transfusion
D. Administer cryoprecipitate

CORRECT ANSWER—B. *Rationales:* Packed red blood cells and stored whole blood do not contain coagulation factors. One unit of fresh frozen plasma and six platelet packs are recommended for every 5 to 10 units of blood transfused. Hypothermia may also alter the coagulation cascade, so blood should be warmed to 98.6° F (37° C). There is no need to discontinue further blood transfusions; pelvic fractures and retroperitoneal hemorrhages may deplete all the circulating volume if they do not tamponade. Cryoprecipitate could be infused if more than 20 units of blood are administered. Cryoprecipitate contains clotting factors that may be lacking in a patient requiring multiple transfusions.
Nursing process step: Intervention

52. Which nursing diagnosis best describes an anaphylactic reaction with generalized erythema and labored respirations?
A. Risk for infection
B. Altered cerebral tissue perfusion
C. Ineffective breathing pattern
D. Decreased cardiac output

CORRECT ANSWER—C. *Rationales:* The patient is experiencing an antigen-antibody reaction that results in generalized erythema and labored respirations. The nursing diagnosis that best describes the allergic reaction is ineffective breathing pattern as evidenced by labored respirations. Angioedema of the upper airway may result in airway obstruction. The patient is not at high risk for infection. During the initial phase of anaphylaxis, the stress response is initiated and the heart rate increases. That in turn increases cardiac output. An alteration in cerebral tissue perfusion is not evident in the initial phase because cardiovascular compensatory mechanisms maintain perfusion to the heart and brain.
Nursing process step: Analysis/Nursing diagnosis

53. A trauma patient is transferred from another hospital where the patient's initial hematocrit was 40%. After receiving 4 L of lactated Ringer's solution, the hematocrit is 32%. This decrease is probably related to which of the following conditions?

A. Additional blood was lost

B. Hemodilution occurred from the infusion of crystalloids

C. Specimen was drawn above the I.V. site

D. A hemolyzed blood specimen was spun

CORRECT ANSWER—B. *Rationales:* Hemodilution from an infusion of crystalloid solution has caused the hematocrit decrease from 40% to 32%. Hemodilution occurs when the ratio of plasma to red cells increases. Additional blood loss may decrease the hematocrit level, but given the situation, this decrease is probably caused by hemodilution. Specimens drawn above the I.V. site would increase the hematocrit level. Even though a specimen may be hemolyzed, a hematocrit level can be obtained.
Nursing process step: Evaluation

54. Children may lose up to which percentage of their circulating volume before clinical manifestations occur?

A. 5%

B. 15%

C. 25%

D. 35%

CORRECT ANSWER—C. *Rationales:* Children may lose up to 25% of their circulating volume before they manifest signs of shock. The normal blood volume for children is 80 to 85 ml/kg (higher in infants). Increased physiologic reserves enable children to stabilize their vital signs. When fluid losses occur, intrinsic compensatory mechanisms initiate changes to augment circulation: venous capacitance decreases, fluid shifts from the interstitial to the intravascular compartments, and arteriolar constriction increases.
Nursing process step: Assessment

55. Which compensatory mechanisms are a response to shock?

A. Increased renal perfusion and retention of sodium and water

B. Decreased renal perfusion and excretion of sodium and water

C. Increased renal perfusion and excretion of sodium and water

D. Decreased renal perfusion and retention of sodium and water

CORRECT ANSWER—D. *Rationales:* Vasoconstriction in response to a low-flow state decreases renal perfusion. Reduction of renal blood flow and stimulation of the renin-angiotensin-aldosterone system increase reabsorption of sodium and water and thereby decrease urine output. None of the other options reflects the compensatory state of shock.
Nursing process step: Evaluation

56. What is the normal range for serum lactate levels?

A. 5 to 15 mg/dl

B. 0 to 4 mg/dl

C. 8 to 20 mg/dl

D. 20 to 32 mg/dl

CORRECT ANSWER—A. *Rationales:* The normal range for serum lactate levels is 5 to 15 mg/dl. In the absence of adequate tissue oxygenation, anaerobic metabolism occurs and results in an accumulation of lactic acid. Marked elevations in serum lactate levels occur late in the shock syndrome.
Nursing process step: Assessment

57. Treatment for a patient in anaphylactic shock includes administering antihistamines, bronchodilators, and epinephrine. Which other histamine₂ (H₂) blocker could be administered?

   A. Atenolol (Tenormin)

   B. Methylprednisolone (Solu-Medrol)

   C. Diphenhydramine (Benadryl)

   D. Cimetidine (Tagamet)

CORRECT ANSWER—D. *Rationales:* Initial treatment of anaphylactic shock includes administering antihistamines, bronchodilators, and epinephrine. It also includes administering H_2 blockers and cimetidine 300 mg I.V. Administration of H_2 blockers and cimetidine is repeated every 6 to 8 hours. Atenolol is a beta blocker. Patients on atenolol may require higher doses of epinephrine to counteract the effects of the mediators released from the mast cells and basophils. Diphenhydramine is an antihistamine. An initial dose of 50 mg is administered I.V. and may be repeated every 6 to 8 hours. Methylprednisolone is a glucocorticoid and may prevent or lessen the delayed reactions from the antigen-antibody reaction.
Nursing process step: Intervention

58. Which nursing diagnosis best describes a patient with a urine specific gravity greater than 1.050?

   A. Risk for infection

   B. Risk for hypervolemia

   C. Altered renal tissue perfusion

   D. Risk for hypothermia

CORRECT ANSWER—C. *Rationales:* Normal urine specific gravity ranges from 1.003 to 1.040. A urine specific gravity greater than 1.050 indicates dehydration with altered renal tissue perfusion. The compensatory mechanism during a low-flow state is to shunt blood from the skin and the GI and renal systems to maintain heart and brain functions. Decreased renal perfusion results in decreased water excretion and reabsorption of sodium. The patient does not have an increased risk for infection but rather for acute tubular necrosis. Hypervolemia is usually evidenced by a decrease in urine specific gravity. Risk for hypothermia does not best describe this condition.
Nursing process step: Analysis/Nursing diagnosis

59. A patient with blunt trauma to the abdomen has received 2 L of lactated Ringer's solution. Which is the most appropriate intervention in response to the following arterial blood gas values: pH 7.21, $PaCO_2$ 45, PaO_2 84, HCO_3- 15?
   A. Infuse lactated Ringer's solution at a keep-vein-open rate
   B. Infuse a bolus with lactated Ringer's solution at 40 ml/kg
   C. Infuse whole blood or packed red cells
   D. Administer sodium bicarbonate

CORRECT ANSWER—C. *Rationales:* The arterial blood gas values reveal that the patient is in metabolic acidosis because of decreased tissue perfusion from hemorrhage. Blunt trauma to the abdomen may result in injury to the solid viscera (spleen and liver) and produce severe loss of circulating volume and oxygen. When tissues do not have adequate oxygenation, an anaerobic environment occurs and produces a buildup of lactic acid. The replacement of red blood cells decreases the anaerobic environment. Replacement may be with whole blood or packed red blood cells. The infusion of crystalloids, such as lactated Ringer's solution or normal saline, will replace circulating volume; however, hemodilution of existing red blood cells will occur. During the initial shock phase, metabolic acidosis is treated with blood and fluid replacement. If acidosis continues, sodium bicarbonate may be administered.
Nursing process step: Intervention

60. Which nursing diagnosis is most appropriate for a patient with obstructive shock from a pulmonary embolus?
   A. Risk for infection
   B. Impaired gas exchange
   C. Potential for hypothermia
   D. Ineffective airway clearance

CORRECT ANSWER—B. *Rationales:* Pulmonary embolus occurs when a venous clot lodges in the pulmonary artery or one of its branches. The nursing diagnosis most appropriate for this patient is impaired gas exchange. There is no risk for infection or a potential for hypothermia. Ineffective airway clearance is not appropriate.
Nursing process step: Analysis/Nursing diagnosis

61. Which is the best unit of measure for identifying early shock in a trauma patient?
   A. Hemoglobin and hematocrit
   B. Central venous pressure (CVP)
   C. Blood pressure
   D. Heart rate

CORRECT ANSWER—B. *Rationales:* Central venous pressure is the best unit of measure for identifying shock in a trauma patient. CVP measures the right-sided heart pressure, which reflects blood and fluid status. A normal CVP measurement is 4 to 10 cm H_2O pressure. A value less than 4 cm may indicate hypovolemia or vasodilation. Hemoglobin and hematocrit are not the best indicators of early shock in a trauma patient because they may be normal in early shock unless there has been massive blood loss. It normally takes 4 to 6 hours for blood loss to be reflected in hemoglobin and hematocrit levels.
Nursing process step: Assessment

62. After having a leg accidentally amputated in an industrial mishap, an 80-kg patient is treated in the emergency department. Treatment is immediately initiated to correct symptoms of hypovolemic shock. Which of the following findings indicate improved fluid volume status?
A. Capillary refill time of 4 seconds
B. Central venous pressure (CVP) of 4 cm H_2O
C. Hourly urine output of 10 ml
D. Cardiac output of 3 L/minute

CORRECT ANSWER—B. *Rationales:* A person in decompensated shock shows signs of decreased blood pressure, increased pulse rate, narrowed pulse pressure, and poor skin perfusion. Additionally, the patient has decreased urine output, CVP, cardiac output, hematocrit, and tidal volume. It is important to recognize the signs associated with hypovolemic states as well as the abnormal values of these signs. CVP directly reflects the filling pressure of the right ventricle. Indirectly, it reflects vascular tone, the efficiency of the heart as a pump, and fluid volume status. A normal range for CVP is 4 to 10 cm H_2O. Capillary refill is normally less than 3 seconds. A delayed response indicates vasoconstriction that occurs when the body shunts blood away from the periphery to the central core. Adequate urine output occurs if the flow is 1 ml/kg/hour or about 20 ml/hour. A flow less than this indicates inadequate renal perfusion. Normal cardiac output ranges between 4 and 8 L/minute. Decreases in this value occur when the heart fills inadequately and pulse pressure narrows.
Nursing process step: Evaluation

63. A patient who is receiving beta blockers shows which response to a shock state?
A. Increased pulse rate and hypotension
B. Bradycardia, hypotension, and decreased renin secretion
C. Increased pulse rate and hypertension
D. Bradycardia and hypertension

CORRECT ANSWER—B. *Rationales:* Beta blockers may mask the signs of shock. The sympathetic stimulation causing an increase in heart rate is blocked by beta blockers. The patient may show bradycardia and hypotension with a decrease in renin secretion.
Nursing process step: Evaluation

SUBSTANCE ABUSE AND TOXICOLOGIC EMERGENCIES

CHAPTER 16

Substance Abuse and Toxicologic Emergencies

1. An alcoholic patient presents to the emergency department 12 hours after the last drink with anxiety, mild tachycardia, and tremors. Which is the highest priority nursing diagnosis for this patient?
A. Anxiety related to alcohol withdrawal
B. Altered thought processes related to confusion
C. Risk for injury related to seizures
D. Impaired memory related to blackouts

CORRECT ANSWER—C. *Rationales:* Alcohol withdrawal symptoms begin 6 to 8 hours after the last drink and include anxiety, irritability, insomnia, tremors, mild tachycardia, seizures, and hallucinations. Altered thought processes related to confusion is present in alcohol withdrawal syndrome, and impaired memory related to blackouts occurs during the drinking period.
Nursing process step: Analysis/Nursing diagnosis

2. A 20-year-old patient with a complaint of substernal chest pain presents to the emergency department triage desk. Breath sounds are clear, and the patient is negative for a history of medical problems. The nurse should ask specifically about the use of which of these drugs?
A. Tricyclic antidepressants
B. Benzodiazepines
C. Opioids
D. Cocaine

CORRECT ANSWER—D. *Rationales:* Cocaine has direct effects on the heart that include increased myocardial oxygen consumption, coronary artery spasm, ischemia, and myocardial infarction. Tricyclic antidepressants cause arrhythmias in overdoses. Benzodiazepines cause drowsiness and confusion in overdoses. Opioids cause respiratory depression.
Nursing process step: Assessment

3. Appropriate nursing interventions for a patient who is actively hallucinating and agitated after ingesting D-lysergic acid diethylamide (LSD) include all except which of the following?
A. Instruct the patient to keep the eyes closed
B. Keep the room well lighted
C. Reassure the patient
D. Explain to the patient what is happening

CORRECT ANSWER—A. *Rationales:* Keeping the eyes open helps to reduce the intensity of the hallucinations. Explain to the patient what is happening. Reassure the patient that he or she is not losing the mind and that the effects of the drug will wear off. Keeping the room well lighted reduces shadows that may be misinterpreted by the patient.
Nursing process step: Intervention

4. When planning care for a patient who has ingested phencyclidine (PCP), which of the following is the highest priority?
A. Patient's physical needs
B. Patient's safety needs
C. Patient's psychosocial needs
D. Patient's medical needs

CORRECT ANSWER—B. *Rationales:* The highest priority for a patient who has ingested PCP is meeting safety needs of the patient as well as the staff. Drug effects are unpredictable and prolonged, and the patient may lose control easily. Once safety needs have been met, the patient's physical, psychosocial, and medical needs can be met.
Nursing process step: Planning/Intervention

5. Which of the following drugs should the nurse prepare to administer to a patient with a toxic acetaminophen (Tylenol) level?
A. Deferoxamine mesylate (Desferal)
B. Succimer (Chemet)
C. Flumazenil (Romazicon)
D. Acetylcysteine (Mucomyst)

CORRECT ANSWER—D. *Rationales:* The antidote for acetaminophen toxicity is acetylcysteine. It enhances conversion of toxic metabolites to nontoxic metabolites. Deferoxamine mesylate is the antidote for iron intoxication. Succimer is an antidote for lead poisoning, and flumazenil reverses the sedative effects of benzodiazepines.
Nursing process step: Intervention

6. To evaluate the effectiveness of interventions for a hydrofluoric acid burn, the nurse should note the absence of which of these conditions?
A. Dilated pupils
B. Chvostek's sign
C. Seizures
D. Hypertension

CORRECT ANSWER—B. *Rationales:* Fluoride ions in hydrofluoric acid bind with calcium and cause severe hypocalcemia, which can lead to tetany and death. Chvostek's sign is elicited by tapping the side of the face over the facial nerve. If hypocalcemia is present, the patient's facial muscles will contract.
Nursing process step: Evaluation

7. An inebriated patient is brought to the emergency department by the police. The nurse suspects that the patient has ingested methanol after she notes which of the following odors on the patient's breath?
A. Bitter almond
B. Moth balls
C. Formalin
D. Garlic

CORRECT ANSWER—C. *Rationales:* A number of poisons have characteristic breath odors. One of the metabolites of methanol is formic acid. The patient's urine may also have a formalin odor. Bitter almond is characteristic of cyanide. Moth balls is characteristic of camphor and naphthalene. Garlic is characteristic of arsenic, organophosphates, phosphorous, selenium, and thallium.
Nursing process step: Analysis

8. Nursing assessment of the patient undergoing therapy for ethylene glycol ingestion includes monitoring for which of the following?
   A. Hypercalcemia
   B. Hypokalemia
   C. Hypertension
   D. Ethanol levels

CORRECT ANSWER—D. *Rationales:* Medical therapy for ethylene glycol ingestion includes blocking the metabolism of the drug by saturating alcohol dehydrogenase sites with ethanol to prevent the production of toxic metabolites. The dehydrogenase sites are saturated when ethanol levels are 100 mg/dl. Hypercalcemia is not present because ethylene glycol toxicity causes hypocalcemia from chelation of calcium by oxalates. Hypokalemia is not present because metabolites cause severe acidosis and hyperkalemia. Ethylene glycol toxicity does not cause hypertension although the patient may become hypotensive 4 to 12 hours after ingestion.
Nursing process step: Assessment

9. Which nursing diagnosis is a priority for the patient with methanol toxicity?
   A. Sensory or perceptual alteration (visual)
   B. Inability to sustain spontaneous ventilation
   C. Acute confusion
   D. Decreased cardiac output

CORRECT ANSWER—B. *Rationales:* The priorities when caring for all patients are airway, breathing, and circulation. Patients with methanol intoxication are at risk for sudden respiratory arrest because methanol and its metabolites depress the brain stem. Options A, C, and D are also correct but have lower priority.
Nursing process step: Analysis/Nursing diagnosis.

10. Which of the following should the nurse assess in a patient with a known amphetamine overdose?
    A. Hypotension
    B. Tachycardia
    C. Hot, dry skin
    D. Constricted pupils

CORRECT ANSWER—B. *Rationale:* Amphetamines are central nervous system stimulants. They cause sympathetic stimulation, including hypertension, tachycardia, vasoconstriction, and hyperthermia. Hot, dry skin is seen with anticholinergic agents such as jimsonweed. Pupils will be dilated not constricted.
Nursing process step: Assessment

11. A comatose patient with a suspected barbiturate overdose is admitted to the emergency department. Gastric lavage is ordered for the patient. How does the nurse perform this procedure correctly in an adult patient?
    A. By instilling 300 ml of fluid
    B. By placing the patient in the right lateral Trendelenburg position
    C. By inserting an 18 French gastric tube
    D. By instilling activated charcoal before lavage

CORRECT ANSWER—A. *Rationales:* A patient receiving gastric lavage should have 100 to 300 ml of fluid instilled. The fluid should then be removed by gravity or gentle suction. Larger amounts may cause the pyloric sphincter to open and force the toxins into the intestine. The patient should be placed in the left lateral Trendelenburg position. A large-bore gastric tube (22 to 36 French) should be used. The average size for an adult is 32 to 36 French. Activated charcoal is usually instilled after lavage has been completed.
Nursing process step: Intervention

12. Which nursing diagnosis is a priority for a conscious but confused patient with carbon monoxide poisoning?
A. Altered thought processes
B. Ineffective airway clearance
C. Acute confusion
D. Impaired gas exchange

CORRECT ANSWER—**D.** *Rationales:* The primary problem is impaired gas exchange at the cellular level because carbon monoxide has displaced oxygen on the hemoglobin. This displacement leads to hypoxia, which causes confusion. The highest priority is improvement of gas exchange at the cellular level. Altered thought processes and acute confusion are also present, but impaired gas exchange is the cause. The patient does not exhibit signs of ineffective airway clearance at this time. If the patient becomes comatose, then the patient may be at risk for ineffective airway clearance.
Nursing process step: Analysis/Nursing diagnosis

13. After swallowing evidence during an arrest, a patient with a possible cocaine overdose is brought to the emergency department. Which of the following signs should the nurse assess for cocaine overdose?
A. Hypotension
B. Hypothermia
C. Constricted pupils
D. Tachycardia

CORRECT ANSWER—**D.** *Rationales:* Cocaine is a stimulant drug. It causes hypertension, hyperthermia, dilated pupils, and tachycardia. Seizures also occur in significant overdoses.
Nursing process step: Assessment

14. A patient with a known acute cyanide ingestion is admitted to the emergency department. Which intervention takes highest priority?
A. Administer cyanide antidote
B. Perform gastric lavage
C. Administer activated charcoal
D. Manage seizures

CORRECT ANSWER—**A.** *Rationales:* The cyanide antidote should be administered before decontaminating the GI tract. Because cyanide is rapidly absorbed and causes cellular hypoxia, reversing the hypoxia takes priority over decontamination. The Lilly Cyanide Kit, used to treat cyanide poisoning, contains an amyl nitrite inhaler and sodium nitrite, which create methemoglobin and attract cyanide away from the respiratory enzyme cytochrome oxidase. Sodium thiosulfate is also used; it forms nontoxic thiocyanate. Performing gastric lavage, administering activated charcoal, and managing seizures are correct interventions, but the antidote should be administered first.
Nursing process step: Intervention

15. A patient is admitted to the emergency department with arsenic poisoning. Which of the following medications should the nurse prepare to administer?
   A. Deferoxamine mesylate (Desferal)
   B. Dimercaprol (BAL in Oil)
   C. Calcium EDTA (calcium disodium versenate)
   D. Succimer (Chemet)

CORRECT ANSWER—**B.** *Rationales:* Arsenic is a heavy metal. Effective chelating agents for it include dimercaprol and D- penicillamine. Other measures include alkalinization of the urine and hemodialysis. Deferoxamine mesylate is used for iron intoxication. Calcium EDTA and succimer are indicated for lead poisoning.
Nursing process step: Intervention

16. A child is admitted to the emergency department after swallowing his mother's prenatal vitamins. The child has abdominal pain and diarrhea. After determining that the child has ingested more than 20 mg/kg of elemental iron, chelation therapy is started. Which of the following indicates a positive response to deferoxamine mesylate (Desferal)?
   A. Urine color turns orange to red
   B. Diarrhea stops
   C. Acid-base balance returns to normal
   D. Vital signs return to normal

CORRECT ANSWER—**A.** *Rationales:* After deferoxamine chelates iron, it is excreted as pink to orange-red urine. This is the earliest indication of a positive response to chelation therapy. The symptoms displayed by a child with iron poisoning depend on how quickly medical attention is received. Early symptoms are GI irritation, hematemesis, abdominal pain, and lethargy. This is followed by a latent period in which the patient appears to improve. The third phase includes shock, acidosis, and fever.
Nursing process step: Evaluation

17. A patient with depressed mental status and slowed respirations is brought to the emergency department by emergency medical personnel. They state that no pill bottles or needles were found at the scene, but they did find a white powder substance and a pipe that the patient appeared to have been inhaling. What should the nurse assess for next?
   A. Hypertension
   B. Tachycardia
   C. Pinpoint pupils
   D. Hot, dry skin

CORRECT ANSWER—**C.** *Rationales:* This patient shows signs of a possible opioid overdose. Opioids, except for meperidine, cause pinpoint pupils. The nurse should rapidly assess the patient's pupils before taking the patient's blood pressure and pulse. Hypertension and tachycardia are not present because opioids cause bradycardia and hypotension. Hot, dry skin is seen with an anticholinergic overdose.
Nursing process step: Assessment

18. The nurse should prepare to administer which of the following drugs to the patient with symptoms of organophosphate overdose?
   A. Physostigmine (Antilirium)
   B. Flumazenil (Romazicon)
   C. Glucagon
   D. Atropine

CORRECT ANSWER—**D.** *Rationales:* The symptoms of organophosphate poisoning result from cholinergic overactivity. The antidote is the anticholinergic agent atropine. Physostigmine is a cholinergic agent and will worsen symptoms. Flumazenil reverses the sedative effects of benzodiazepines. Glucagon is the antidote for beta blockers.
Nursing process step: Intervention

19. When evaluating the effectiveness of antidote therapy for organophosphate poisoning, the nurse should prepare to administer additional antidote if the patient continues to display which of the following signs or symptoms?
A. Hot, dry skin
B. Pinpoint pupils
C. Tachycardia
D. Drying of mucous membranes

CORRECT ANSWER—**B.** *Rationales:* Atropine, the antidote for organophosphate poisoning, is an anticholinergic agent. The nurse will find pupil dilation if the patient has received an adequate dose of atropine. Hot, dry skin as well as tachycardia and dry mucous membranes are signs that the atropine has been effective.
Nursing process step: Evaluation

20. A teenager is brought to the hospital by friends after accidentally ingesting gasoline while siphoning it from a car. Based on the nurse's knowledge of petroleum distillates, which system should be the priority assessment?
A. GI system
B. Respiratory system
C. Neurologic system
D. Cardiovascular system

CORRECT ANSWER—**B.** *Rationales:* The primary concern with petroleum distillate ingestion is its effect on the pulmonary system. Aspiration or absorption of petroleum distillates can cause severe chemical pneumonitis and impaired gas exchange. The GI, neurologic, and cardiovascular systems may also be affected if the petroleum contains additives such as pesticides.
Nursing process step: Assessment

21. A patient who is actively hallucinating is brought to the emergency department by friends. They say that the patient used either LSD (D-lysergic acid diethylamide) or angel dust (phencyclidine [PCP]) at a concert. During triage, which of the following assessment findings indicates that the patient may have ingested PCP?
A. Dilated pupils
B. Nystagmus
C. Paranoia
D. Altered mood

CORRECT ANSWER—**B.** *Rationales:* Phencyclidine is an anesthetic with severe psychological effects. It blocks the reuptake of dopamine and directly affects the midbrain and thalamus. Nystagmus and ataxia are common physical findings of PCP use. Dilated pupils are evidence of LSD ingestion. Paranoia and altered mood occur with both PCP and LSD ingestion.
Nursing process step: Assessment

22. After chewing rhubarb leaves in the garden, a 3-year-old child is brought to the emergency department by her parents. The nurse should assess for which of the following conditions?
A. Lethargy
B. Bradycardia
C. Hypertension
D. Dysphagia

CORRECT ANSWER—**D.** *Rationales:* Rhubarb leaves contain oxalic acid, a toxin that irritates the mouth and throat. The acid may cause edema of the mouth and throat, dysphagia, and increased salivation. Systemic effects include hypocalcemia. Calcium oxalate crystals may be found in the urine. Lethargy may occur after ingestion of a number of plants, especially of the amygdalin-glycoside-cyanide category. Bradycardia is found after ingestion of plants that contain cardiac glycosides. Hypertension occurs after ingestion of plants that contain anticholinergic agents.
Nursing process step: Assessment

23. A patient is brought to the emergency department after ingesting seeds from jimsonweed. Which is the priority nursing diagnosis?
   A. Ineffective airway clearance
   B. Altered thought processes
   C. Hypothermia
   D. Fluid volume deficit

CORRECT ANSWER—B. *Rationales:* Jimsonweed, which has anticholinergic properties, may be ingested for its hallucinogenic effects. The nurse should provide a safe environment for the patient until the effects subside. Patients have warm, dry, flushed skin as well as dilated pupils and tachycardia. They usually do not have airway problems. Their temperature may be elevated, but their fluid volume is usually not affected. **Nursing process step:** Analysis/Nursing diagnosis

24. The doctor orders physostigmine (Antilirium) 1 mg slow I.V. push for a patient who has ingested deadly nightshade. After administering the medication, the nurse should look for which change to determine if the medication has been effective?
   A. Heart rate increases
   B. Blood pressure rises
   C. Hallucinations subside
   D. Pupils dilate

CORRECT ANSWER—C. *Rationales:* Deadly nightshade has anticholinergic properties like jimsonweed, and physostigmine is given to reverse the effects of severe poisoning. Increased heart rate and blood pressure and dilated pupils are all signs of an anticholinergic effect. **Nursing process step:** Evaluation

25. An elderly patient presents to the triage desk and complains of arthritis pain and tinnitus. The patient has been taking nonprescription medications for pain relief. Based on the patient's chief complaints, the nurse should ask the patient about the use of which nonprescription medication?
   A. Ibuprofen (Motrin)
   B. Acetaminophen (Tylenol)
   C. Naproxen sodium (Aleve)
   D. Aspirin

CORRECT ANSWER—D. *Rationales:* Tinnitus is the most common central nervous system sign of mild salicylate toxicity. Patients taking medications that contain salicylates at doses prescribed for arthritis may develop mild toxicity (salicylism). Ibuprofen usually causes GI upset and blurred vision. Acetaminophen toxicity causes liver failure. Naproxen may cause GI bleeding without other GI symptoms. It may also mask infection. **Nursing process step:** Assessment

26. Flumazenil (Romazicon) has been ordered for a patient who has overdosed on oxazepam (Serax). Before administering the medication, the nurse should be prepared for which of the following potential immediate outcomes?
   A. Seizures
   B. Shivering
   C. Anxiety
   D. Chest pain

CORRECT ANSWER—A. *Rationales:* The most common serious side effect of using flumazenil to reverse benzodiazepine overdose is seizures. The effect is magnified if the patient has a combined tricyclic antidepressant and benzodiazepine overdose. Less common side effects include shivering, anxiety, and chest pain. **Nursing process step:** Evaluation

27. An awake, alert patient is brought to the emergency department by family members. Fifteen minutes earlier, the patient ingested the entire contents of a new prescription for the tricyclic antidepressant amitriptyline (Elavil). Which of the following orders should the nurse question?
A. Activated charcoal, 50 g
B. Ipecac, 30 ml
C. Gastric lavage
D. ECG

CORRECT ANSWER—**B.** *Rationales:* Ipecac is contraindicated in tricyclic antidepressant overdose. Rapid deterioration with cardiovascular collapse and seizures can occur in a patient who is initially awake and alert. Airway compromise may occur from aspiration. Gastric lavage may be ordered with appropriate airway management. Administration of activated charcoal may be delayed. A baseline ECG may be ordered. The patient should be placed on a cardiac monitor because arrhythmias and cardiac conduction delays are common.
Nursing process step: Intervention

28. A comatose patient, who had ingested the tricyclic antidepressant doxepin (Sinequan), is brought to the emergency department. In addition to supportive measures, the nurse administers ordered sodium bicarbonate I.V. push. When evaluating the effectiveness of the medication, the nurse should monitor which of the following?
A. Neurologic status
B. Respiratory status
C. Acid-base status
D. Cardiovascular status

CORRECT ANSWER—**D.** *Rationales:* Management of tricyclic antidepressant overdose is focused on reversing cardiotoxicity. The primary effect of administering sodium bicarbonate is to reverse QRS prolongation and hypotension. The actual mechanism of action is unclear. Sodium bicarbonate may inhibit binding of tricyclic antidepressants to the myocardial sodium channels. Seizures may occur, but administration of benzodiazepines will suppress them. The administration of sodium bicarbonate does not directly affect respiratory status. Acid-base status should also be monitored, but effectiveness is based on cardiac response.
Nursing process step: Evaluation

Questions 29 and 30 refer to the following information:
A mother brings her 3-year-old child and a can of crystalline Drano with her to the emergency department. The mother states that she thinks the child may have ingested some of the crystals.

29. What should the triage nurse do first?
  A. Ask the mother how full the Drano container had been
  B. Note whether the child is drooling
  C. Contact the poison control center immediately
  D. Give the child milk to dilute the poison

CORRECT ANSWER—**B.** *Rationales:* Crystalline Drano is an alkaline substance and causes severe tissue necrosis. Signs of tissue necrosis include dysphagia and drooling from burns to the oral mucosa and esophagus. The priority is to assess the child for signs of poisoning and airway compromise. Even small amounts of alkali can cause severe burns. The poison control center should be contacted if the patient care team is unfamiliar with the treatment of alkali poisoning. Milk or water may be used to dilute the poison if there are no signs of drooling and dysphagia. If such signs are present, the child may have a severe burn. In that case, more damage may occur if the child's esophagus has perforated and water or milk enters the mediastinum.
Nursing process step: Assessment

30. Which nursing diagnosis best describes the greatest long-term risk for the child?
  A. Impaired swallowing
  B. Pain
  C. Impaired gas exchange
  D. Impaired tissue integrity

CORRECT ANSWER—**A.** *Rationales:* Scarring of the esophagus, which occurs during the healing phase of esophageal burns caused by alkalis, leads to strictures and narrowing of the esophagus. Pain and impaired gas exchange are generally early problems of alkali ingestion. Pulmonary edema may occur from exposure to acids.
Nursing process step: Analysis/Nursing diagnosis

31. During the past 2 to 3 hours, several adult patients with similar GI symptoms have arrived at the emergency department. Symptoms include vomiting, severe diarrhea, and abdominal cramps. Each of these patients ate at the same restaurant the evening before. None has anything else in common. Based on this information, the triage nurse suspects that these patients are suffering from which type of food poisoning?
  A. Staphylococcal
  B. Listeriosis
  C. Botulism
  D. Salmonella

CORRECT ANSWER—**D.** *Rationales:* Signs of salmonella poisoning appear from 12 to 24 hours after the ingestion of contaminated food. Common foods contaminated with salmonella include milk, custards and other egg dishes, salad dressings, sandwich fillings, polluted shellfish, and poultry. Staphylococcal symptoms appear suddenly 1 to 6 hours after exposure and also include headache and fever. Listeriosis occurs 3 to 21 days after exposure and, in addition to diarrhea, fever, and headache, may result in pneumonia, meningitis, and endocarditis. Botulism does not usually cause diarrhea.
Nursing process step: Analysis

32. A child is brought to the emergency department after ingesting oleander. The nurse should monitor the patient for which of the following?
   A. Dysarthria
   B. Drooling
   C. Bradycardia
   D. Diarrhea

CORRECT ANSWER—**C.** *Rationales:* Oleander is a plant that can produce cardiac glycoside effects. Symptoms of toxicity are similar to those of digoxin toxicity, so bradycardia may be evident. Dysarthria, drooling, and diarrhea are not associated with oleander toxicity.
Nursing process step: Assessment

33. Two hours after taking an overdose of acetaminophen (Tylenol), a patient arrives at the emergency department. Based on the nomogram for acute ingestion, when can the nurse expect to draw which blood acetaminophen level?
   A. Immediately
   B. In 1 hour
   C. In 2 hours
   D. In 4 hours

CORRECT ANSWER—**D.** *Rationales:* Based on the nomogram for acute ingestion, serum acetaminophen levels should be drawn 4 hours after ingestion. Levels drawn sooner would not reflect the peak acetaminophen level. An acetaminophen level greater than 150 g/ml 4 hours after ingestion indicates toxicity.
Nursing process step: Planning/Intervention

34. After ingesting 10 mg of the antihypertensive drug clonidine hydrochloride (Catapress) in a suicide attempt, a patient comes to the emergency department with a depressed level of consciousness. After the airway is secured and I.V. access has been obtained, the nurse should anticipate administering which of the following?
   A. Naloxone (Narcan)
   B. Calcium chloride (Calciject)
   C. Magnesium sulfate
   D. Sodium bicarbonate

CORRECT ANSWER—**A.** *Rationales:* Clonidine is an imidazoline antihypertensive agent that stimulates alpha-adrenergic receptors in the central nervous system. Clonidine may also stimulate the production of an opioid-like substance. Investigational uses include detoxification of opioid dependence. Calcium chloride, magnesium sulfate, and sodium bicarbonate are not indicated.
Nursing process step: Intervention

35. A patient is brought to the emergency department after ingesting an overdose of the beta blocker propranolol (Inderal). The nurse should prepare to administer which of the following medications to reverse the effects of the propranolol?
   A. Calcium chloride
   B. Glucagon
   C. Furosemide (Lasix)
   D. Sodium bicarbonate

CORRECT ANSWER—**B.** *Rationales:* Glucagon is first-line therapy for beta blocker overdose. It reverses bradycardia as well as the cardiac depression that beta blockers cause. Adverse effects of glucagon therapy include nausea and vomiting. Calcium chloride may be given in calcium channel blocker overdose. Furosemide does not reverse the effects of propranolol. Sodium bicarbonate does not reverse the effects of beta blocker toxicity.
Nursing process step: Intervention

36. A patient has been admitted to the emergency department after ingesting an overdose of sustained-release theophylline. Theophylline levels continue to rise after administration of activated charcoal, and the doctor orders whole bowel irrigation with isotonic polyethylene glycol and electrolyte solution (GoLYTELY). The patient will no longer require administration of the solution when which of the following occurs?

A. Serum levels return to normal
B. The patient has a bowel movement
C. Pulse rate returns to normal
D. The patient has clear rectal effluent

CORRECT ANSWER—D. *Rationales:* Whole bowel irrigation is a safe technique for treatment of overdoses of sustained-release products that are absorbed in the intestine. The technique is also safe for lithium, lead, and iron overdose. To confirm that all the pills have been removed, treatment should continue until rectal effluent is clear. Stopping after the first bowel movement is too soon. This treatment does not directly affect serum levels or pulse rate.

Nursing process step: Evaluation

WOUND MANAGEMENT

Wound Management

1. Rabies is least likely to be transmitted to humans through bites from which of the following animals?
A. Dogs
B. Bats
C. Rats
D. Skunks

CORRECT ANSWER—**C.** *Rationales:* Rabies is not generally transmitted through the bites of rodents. Members of the rodent family include rats, mice, hamsters, gerbils, squirrels, and chipmunks. Rabies is primarily transmitted through the saliva of carnivorous animals. All wild carnivorous animals should be considered rabid unless proven otherwise by laboratory analysis. Domestic animals that do not have veterinary documentation of immunization should be observed for 10 days for development of symptoms.
Nursing process step: Assessment

2. Pharmacologic interventions for a patient who has been bitten by a wild animal should include all except which of the following?
A. Administration of corticosteroids
B. Administration of tetanus toxoid
C. Administration of rabies immune globulin
D. Administration of human diploid cell vaccine (HDCV)

CORRECT ANSWER—**A.** *Rationales:* Corticosteroids should not be given to a patient who is receiving rabies immunization. The anti-inflammatory properties of corticosteroids interfere with active immunity. Administering tetanus toxoid is an appropriate choice for a break in skin integrity from a potentially contaminated source. Rabies immune globulin and the HDCV should be administered as soon as possible after the bite.
Nursing process step: Intervention

3. To which classification is coral snake venom assigned?
A. Neurotoxic
B. Hemotoxic
C. Proteolytic
D. Coagulopathic

CORRECT ANSWER—**A.** *Rationales:* The coral snake is an elapid, and its venom is neurotoxic. The effects are primarily systemic; local wound signs or symptoms are few or absent. Hemotoxic and proteolytic venoms are associated with pit vipers. Coagulopathic venom is not a category of snake venom.
Nursing process step: Analysis

4. A patient who has been bitten by a copperhead snake is at risk for developing which of the following conditions?
  A. Slurred speech
  B. Compartment syndrome
  C. Respiratory paralysis
  D. Muscle weakness

CORRECT ANSWER—**B.** *Rationales:* Pit viper bites (copperheads, water moccasins, and rattlesnakes) are associated with proteolytic and hemotoxic reactions. Their bites are painful, and blood usually oozes from visible fang marks. Edema of the affected area can lead to compartment syndrome. Other signs and symptoms include erythema, ecchymosis, blisters, hypotension, shock, and coagulopathies. Slurred speech, respiratory paralysis, and muscle weakness are associated with the neurotoxic venom of elapids (coral snakes and cobras).
Nursing process step: Assessment

5. If the patient will not receive antivenin for more than 2 hours, which of the following interventions should be taken?
  A. Immobilize the affected extremity
  B. Elevate the affected extremity above the level of the heart
  C. Apply a tightly constricting band above the site of envenomation
  D. All of the above

CORRECT ANSWER—**A.** *Rationales:* Because venom is spread through the lymphatic system, immobilization of the extremity reduces lymph production. The affected extremity should be placed slightly lower than the heart to decrease the spread of the venom. Applying tight or constricting bands is not recommended. Instead, a moderately constricting band may be placed about 4 inches proximal to the bite. The purpose of the band is to slow lymphatic flow. Care should be taken to avoid impeding arterial or venous flow.
Nursing process step: Intervention

6. Which of the following is the initial intervention for a patient with external bleeding?
  A. Elevation of the extremity
  B. Pressure point control
  C. Direct pressure
  D. Application of a tourniquet

CORRECT ANSWER—**C.** *Rationales:* Applying direct pressure to an injury is the initial step in controlling bleeding. For severe or arterial bleeding, pressure point control can be used. Pressure points are those areas where large blood vessels can be compressed against bone: femoral, brachial, facial, carotid, and temporal artery sites. Elevation reduces the force of flow, but direct pressure is the first step. A tourniquet may further damage the injured extremity and should be avoided unless all other measures have failed.
Nursing process step: Intervention

7. After receiving treatment for multiple human bites, a patient is discharged with a prescription for tetracycline (Achromycin). Which of the following statements indicate that the patient understands the antibiotic treatment?
A. "I should limit my exposure to the sun because I now have an increased risk of burning."
B. "I should take the medication with food so I do not irritate my stomach."
C. "Rash and itching are expected side effects. I can still continue my medications."
D. "I can take Mylanta to prevent nausea."

CORRECT ANSWER—**A.** *Rationales:* Patients taking tetracycline are photosensitive and have exaggerated sunburn reaction. At the first sign of skin erythema, patients should stop taking the drug and notify their doctors; rash and itching are signs of a hypersensitivity reaction. Tetracycline should be taken with a full glass of water 1 hour before or 2 hours after meals because taking it with food or milk interferes with its absorption. Antacids that contain aluminum, calcium, or magnesium impair absorption of tetracycline.
Nursing process step: Evaluation

8. Which of the following medications is used in the treatment of tetany?
A. Tetanus immune globulin
B. Anticonvulsants
C. Narcotic analgesics
D. Cephalosporins

CORRECT ANSWER—**A.** *Rationales:* Tetanus immune globulin should be administered I.M. (in 3,000 to 5,000 units) along with tetanus toxoid. Seizures are not associated with tetany. Sedatives and muscle relaxants can be used to reduce pain. Because of their effect against *Clostridia*, penicillin and tetracycline are the antibiotics of choice.
Nursing process step: Intervention

9. Prophylaxis for exposure to rabies includes administration of which of the following medications?
A. 20 IU/kg of rabies immune globulin (Hyperab) in one I.M. injection
B. Tetanus toxoid, regardless of date of last immunization
C. Human diploid cell vaccine (Imovax), 1 ml I.M. on days 0, 3, 6, and 14
D. Human diploid cell vaccine, 1 ml I.M. on days 0, 3, 7, 14, and 28

CORRECT ANSWER—**D.** *Rationales:* Postexposure rabies prophylaxis includes administration of human diploid cell vaccine, 1 ml I.M. on days 0, 3, 7, 14, and 28. If human diploid cell vaccine is being administered as a preexposure immunization, only days 0 and 3 are necessary. Rabies immune globulin is administered in a dose of 20 IU/kg, but one half of the total dose is administered I.M. and one half of the dose is administered locally in the wound. Option C is an incorrect schedule for administering this immunization.
Nursing process step: Intervention

Questions 10 through 13 refer to the following information:
A hiker with complaints of fever, headache, abdominal pain, and generalized muscle discomfort presents to the emergency department. Symptoms began 1 week after returning from a summer camping trip in Virginia. Physical exam reveals a 3-day-old deep-red rash on the ankles, soles, wrists, and palms. The rash now appears petechial and purpuric.

---

10. Based on the information above, the patient is diagnosed with which of the following conditions?
A. Meningococcemia
B. Rocky Mountain spotted fever
C. Poison ivy
D. Measles

CORRECT ANSWER—B. *Rationales:* Found in every state, Rocky Mountain spotted fever has the highest incidence in North Carolina, South Carolina, Oklahoma, and Virginia. The disease is primarily seen in the warmer months of late spring, summer, and early fall. Symptoms of the fever appear 2 to 14 days after contact with infected ticks, and a rash develops over the soles, palms, hands, feet, wrists, and ankles on the 2nd to 5th day. The rash becomes petechial and eventually spreads to the rest of the body. The patient may develop edema, hypotension, and delirium. Meningococcemia often follows a mild upper respiratory tract infection. A petechial rash appears on the trunk and lower portion of the body. Poison ivy erupts in linear streaks that correspond to the areas that have come in contact with the vines or stems of the ivy. Additional lesions can spread to new locations and may have accompanying blisters and edema. Measles begins as a red maculopapular rash on the face that rapidly spreads over the trunk and arms.
Nursing process step: Assessment

11. Which is the best method for removing a tick?
A. Grasping the tick close to the skin with tweezers and then pulling the tick away from the skin
B. Applying nail polish to the tick's body
C. Applying isopropyl alcohol to the tick's body.
D. Touching a hot match to the tick's body

CORRECT ANSWER—A. *Rationales:* The best method for removing a tick is to grasp it gently with a tweezer close to the skin. Then slowly pull it away from the skin while applying gentle traction. Take care not to squeeze the tick because toxins or viruses could be injected into the patient. Options B, C, and D are not recommended because they may cause the tick to regurgitate or salivate into the wound.
Nursing process step: Intervention

12. The most effective treatment of Rocky Mountain spotted fever is early administration of which antimicrobial?
A. Amoxicillin/clavulanate potassium (Augmentin)
B. Tetracycline hydrochloride
C. Co-trimoxazole (Bactrim)
D. Erythromycin base (E-Mycin)

CORRECT ANSWER—B. *Rationales:* Tetracycline hydrochloride (25 to 50 mg/kg/day) or chloramphenicol (Antibiopto) (50 to 100 mg/kg/day) can be given orally divided into four equal doses. Amoxicillin, co-trimoxazole, and erythromycin, although antimicrobials, are not effective for treating *Rickettsia rickettsii* (Rocky Mountain spotted fever).
Nursing process step: Intervention

13. Which of the following nursing diagnoses is appropriate for a patient who is showing neurotoxic signs from the female dog tick?
  A. Risk for aspiration related to reduced level of consciousness
  B. Impaired physical mobility related to ascending motor paralysis
  C. Altered cerebral tissue perfusion related to cerebral edema
  D. Risk for fluid volume deficit related to hemorrhage

CORRECT ANSWER—B. *Rationales:* Tick paralysis is a rapidly ascending motor condition caused by neurotoxins from wood and dog ticks. Symptoms begin 5 to 7 days after a tick becomes attached to the patient. The patient exhibits ataxia and lower-extremity weakness that progresses to the upper extremities. Respiratory cessation may occur. Within hours of removing the tick, the patient improves. Complete resolution of paralysis occurs within a few days to a few weeks.
Nursing process step: Analysis

14. What is the recommended treatment for scabies in a child who is under 1 year of age?
  A. Lindane (Kwell)
  B. Tolnaftate (Tinactin)
  C. Thiabendazole (Mintezol)
  D. Permethrin (Elimite)

CORRECT ANSWER—D. *Rationales:* Permethrin is supplied in a cream. It should be massaged into the skin from the head to the soles. Although permethrin is the treatment of choice for children younger than 1 year of age, its safety has not been established for patients younger than 2 months. Lindane, a treatment for scabies, is not recommended for children younger than 1 year of age, and it should not be used on children older than 1 year if they will not be supervised. The hands and feet of a child should be covered during treatment to prevent the child from sucking the cream or lotion. Young children may be more sensitive to central nervous system toxicity from the drug. Tolnaftate is used to treat ringworm. Thiabendazole is used to treat hookworm, roundworm, threadworm, and whipworm.
Nursing process step: Intervention

15. Which of the following statements shows that a patient diagnosed with scabies does not have an understanding of discharge instructions?
  A. "My symptoms might not disappear for 1 to 2 weeks after I begin my treatment."
  B. "It is not necessary to treat my family members if they do not have symptoms."
  C. "I should apply the prescribed lotion to all body areas below my neck."
  D. "I should machine wash all clothing and bed linen in very hot water."

CORRECT ANSWER—B. *Rationales:* Because scabies is transmitted through prolonged contact, it frequently affects all family members. Most patients are infested before obvious symptoms appear. Options A, C, and D represent information that should be included in discharge instructions.
Nursing process step: Evaluation

16. Which characteristic identifies the brown recluse spider?
A. Violin-shaped mark anterodorsally
B. Hourglass shape ventrally
C. Velvety black abdomen with brushes of red hair
D. Two circular black markings on a brown anterodorsal area

CORRECT ANSWER—A. *Rationales:* The brown recluse spider is commonly found in southern portions of the United States. It commonly has a light brown color with a darker brown violin shape on its back. Circular black markings and a velvety black abdomen with brushes of red hair are not found on the brown recluse spider. The black widow spider can be identified by its black body and a bright red hourglass on its abdomen.
Nursing process step: Analysis

17. Which skin reaction can be expected several hours after a bite by a brown recluse spider?
A. Slight erythema with tiny visible punctum
B. Eschar
C. Reddish blue halo surrounding the area
D. Petechiae on the affected extremity

CORRECT ANSWER—C. *Rationales:* Initially, there is a mild stinging sensation at the site of the brown recluse's bite. Next, a reddish blue halo and local edema appear. Erythema and necrosis of the tissue follow by the end of the 4th day. Eschars form by day 14, and healing is completed by day 21. The patient experiences joint pain, malaise, nausea, and vomiting. Treatment includes corticosteroids and antibiotics. Slight erythema with tiny visible punctum is a sign of the black widow spider's bite. An eschar is a later symptom and forms on the 14th day after the bite. Petechiae on the same extremity as a bite injury indicates Rocky Mountain spotted fever.
Nursing process step: Assessment

18. Which of the following is the primary intervention for a patient who is having a severe reaction to a black widow's bite?
A. Administration of black widow spider antivenin
B. Application of ice to the injury site
C. Administration of narcotics for pain relief
D. Administration of oxygen

CORRECT ANSWER—D. *Rationales:* Maintaining an airway should always be the primary focus in an emergency. The nurse should prepare to intubate if the patient develops severe respiratory distress or signs and symptoms of anaphylaxis. Black widow spider antivenin (one ampule in 10 to 50 ml of saline in a slow I.V.) can be administered after skin testing. Applying ice slows the venom's absorption rate, but this action should be taken after airway, breathing, and circulation have been assessed and maintained. Narcotics are helpful in pain management but should be used cautiously to prevent respiratory depression.
Nursing process step: Intervention

19. A patient presents to the emergency department after being stung by a Portuguese man-of-war. The patient is wheezing and tachycardic and has diffuse edema at the site of injury. Which of the following indicates that interventions have decreased the potential for poisoning?
A. Minimal edema progression
B. Positive response to antivenin sensitivity testing
C. Quiet breath sounds
D. All of the above

CORRECT ANSWER—A. *Rationales:* Treatment is effective in a hazardous marine life poisoning if the patient has stable vital signs, minimal edema, a negative response to antivenin sensitivity testing, and slowed symptom progression. A positive response to antivenin sensitivity testing indicates that this is an incompatible alternative for this patient. Wheezing that progresses to quiet breath sounds is an ominous finding. This indicates that air exchange in the lungs is decreasing.
Nursing process step: Evaluation

20. A patient presents to the emergency department after sustaining an injury while operating a table saw. The first and third digits have been amputated below the distal phalanx and another digit has a tip avulsion. Which of the following interventions is appropriate?
A. Wrap the amputated parts in a sterile dressing and place them on dry ice
B. Wrap the amputated parts in povidone iodine–soaked dressings
C. Wrap the amputated parts in gauze moistened with normal saline, place this in a sealed plastic bag, and submerge the bag in ice water
D. Wrap the amputated parts in sterile gauze and place in a bath of sterile saline.

CORRECT ANSWER—C. *Rationales:* Sterile technique should be used whenever handling amputated parts. The part should be cleaned of debris by gently irrigating with sterile saline, water, or Ringer's lactate. It should then be wrapped in gauze (dry or moistened) and placed in a plastic bag. The bag should then be submerged in a container of ice water until reimplantation occurs. Placing the amputated part on dry ice increases tissue damage (necrosis) because of the excessively cold temperature. Wrapping the part in povidone iodine–soaked dressings causes the subcutaneous tissue to dry out. Placing the amputated parts directly in a solution leads to tissue sloughing and maceration.
Nursing process step: Intervention

21. Bites from which of the following has the highest rate of infection?
A. Cats
B. Dogs
C. Humans
D. Scorpions

CORRECT ANSWER—C. *Rationales:* Human bites have the highest infection rate. Human saliva contains *Staphylococcus aureus*, *Streptococcus*, *Proteus*, *Klebsiella*, and *Escherichia coli*. Often there is an open wound that presents as a laceration, puncture, tear, crush injury, avulsion, or amputation. Cat bites are second in infection rate because of their frequent mouth contact with rodents. Dogs are more a source of disfigurement than of infection. There is no evidence that scorpion bites are an infection risk.
Nursing process step: Analysis

22. A patient who presents with a scorpion sting may initially exhibit which of the following symptoms?
   A. Bradycardia
   B. Hypotension
   C. Decreased respiratory drive
   D. Wheezing

CORRECT ANSWER—**D.** *Rationales:* Signs and symptoms of scorpion stings include pain and swelling at the sting site, tachycardia, hypertension, tachypnea, wheezing, ataxia, visual disturbances, and anaphylaxis.
Nursing process step: Assessment

23. Treatment of stings caused by a Portuguese man-of-war should include which of the following?
   A. Immediate rinsing with fresh water
   B. Soaking the wound in salt water
   C. Applying ice to the sting sites
   D. Options A and C

CORRECT ANSWER—**B.** *Rationales:* Treatment of a Portuguese man-of-war sting consists of soaking the wound in salt water. To prevent discharge of additional venom into the patient, any tentacles still clinging to the skin should be inactivated by rinsing with acetic acid. Tentacles can then be scraped off the skin. Ice should not be applied because of vasoconstriction.
Nursing process step: Intervention

24. During trauma resuscitation, clothing saturated with blood is cut from the victim of a gunshot wound. The patient is pronounced dead after efforts at resuscitation are unsuccessful. Proper handling of the patient's belongings should include which of the following procedures?
   A. Disposal with other biohazardous materials
   B. Release to family members at their request
   C. Release of clothing to police
   D. Clothing kept with the victim

CORRECT ANSWER—**C.** *Rationales:* A gunshot wound should be reported to law enforcement agencies. The victim's clothing should be treated as evidence from the moment the victim arrives in the emergency department. Care should be taken not to cut clothing through bullet holes. While handling clothing, gloves should be worn for standard precautions as well as for preserving evidence. When a suspect dies, the coroner can claim the body. At that time, police are free to gather any evidence that will not mutilate the body. A dead body has no constitutional rights. Disposal of the clothing will destroy the evidence in this case. The family cannot claim the victim's belongings until they are released from the coroner. Sending belongings to the morgue along with the victim does not guarantee safekeeping of the evidence. Suspects and victims of crime should remain secured in the emergency department until released to the morgue by the coroner or released to a law enforcement agency.
Nursing process step: Intervention

25. Which of the following is the classification of a degloving injury?
   A. Burn
   B. Laceration
   C. Avulsion
   D. Abrasion

CORRECT ANSWER—C. *Rationales:* An avulsion is full-thickness skin loss that does not allow for reapproximation of the skin. In a degloving injury, the skin is pulled away from the remainder of the extremity, usually a hand or foot. Burns are tissue injuries that occur as a result of prolonged exposure to thermal, chemical, radioactive, or electrical agents. A laceration is a tear in the flesh. Abrasions are caused by friction that may remove the epithelial or epidermal layers of the skin.
Nursing process step: Analysis

26. After a fall, what is the intervention for a patient with a contusion to the lower leg?
   A. Application of dry sterile dressing
   B. Administration of tetanus toxoid if it has been more than 5 years since the last immunization
   C. Application of a firm pressure bandage
   D. Application of cold

CORRECT ANSWER—D. *Rationales:* Applying cold to a contused area helps to decrease swelling and discomfort. Applying a dry sterile dressing and administering tetanus toxoid are unnecessary because the skin remains intact and the chance of the area becoming infected is minimal. Applying a pressure dressing should be avoided; prolonged pressure to an area with edema can lead to compartment syndrome.
Nursing process step: Intervention

27. In gunshot wounds, yaw refers to which of the following?
   A. The mass of the bullet
   B. The length of the gun barrel
   C. The rotation of the missile
   D. The missile's angle of entry into the body

CORRECT ANSWER—D. *Rationales:* Yaw is the deviation of the bullet from a straight path. The degree of wound produced from a gunshot varies, depending on the bullet mass, gun barrel length, missile velocity, and angle of yaw. The longer the gun barrel, the higher the velocity of the bullet. This usually results in a small entrance wound and a large exit wound. When the bullet strikes a soft surface (a person), the degree of deformation is influenced by the size of the bullet, the yaw, and the rotation of the bullet (tumbling).
Nursing process step: Analysis

28. A patient is being treated for a lower-leg laceration sustained from a metal bar. He states that he has never received tetanus immunization. Considering this information, the nurse should anticipate an order for which of the following drugs?
A. 0.5 ml of adsorbed tetanus toxoid
B. 250 units of tetanus immune globulin
C. 1 ml of adsorbed tetanus toxoid
D. 0.5 ml of adsorbed tetanus toxoid and 250 units of tetanus immune globulin

CORRECT ANSWER—D. *Rationales:* A patient who has never received tetanus immunization or has received only a partial series of injections (one or two) should receive 0.5 ml of adsorbed tetanus toxoid and 250 units of tetanus immune globulin. For a patient who has received two or more tetanus injections or who received a dose 10 or more years ago, 0.5 ml of adsorbed tetanus toxoid is recommended. Tetanus immune globulin (250 units) is delivered as an adjunct to adsorbed tetanus toxoid. Option C, 1 ml, is an incorrect dose for adsorbed tetanus toxoid.
Nursing process step: Intervention

29. A patient with a laceration to his upper arm is now unable to extend his thumb into a hitchhiker's sign. This indicates damage to which nerve?
A. Pilomotor nerve
B. Median nerve
C. Radial nerve
D. Ulnar nerve

CORRECT ANSWER—C. *Rationales:* Damage to the radial nerve results in the patient's inability to extend his thumb. The pilomotor nerve innervates the pilorum muscles of hair follicles. Damage to the median nerve results in an inability to sense pain in the tip of the index finger. Ulnar nerve damage results in the patient's inability to sense pain in the tip of the little finger.
Nursing process step: Assessment

30. A child received multiple lacerations and puncture wounds to the face, arms, and legs after being attacked by a dog. Conscious sedation was used to assist in reducing pain and anxiety in the child during repair. When alert and oriented, the child is discharged with parents. This level of consciousness is associated with which of the following Ramsey scores?
A. Ramsey score of 1
B. Ramsey score of 2
C. Ramsey score of 6
D. Ramsey score of 10

CORRECT ANSWER—B. *Rationales:* The Ramsey score is an evaluation of the level of sedation. Scores are as follows: 1, irritable and anxious; 2, alert and oriented; 3, responds to verbal stimuli; 4, responds to tactile stimuli; 5, responds to noxious stimuli; and 6, does not respond to stimuli. After receiving conscious sedation, a patient should be alert and oriented, have the ability to ambulate, and be able to tolerate fluids.
Nursing process step: Evaluation

31. A 5-year-old child is brought to the emergency department after being stung multiple times on the face by yellow jackets. Which of the following symptoms of anaphylaxis requires priority medical intervention?
A. Blood pressure of 90/52 mm Hg
B. Diffuse facial urticaria
C. Respiratory rate of 28 breaths/minute
D. Pulse rate of 60 beats/minute

CORRECT ANSWER—D. *Rationales:* Bradycardia is an ominous sign in children. Older children initially demonstrate tachycardia in response to hypoxemia. When tachycardia can no longer maintain tissue oxygenation, bradycardia follows. The development of bradycardia usually precedes cardiopulmonary arrest. The average systolic blood pressure of a child older than age 1 can be determined by this formula: 80 mm Hg + (2 × the age). Thus, an average systolic blood pressure for a 5-year-old child is 80 mm Hg + (2 × 5) = 90 mm Hg. Urticaria should be treated after airway control has been established. The normal respiratory rate for a 5-year-old is 20 to 25 breaths/minute.
Nursing process step: Assessment

32. Verbal understanding of discharge instructions for a patient who exhibits anaphylactic reactions to bee stings should include all except which of the following?
A. "I don't want to use the Epi-Pen unless I have trouble breathing."
B. "I should avoid wearing bright colors when I go outside."
C. "I should avoid using perfumed soaps and shampoos."
D. "I should wear long pants and shirts when I'm around flowers."

CORRECT ANSWER—A. *Rationales:* The patient with severe anaphylactic reactions to bee stings should be advised to use the Epi-Pen immediately after being stung. The nurse should instruct the patient that waiting until dyspnea develops may put the patient at risk for respiratory arrest. Options B, C, and D are correct responses.
Nursing process step: Evaluation

33. Which of the following is an early sign associated with Lyme disease?
A. Synovitis
B. Arthritic pain
C. Reddened lesion with central clearing
D. Myocarditis

CORRECT ANSWER—C. *Rationales:* Lyme disease is a tick-borne disease that progresses through distinctly separate stages. In the first stage, the disease presents with red-ringed circular skin lesions, called erythema chronicum migrans. At the same time the lesions appear, the patient often experiences headache, stiff neck, fever, and malaise. During stage two, cardiomegaly, neuritis, and myopericarditis may appear. The final stage includes arthritic pain, chronic synovitis, lack of coordination, facial palsy, paralysis, and dementia. Tetracycline, penicillin, and ceftriaxone sodium (Rocephin) help to relieve early symptoms and can possibly prevent later occurrences.
Nursing process step: Assessment

34. Which of the following is true about dog bites?
A. Most dog bites occur in adults.
B. A large dog can exert a maximum of 100 lb of pressure per square inch.
C. Osteomyelitis is a potential complication of dog bites.
D. Most dog bites occur in rural areas.

CORRECT ANSWER—C. *Rationales:* Potential complications of dog bites include osteomyelitis, cellulitis, infection, and neurovascular compromise. Most dog bites occur in urban areas and in children. Large dogs can exert up to 400 lb of pressure per square inch.
Nursing process step: Assessment

35. Black widow spider bites can be identified by which of the following signs?
A. A blue-red halo at the site of venom entry
B. Tiny red marks at the point of venom entry
C. Petechiae formation in the area of the bite
D. Wheal formation and edema

CORRECT ANSWER—B. *Rationales:* Black widow bites can be identified by edema and tiny red fang marks at the point of venom entry. Brown recluse spider bites can be identified by a blue-red halo surrounding the area of venom entry. Petechiae formation is associated with Rocky Mountain spotted fever. Wheal formation and edema are associated with wasp and hornet stings.
Nursing process step: Assessment

36. Which of the following statements about wood splinters as foreign bodies is true?
A. They cannot be seen on radiologic examination.
B. The wounds should be soaked in Betadine to reduce the risk of infection.
C. Wood splinters do not need to be removed because scar tissue will encrust the object.
D. Wood splinters do not put the patient at risk for developing tetanus.

CORRECT ANSWER—A. *Rationales:* Wood splinters are not radiopaque unless the wood has been painted. Paint creates a shadow. Wounds that involve wood should not be soaked in liquid. The wood tends to absorb the liquid and disintegrates when removal is attempted. Occasionally, metal objects may be left in place if removal is difficult. Wood, however, should always be removed because of its tendency to swell. It can also carry *Clostridium tetani*. A tetanus immunization should be considered for any injury that breaks skin integrity.
Nursing process step: Evaluation

37. A patient is treated for a laceration to his wrist from a human bite. Which of the following is not an appropriate treatment for the patient's altered skin integrity?
A. The laceration is scrubbed and irrigated
B. The site of injury is splinted
C. Antibiotic therapy is prescribed
D. The laceration is surgically closed and a sterile dressing applied

CORRECT ANSWER—D. *Rationales:* Human bites carry the highest rate of infection of all bite injuries. Intervention should include thorough cleansing of the site, antibiotic therapy, splinting of lacerations that occur over joints to minimize movement, and application of an appropriate dressing. Because of the extremely high risk for infection, the wound should not be surgically closed.
Nursing process step: Evaluation

38. Which of the following is true about cat bite injuries?
   A. The bacteria primarily associated with cat bites is *Bacillus cereus*
   B. Treatment of wounds from cat bites is penicillin V potassium (Pen Vee K) 500 mg by mouth four times a day for 5 to 7 days
   C. Primary closure of lacerations from cat bites and scratches is always recommended
   D. None of the above

CORRECT ANSWER—**B.** *Rationales:* Prophylactic antibiotics should be prescribed for all extensive wounds from cats. Initially penicillin V potassium is prescribed. Wounds that are not initially seen and that develop infection after 24 hours should be treated with a first-generation cephalosporin. *Bacillus cereus* is associated with food poisoning. Primary closure of wounds from cat bites is not recommended except in low-risk, cosmetically disfiguring facial bites.
Nursing process step: Assessment

39. Which of the following is a symptom of rabies?
   A. Hydrophobia
   B. Photosensitivity
   C. Manic behavior
   D. All of the above

CORRECT ANSWER—**D.** *Rationales:* A patient with rabies presents with dysphagia, excessive salivation, dyspnea, seizures, and extreme anxiety. Painful spasms occur whenever the patient swallows; as a result, the patient becomes hydrophobic. Additionally, the patient develops irritability, fever, and a sensitivity to light and noise.
Nursing process step: Assessment

40. An 80-kg patient is treated in the emergency department after amputating his leg in an industrial accident. Treatment was immediately initiated to correct symptoms of hypovolemic shock. Which of the following findings indicate improved fluid volume status?
   A. Capillary refill time of 4 seconds
   B. Central venous pressure of 4 cm H_2O
   C. Hourly urine output of 10 ml
   D. Cardiac output of 3 L/minute

CORRECT ANSWER—B. *Rationales:* A patient with decompensated shock presents with decreased blood pressure, increased pulse rate, narrowed pulse pressure, and poor skin perfusion. Additionally, the patient has decreased urine output, central venous pressure, cardiac output, hematocrit, and tidal volume. The nurse should recognize the signs associated with hypovolemic states as well as the abnormal values of these signs. Central venous pressure directly reflects the filling pressure of the right ventricle. Indirectly, it reflects vascular tone, the efficiency of the heart as a pump, and fluid volume status. A normal range for central venous pressure is 4 to 10 cm H_2O. Capillary refill is normally less than 3 seconds. A delayed response indicates vasoconstriction, which occurs when the body shunts blood away from the periphery and to the central core. Adequate urine output occurs if the flow is 1 ml/kg/hour or about 20 ml/hour; less than this indicates inadequate renal perfusion. Normal cardiac output ranges between 4 and 8 L/minute. Decreases in this value occur when there is inadequate filling of the heart and narrowed pulse pressure.
Nursing process step: Evaluation

41. After airway, breathing, and circulation have been assessed, the next intervention for a patient with an impaled object in the chest is which of the following?
   A. Obtain chest X-ray
   B. Remove the impaled object
   C. Administer tetanus toxoid
   D. Obtain arterial blood gas analysis

CORRECT ANSWER—A. *Rationales:* After assessing airway, breathing, and circulation, the nurse should obtain a chest X-ray to help determine involvement of vital organs (heart and lungs). An impaled object should not be removed until the patient is in the surgical suite. That's because any severed vessels temporarily tamponaded by the impaled object will need immediate clamping. Tetanus toxoid administration is recommended if the patient's immunization history indicates a need, but this is not the initial intervention in this scenario. Arterial blood gas analysis should be obtained only after respiratory involvement is determined.
Nursing process step: Intervention

STABILIZATION AND TRANSFER

CHAPTER 18

Stabilization and Transfer

1. Which level trauma center must have a trauma surgeon, trauma director, operating suite, and in-house operating room staff on duty 24 hours a day?
A. Level I trauma center
B. Level II trauma center
C. Both I and II
D. Level IV trauma center

CORRECT ANSWER—C. *Rationales:* Both level I and level II trauma centers must have a trauma surgeon, trauma director, and staffed operating room (OR) available around the clock. Level III trauma centers are excused from the staffed OR requirement. Level IV trauma centers are excused from all the requirements above.
Nursing process step: Planning/Intervention

2. What advantage does ground transport hold over helicopter transport?
A. Better radio communications with hospitals
B. More space inside
C. Faster speed
D. Fewer traffic and road factors

CORRECT ANSWER—B. *Rationales:* Ground vehicles have more space inside. However, helicopter transport has the advantages of having better radio communication with hospitals, traveling at faster speeds, and contending with fewer traffic and road factors.
Nursing process step: Analysis

3. The primary member of a transport team for critically ill or injured patients is which of these specially trained personnel?
A. Registered nurse
B. Paramedic
C. Doctor
D. Respiratory therapist

CORRECT ANSWER—A. *Rationales:* A specially trained registered nurse is the primary member of all transport teams. The Emergency Nurses Association position statement holds that "patients should be transported at the same level of care needed within the hospital. If the patient required specialized nursing care just before transport, he or she requires the same care during transport."
Nursing process step: Planning/Intervention

4. A multisystem trauma patient is being transferred to a trauma center. The receiving doctor has requested that the patient be intubated before transfer. Who is legally responsible for assuring that the patient is intubated before transfer?
- A. The receiving doctor
- B. The referring doctor
- C. The referring emergency department nurse
- D. The transport team

CORRECT ANSWER—B. *Rationales:* The transferring hospital is legally responsible for performing those treatment and diagnostic studies requested by the receiving facility. The referring doctor is legally responsible for assuring that tests and procedures are completed.
Nursing process step: Planning/Intervention

5. In-house, 24-hour surgeon availability is not required in which of these centers?
- A. Level IV trauma center
- B. Level III trauma center
- C. Level II trauma center
- D. Level I trauma center

CORRECT ANSWER—A. *Rationales:* Immediate access to definitive care is the hallmark of excellent trauma care. Although surgical coverage is desirable, only level IV trauma centers are excused from the requirement of around-the-clock coverage.
Nursing process step: Planning/Intervention

6. A prehospital unit has placed and inflated a pneumatic antishock garment on a trauma patient. During the climb to altitude in a pressurized aircraft, the air pressure exerted on the patient will do which of the following?
- A. Increase
- B. Decrease
- C. Remain constant
- D. Change relative to altitude

CORRECT ANSWER—A. *Rationales:* As the aircraft climbs, the cabin air pressure decreases and stabilizes at 8,000 feet (the design minimum cabin pressure of most pressurized aircraft). Because the volume of air in the pants remains the same and the outside air pressure decreases, the relative pressure inside the garment increases. The pressure on the patient's tissue, therefore, increases.
Nursing process step: Analysis

7. Which of the following devices are considered unacceptable for interhospital transfers?
- A. Plastic I.V. bags
- B. Pneumatic antishock garment
- C. Heimlich valves
- D. Inflatable splints

CORRECT ANSWER—D. *Rationales:* Inflatable air splints can change internal pressure (immobilization effectiveness) and are, therefore, unacceptable for air transport or ground transport over mountainous terrain. They are also subject to air leaks (decreasing pressure and immobilization effectiveness). Because there are other inexpensive alternatives for immobilization, air splints are not recommended for transfer. Plastic I.V. bags, pneumatic antishock garment, and Heimlich valves are all acceptable for interhospital transfers.
Nursing process step: Intervention

8. Which of the following interventions need not be completed before the transfer of a trauma patient?
   A. Closure of all lacerations
   B. Gastric tube insertion
   C. Indwelling urinary catheter insertion
   D. Splinting fractures

CORRECT ANSWER—A. *Rationales:* Suturing superficial lacerations is time-consuming and can be delayed until the patient is stable. All the other interventions should be completed before transfer.
Nursing process step: Intervention

9. A patient has no medical insurance. The Consolidated Omnibus Budget Reconciliation Act (COBRA) requires which of the following?
   A. The patient be transferred to a teaching hospital that receives federal funds
   B. The initial hospital transfer to a level I trauma center as soon as possible
   C. The patient be transferred if the receiving hospital can provide additional care
   D. The patient be transferred as soon as an ambulance is available

CORRECT ANSWER—C. *Rationales:* COBRA requires hospitals to provide a screening examination and stabilize patients. They are to be transferred only if the receiving hospital can provide additional resources for the patient's care.
Nursing process step: Planning/Intervention

Questions 10 through 12 refer to the following information:
A 16-year-old with a scald burn injury is brought to the emergency department. The patient has full-thickness burns to the anterior chest and anterior arms. Vital signs are blood pressure, 100/60 mm Hg; pulse, 120 beats/minute; and respiratory rate, 30 breaths/minute. The decision is made to transfer the patient to a burn unit 80 miles away.

---

10. Based on the initial assessment of the patient, which nursing diagnosis should take priority?
    A. Fluid volume deficit
    B. Risk for infection
    C. Fear
    D. Pain

CORRECT ANSWER—A. *Rationales:* The patient has suffered loss of skin integrity, and blood pressure is decreased. Fluid loss and shift make fluid volume deficit the initial priority. Because the patient has lost skin integrity, there is a risk for infection. Fear for the future and pain from the injury are both high-risk diagnoses, and both will play a role in the patient's care; however, stabilizing the patient physiologically is the priority.
Nursing process step: Analysis

11. The patient's airway, breathing, and circulation are stabilized. The emergency department nurse should document which additional initial assessment?
   A. Neurologic assessment
   B. Burn percentage calculation
   C. Fluid volume infused
   D. Head-to-toe survey

CORRECT ANSWER—A. *Rationales:* The initial assessment includes ABC and D (airway, breathing, circulation, disability). Disability, or the neurologic assessment, is the missing element in the initial assessment.
Nursing process step: Assessment

12. Which of the following interventions is the highest priority before transport?
   A. Endotracheal intubation
   B. Vascular access
   C. Pneumatic antishock garment placed but not inflated
   D. Blood administration

CORRECT ANSWER—B. *Rationales:* The priority nursing diagnosis is fluid volume deficit. The highest priority intervention after ABCs (airway, breathing, circulation) is vascular access followed by volume resuscitation.
Nursing process step: Intervention

13. How will the emergency nurse recognize that a patient's oxygenation has improved?
   A. Capillary refill time decreases
   B. Heart rate decreases
   C. Respiratory rate decreases
   D. SaO$_2$ increases from 90% to 95%

CORRECT ANSWER—D. *Rationales:* A pulse oximeter value of 95% in a patient who has not been exposed to products of combustion is a sign of improving oxygenation. Changes in capillary refill time are indicative of changes in perfusion. Changes in heart rate and respiratory rate are nonspecific to oxygenation.
Nursing process step: Evaluation

14. Who is responsible for assuring that appropriate personnel and equipment are available to transport a critical patient?
   A. The referring hospital
   B. The receiving hospital
   C. The transport ambulance
   D. The state ambulance regulators

CORRECT ANSWER—A. *Rationales:* The referring hospital is responsible for assuring that appropriate personnel and equipment are available to maintain care during transport. The receiving hospital should be involved in determining the mode of transport. The transport ambulance and the state ambulance regulators are not responsible for assuring that appropriate personnel and equipment are available to transport a critical patient. The state ambulance regulators write broad-based guidelines for patient care.
Nursing process step: Planning/Intervention

15. A child is intubated to treat increasing respiratory compromise. Which device should be used to ventilate the child optimally during transport?

A. Bag-valve-tube

B. T-tube

C. Oxygen-powered, manually triggered breathing device

D. Transport ventilator

CORRECT ANSWER—D. *Rationales:* A transport ventilator will best control ventilation. Bag-valve-tube devices allow for significant changes in respiratory rate and volume. Oxygen-powered, manually triggered breathing devices have the same limitations. A T-tube will assure high-flow oxygen but not ventilation.

Nursing process step: Analysis

PATIENT AND COMMUNITY EDUCATION

CHAPTER 19

Patient and Community Education

Questions 1 and 2 refer to the following information:
A patient presents at the emergency department and complains of tremors, headache, and confusion. The nurse detects a fruity odor about the patient. The patient admits to having diabetes controlled by diet and an oral agent.

---

1. Once physical assessment has been completed, which question should the nurse ask the patient to determine the patient's learning needs?
A. "When was the last time you ate?"
B. "What have you had to eat and drink in the past 24 hours?"
C. "Have you been drinking anything?"
D. "Have you been sticking to your diet?"

CORRECT ANSWER—B. *Rationales:* The confused patient may have difficulty understanding and responding to general questions. Specific time periods and specific information may be easier for the patient to recall. Confusion blurs the patient's ability to think and remember.
Nursing process step: Assessment

2. "I was afraid of getting low sugar so I ate some cereal and drank vodka and coke yesterday." This response indicates to the nurse that the patient has some knowledge about low blood sugar. What conclusion should the nurse draw?
A. This patient has some knowledge but not enough to realize that hypoglycemia and hyperglycemia mimic each other
B. The patient has a knowledge deficit related to the complications and control of diabetes
C. The patient's significant other should be monitoring the patient's diet better
D. The patient is an alcoholic

CORRECT ANSWER—B. *Rationales:* The patient has some knowledge but not enough to fully control the disease condition. Knowledge of hyperglycemia and hypoglycemia and the impact of diet on diabetes is important if the patient is to remain in control. Unless the patient is mentally incompetent, it is not the spouse's responsibility to monitor the patient. Not enough information has been presented to determine if the patient is an alcoholic.
Nursing process step: Analysis

3. Which of the following factors influence a patient's readiness to learn?
   A. Culture
   B. Primary language
   C. Anxiety level
   D. All of the above

CORRECT ANSWER—D. *Rationales:* Some cultures do not permit or encourage patient education because of beliefs and values. Education is best integrated when instruction occurs in the patient's primary language. Some anxiety is necessary for learning to occur, but too high a level interferes with learning.
Nursing process step: Assessment

4. After an acute episode of illness, a patient has resolved to improve self-care actions. How can the emergency department nurse take advantage of this resolve?
   A. Encourage the patient to sign up for educational classes immediately
   B. Offer the patient a list of classes offered by the health care organization
   C. Provide the patient with pamphlets and brochures
   D. Have the nurse educator talk to the patient

CORRECT ANSWER—C. *Rationales:* Educational classes or one-on-one instruction by the nurse educator do not offer the patient hard data. To augment the patient's resolve, printed educational information, such as pamphlets and brochures, can be rapidly provided and reread as often as the patient finds necessary. Encouraging the patient to sign up for classes requires current action with future results. The patient may or may not sign up for classes, and even if the patient signs up, the patient may not attend when the time arrives. Talking to the nurse educator after reading pamphlets and brochures allows for immediate confirmation of information learned or clarification of new information.
Nursing process step: Intervention

5. Learning goals and objectives should be written in measurable terms and should describe whose behavior?
   A. Nurse
   B. Patient
   C. Patient's significant other
   D. All of the above

CORRECT ANSWER—B. *Rationales:* Learning goals and objectives should be established by the patient and nurse to meet the patient's needs. They should describe the patient's learning behavior. While the patient's significant other and the nurse may be involved in establishing goals, ultimately goals must focus on the patient. Only in this way will the patient have learning goals that meet her or his own learning needs.
Nursing process step: Planning/Intervention

6. A patient on nitroglycerin tablets (sublingual) is discharged from the emergency department. Which adverse effect of nitroglycerin should be explained to the patient?
   A. Flushing
   B. Hot flash
   C. Blurred vision
   D. Sudden headache

CORRECT ANSWER—D. *Rationales:* The sudden headache that can result from taking nitroglycerin tablets can be disconcerting and frightening for the patient. Although the flushing and hot flash may be uncomfortable, they are not as frightening as the headache. Nitroglycerin does not often cause blurred vision.
Nursing process step: Assessment

7. One of the Standards of Emergency Nursing Practice explicitly incorporates patient education as an expectation. Where else is the expectation of patient education found?
A. Most state nurse practice acts
B. Accrediting criteria (Joint Commission on Accreditation of Healthcare Organizations)
C. Quality assurance criteria
D. All of the above

CORRECT ANSWER—D. *Rationales:* The need for patient education is recognized and stated in all of the documents cited. Patient education is the responsibility of the emergency department nurse, especially when the patient is discharged.
Nursing process step: Evaluation

8. The ability to assess a patient's motivation for learning is important in order to use available opportunities. Where does the nurse look for clues to the patient's motivational level?
A. In what the patient says (verbal)
B. In what the patient does not say (nonverbal)
C. In what the patient does (behavioral)
D. All of the above

CORRECT ANSWER—D. *Rationales:* Consideration of the behavioral, verbal, and nonverbal clues given by the patient enables the nurse to accurately assess the patient's motivation for learning. Verbal, nonverbal, and behavioral clues alone are not enough to provide insight.
Nursing process step: Assessment

9. Because of the relationship and time frame provided by the emergency department, which kind of learning goals are best established with the patient?
A. Long term
B. Short term
C. Middle range
D. Long-term goals, short-term objectives

CORRECT ANSWER—B. *Rationales:* The relationship between nurse and patient as well as the time the patient spends in the emergency department is short term. Short-term learning goals or objectives are most appropriate in this setting. Long-term and middle-range goals are best met in a setting other than the emergency department.
Nursing process step: Assessment

10. Teaching a patient the symptoms of hyperglycemia and hypoglycemia is an example of which type of learning?
A. Cognitive
B. Affective
C. Psychomotor
D. Social

CORRECT ANSWER—A. *Rationales:* Teaching a patient the signs and symptoms of a disease process involves the patient's use of cognitive learning skills. These skills require thinking and reasoning in order to integrate the learning. Affective learning involves feelings and attitudes. Psychomotor learning requires the coordination of the brain and extremities to complete a task.
Nursing process step: Assessment

11. In which of the following situations is a potential nursing diagnosis of knowledge deficit most likely?
A. Acute dehydration resulting from participation in a Walk for Muscular Dystrophy
B. Digitalis toxicity
C. Chronic renal failure
D. Bacterial pneumonia

CORRECT ANSWER—**A.** *Rationales:* Patients who participate in amateur events for the sake of supporting a cause are probably not athletes; therefore, their knowledge of potential illness may be lacking. A patient can become digitalis toxic, have chronic renal failure, or acquire bacterial pneumonia without having a knowledge deficit.
Nursing process step: Analysis

Questions 12 and 13 refer to the following information:
A truck driver complaining of severe bladder pain and urinary urgency and frequency is admitted to the emergency department. The medical diagnosis is urinary bladder infection. The doctor orders 1 g of sulfisoxazole (Gantrisin) by mouth four times a day. The nurse knows that the medication can cause sulfa salt urinary stones.

---

12. What should the nurse tell the patient to do to prevent the urinary stones?
A. Drink at least 1 quart of water per day
B. Increase fluid intake by twice the normal amount
C. Avoid alkaline foods
D. Urinate every 4 hours

CORRECT ANSWER—**A.** *Rationales:* Increasing daily water intake to 1 quart helps discourage stone formation. Specific instructions are easier for patients to adhere to than general ones. The patient probably does not know which foods form alkaline ash and which foods form acid ash. These byproducts cause changes in urine pH. Consistently acidic or alkaline urine may provide a favorable medium for calculus (stone) formation, especially for magnesium ammonium phosphate or calcium phosphate calculi. The patient should urinate every 2 hours to avoid stone formation and to promote adequate kidney function.
Nursing process step: Intervention

13. Which of the following actions would best serve the truck driver?
A. Provide written instructions on which foods to eat and which to avoid, and suggest carrying an insulated container of water in the truck.
B. Discuss the interaction of food, fluid, and medication, and help the patient figure out how to perform self-care while continuing to work.
C. Encourage the patient to take several days off work until the symptoms clear.
D. Suggest several alternative careers to the patient to prevent chronic bladder infections.

CORRECT ANSWER—**B.** *Rationales:* Interaction between nurse and patient provides opportunities for learning. Patients need help in problem solving, but they still must make their own decisions.
Nursing process step: Intervention

14. Which type of learning takes more time to accomplish?
- A. Cognitive
- B. Psychomotor
- C. Social
- D. Affective

CORRECT ANSWER—D. *Rationales:* Changes in attitudes, beliefs, and values take place over time. Cognitive learning is mental activity to learn some knowledge. Although cognitive material may be complex, it does not necessarily require a change in attitude or values. Psychomotor learning is the accomplishment of a skill requiring physical and mental coordination. **Nursing process step: Intervention**

15. Generally speaking, the content and the learning goal dictate which step in the teaching-learning process?
- A. Audiovisual resources
- B. Teaching method
- C. Time frame
- D. Teacher

CORRECT ANSWER—B. *Rationales:* The goals established by the nurse and patient as well as what is to be learned dictate the teaching method. For example, a patient cannot be taught a diet without learning about the food pyramid and which foods should be eaten and which foods should be avoided. Teaching methods include lecture, self-study, small-group discussion, guided learning manual, one-on-one, and so forth. Time frame is the amount of time required to teach the material. Audiovisual resources are teaching aids that the teacher may use to explain content. The teacher is the person doing the teaching. **Nursing process step: Analysis**

LEGAL ISSUES

CHAPTER 20

Legal Issues

1. The sources of law governing the practice of emergency nursing include which of the following?
   A. U.S. Constitution
   B. Federal and state statutes
   C. Common law
   D. All of the above

CORRECT ANSWER—D. *Rationales:* All three of the options listed can govern the practice of emergency department nursing. The Constitution is the supreme law of the land and cannot be overturned by state or federal statute. In order of hierarchy, the Constitution is first and then federal, state, and common law. Institutional policy is the authority if other legal venues have not addressed the specific issue.

2. Cases involving medical or nursing negligence or malpractice fall into the legal category of tort. Which of the following is the definition of a tort?
   A. Intentional criminal act that can be remedied with money paid to the plaintiff
   B. A civil wrong committed against a person or property that can be remedied with money paid to the plaintiff
   C. Unintentional criminal act that can be remedied with money paid to the plaintiff
   D. A civil wrong committed against property

CORRECT ANSWER—B. *Rationales:* As defined in Black, H. C. (1979). *Black's Legal Dictionary*, 5th ed. St. Paul: West Publishing. Answers A, C, and D describe other legal categories. A tort is neither an intentional nor an unintentional criminal act, but rather a civil wrong against a person.

3. Which of the following is the best method for the emergency department staff to protect themselves against possible negligence or malpractice litigation?
   A. Document their actions with a difficult patient
   B. Document the staff and nurse–client ratio on a daily basis
   C. Provide and document care within accepted standards
   D. Provide care to the best of one's abilities, and document what was not done for specific patients

CORRECT ANSWER—C. *Rationales:* Meeting the standards of care and documenting them may not prevent litigation, but these actions will certainly provide support that the standards of care were known and adhered to. Actions should be documented for all patients, not just for difficult ones. Documentation of staffing and nurse–client ratios does not relieve the nurse of the responsibility to provide care within accepted standards. Accepted practice is to document what was done for a patient, not the opposite.

4. What does the plaintiff have to prove in ligation for negligence?
   A. Intent to cause harm
   B. Substandard care delivery
   C. Mitigating circumstances
   D. Lack of intent

CORRECT ANSWER—B. *Rationales:* The plaintiff must prove that the care received was substandard; it is not necessary to prove intent to cause harm. Mitigating circumstances are issues that would be brought up by the defendant, not the plaintiff. Negligence is by definition an unintentional tort. It is a civil wrong done without intent by the defendant. Therefore it is not necessary to demonstrate lack of intent.

5. Which of the following is the most common unintentional tort involving health care personnel?
   A. Malpractice
   B. Negligence
   C. Assault
   D. Battery

CORRECT ANSWER—B. *Rationales:* Negligence is the most common unintentional tort involving health care personnel. Malpractice is a more restricted, specialized kind of negligence, defined as a violation of professional duty to act with reasonable care and in good faith. Assault and battery are *intentional* torts (note that intentional here means that the plaintiff meant to perform the complained of action).

6. Which of the following actions is most likely to lead to a claim of battery?
   A. Leaving foreign objects in a patients body after surgery
   B. Failing to obtain informed consent
   C. Threatening a patient
   D. Treatment of nonemergent conditions without informed consent

CORRECT ANSWER—D. *Rationales:* Battery is the touching of a person without that person's consent. A nurse who treats a patient beyond what the patient has consented to has committed battery (the theory of implied consent does not apply to nonemergent conditions). Leaving foreign objects in a patient's body after surgery and failing to obtain informed consent are examples of negligence. Threatening a patient is an example of assault.

7. What is breach of duty?
   A. Willful violation of an oath or code of ethics
   B. Failure to meet accepted standards in providing care for a patient
   C. Threatening a patient
   D. Confining a patient to a psychiatric unit without a doctor's order

CORRECT ANSWER—B. *Rationales:* If a patient sues a nurse for negligence, the patient must prove that the nurse owed him a specific duty and that she breached this duty. A breach of duty in this case means that the nurse did not provide the patient with care within the accepted standard. A breach is not always willful, as implied in answer A. Threatening a patient is assault, more accurately described as a direct invasion of a patient's rights rather than a breach of duty. Confining a patient to a psychiatric unit without a doctor's order is false imprisonment, another example of direct invasion of a patient's rights.

8. It is the plaintiff's responsibility to prove four elements in a negligence lawsuit. Which of the following is not one of the four elements?
A. A duty was owed to the patient
B. The defendant breached the duty
C. The breach of duty was the cause of the plaintiff's injury
D. The plaintiff was at risk for sustaining an injury as a result of the breach of duty

CORRECT ANSWER—D. *Rationales:* The plaintiff must prove that the injuries sustained were real or actual. The plaintiff must prove that the defendant owed him a specific duty; that the defendant breached this duty; that the plaintiff was harmed physically, mentally, emotionally, or financially; and that the defendant's breach of duty caused this harm.

Questions 9 and 10 refer to the following situation:
"The protective privilege ends where the public peril begins" is a phrase that indicates the duty of the emergency department nurse when a patient threatens another person with bodily injury or harm.

---

9. What does the quoted statement mean?
A. The confidentiality enjoyed between patient and nurse or doctor does not relieve the emergency department personnel of the duty to warn the threatened person and authorities
B. Confidentiality between nurse or doctor and patient is as sacred as the attorney-client privilege
C. Emergency department personnel must weigh the seriousness of the threat to another person before breaking the confidentiality between patient and nurse or doctor
D. Warning the patient not to commit a felony is relief from the duty to warn

CORRECT ANSWER—A. *Rationales:* Confidentiality between patient and nurse or doctor should be breached to alleviate a threat to another person. Medical personnel have a duty to warn the intended victim (if known) and the authorities. Warning the patient not to commit a felony or weighing the seriousness of the threat is not sufficient grounds for relief from the duty to warn.

10. Which patient situation would be subject to the quoted phrase?
A. The discharge of a drunk driver who intends to drive home
B. The discharge of a commercial driver with an onset of seizure disorder
C. A psychiatric patient threatening to kill a family member
D. All of the above

CORRECT ANSWER—D. *Rationales:* Confidentiality between patient and nurse or doctor should be breached to alleviate a threat to another person. The medical personnel have a duty to warn the intended victim (if known) and the authorities. In all three options, there is potential for harm to others. Even though the medical personnel may not know who the victim might be, there is an obligation to tell the authorities about the condition of the patient.

11. Which type of assessment data should be recorded in the emergency department record about every woman of child-bearing age who presents to the emergency department?
A. Number of pregnancies and live births (para, gravida)
B. Date of last menstrual period
C. Known sexual partners
D. Birth name

CORRECT ANSWER—B. *Rationales:* The date of the last menstrual period provides information about the likelihood of a first-trimester pregnancy. This information may affect medications ordered and radiographic procedures performed. The number of pregnancies and live births is important historical information and indicates the health of the client, but it has no impact on ordered medications or radiographic procedures. Information about known sexual partners is only important in the presence of a sexually transmitted infection.

Questions 12 and 13 refer to the following patient and situation:
S. K. is 3 years old. The mother is bringing the child to the emergency department because of blood in the child's underwear. A physical exam reveals sexual assault and felonious penetration. The mother does not want the police notified because of the potential publicity.

12. Which action should the nurse take?
A. No action is necessary because the mother is the child's legal guardian and her decisions are final
B. Report the findings to the police and have a social worker talk with the mother
C. Encourage the mother to reconsider her decision and give the telephone number of a child psychologist
D. Have the emergency department doctor talk to the mother

CORRECT ANSWER—B. *Rationales:* The nurse has a duty of care to the patient and to the public to report the crime to the authorities. Regardless of the mother's wishes, the child has been harmed and a report to the authorities is necessary. Even though the emergency department doctor may talk to the mother and the mother may be encouraged to reconsider her wishes, the fact remains that the crime must be reported and evidence must be collected.

13. The mother becomes upset and is afraid the child's father will beat her. The nurse can refer the mother to several social service agencies. Which one would be most appropriate?

A. A women's shelter

B. The welfare bureau

C. Children's Protective Services

D. A homeless shelter

CORRECT ANSWER—A. *Rationales:* A women's shelter can provide services that are necessary for both mother and child and keep them together. The other alternatives may result in separation of the child from the mother and cause further trauma. The welfare bureau is a state agency that provides money, food, or shelter for people who need it. It does not necessarily deal with children who are victims of sexual abuse. The Children's Protective Services will investigate the crime and may want to place the child in a foster home or with other relatives during the investigation. Homeless shelters are voluntary organizations for people in need of shelter and food. They do not necessarily have resources to accommodate women and children or for handling sexual abuse.

14. Which of the following does the Consolidated Omnibus Budget Reconciliation Act mandate for a patient having labor contractions?

A. If the contractions are 5 or more minutes apart, the patient can be referred to a hospital that offers maternity services

B. All patients having contractions must be medically screened and stabilized before transport to another facility

C. Only patients in obvious active labor need to be medically screened before transport to another facility

D. The emergency department has the right to refuse patients for whom it does not offer the needed services

CORRECT ANSWER—B. *Rationales:* All patients experiencing contractions must be medically screened before transport. Whether it is obvious that the patient is in labor or not, the patient must be medically screened and examined before the decision is made to transport the patient to another facility. The emergency department does not have the right to refuse treatment to a patient before medically screening the patient.

15. Which of the following does the Consolidated Omnibus Budget Reconciliation Act mandate for a patient presenting without insurance?

A. Medical screening of patients cannot be delayed until insurance coverage or the ability to pay has been determined

B. The patient must present proof of ability to pay before services are rendered

C. Every urban area must maintain hospital beds for patients who are not able to pay for services

D. The ability to pay for services should not be part of the admission procedure

CORRECT ANSWER—**A.** *Rationales:* To assure that patients are not denied care based on their ability to pay, patients must be medically screened and stabilized before their ability to pay is determined. Failure of a hospital to comply may result in denial of Medicare funding. Only hospitals accepting Medicare funding are required to have some beds available for the indigent. The Consolidated Omnibus Budget Reconciliation Act does not address payment for services as part of the admission procedure. It only addresses medical screening and stabilization of patients before transport or the determination of ability to pay for services rendered.

ORGANIZATIONAL ISSUES AND QUALITY IMPROVEMENT

CHAPTER 21

Organizational Issues and Quality Improvement

1. When conflict arises among the staff, which response by a nurse manager is the most helpful?
A. To delegate the issue to assistants or clinical specialists
B. To invite an outside mediator to assist
C. To bring all conflicting parties together to resolve the problem with ample notification for each side to build coalitions
D. To help the staff clarify the issues and confront one another assertively and respectfully

2. To arrive at an appropriate nursing staff pattern in an emergency department, the manager must do which of the following?
A. Know the patient volume and acuity levels by hour of the day, and take into consideration variability according to day of the week or time of year
B. Be aware of the Joint Commission on Accreditation of Healthcare Organizations (JCAHO) standard that emergency services shall be appropriately integrated with other units and departments within the organization
C. Realize that patient visits are so unpredictable that a different staffing pattern will have to occur every day according to need
D. For the sake of standardization, arrange staffing so that it closely corresponds with the rest of the organization

CORRECT ANSWER—D. *Rationales:* Assisting the staff to resolve conflicts falls within the role of a nurse manager. Encouraging confrontation and clarifying issues are the most helpful interventions. A response that overemphasizes the problem or leads to increased conflict and division of staff is not helpful. For most staff conflicts, the resolution of a problem best lies with the people who identified it. Nothing in the question suggests the need for a mediator.

CORRECT ANSWER—A. *Rationales:* Although exact volume and acuity levels can be somewhat unpredictable, the manager should track both over time so that numbers and type of staff are appropriately placed. Staffing patterns are unit-specific and standardization is irrelevant. The JCAHO standard for integrating emergency services is not directly related to the question.

3. A team of nurses, doctors, and registration clerks met to address a departmental goal of decreasing total patient time in the department. First, they collected data (sorted by triage category) on the length of time patients wait to be seen. The activity described above is an early step in which of the following?
A. Descriptive research
B. Indicator relevance testing
C. Collaborative research
D. Quality improvement process

CORRECT ANSWER—D. *Rationales:* The scenario describes a quality improvement process. This reflects an interdisciplinary approach to process improvement for better patient experience or outcome. It is not intended to generate or validate a scientific knowledge base. The element of data collection is found in research also. In the research process, however, data collection occurs later (after a literature review and after decisions have been made regarding conceptual or theoretical framework and research design). Indicator relevance testing is not a recognized entity in either process.

4. When interviewing a prospective staff member, the manager or peer recruitment team should be certain to do which of the following?
A. Ascertain whether the applicant has health problems that have ever resulted in a workers' compensation claim
B. Verify experience and qualifications by checking references
C. Ask primarily open-ended questions
D. Verify that the applicant has appropriate child care arrangements

CORRECT ANSWER—B. *Rationales:* Ascertaining whether the applicant has health or child care problems is prohibited by federal laws addressing gender bias and disabled workers. Open-ended questions are useful for gleaning clues to personality and style. Direct questions, which have specific answers, are an efficient means of learning whether an applicant has the knowledge, experience, and attitude being sought. Checking references and verifying experience and education are common ways of ensuring that an applicant has the background for the job.

5. An emergency department lobbies for a departmental pharmacist to function as a resource and consultant in toxicology and medication issues. Which is the correct budget for such a request?
A. Operational
B. Capital
C. Manpower or personnel
D. Overhead

CORRECT ANSWER—C. *Rationales:* Manpower or personnel budgets cover wages and benefits for regular and temporary workers and are sometimes a subset of an operational budget. An operational budget covers supplies, unit equipment, repairs, and overhead. Capital budgets cover land, buildings, and expensive durable equipment (usually costing more than $500).

6. A patient classification system that is reliable, valid, and consistently used can be a management tool for determining which of the following?
A. Staffing levels based on nursing workload
B. Quality of care rendered by individuals or groups of nurses
C. Problem solving and conflict resolution
D. Mix of paying and nonpaying patients and thereby improve the budget

CORRECT ANSWER—A. *Rationales:* Patient classification systems are a means of measuring workload and thereby determining staffing needs. They do not measure comparative quality or relate to patient payment and are not part of conflict resolution.

7. Brainstorming is a problem-solving method whereby a group rapidly generates which type of solutions?
  A. As many as possible
  B. As practical as possible
  C. As wild and crazy as possible
  D. As high quality as possible

CORRECT ANSWER—A. *Rationales:* Brainstorming is a problem-solving method in which a group rapidly generates a large number of alternatives. Quality and practicality are unimportant. Some wild and crazy solutions emerge and make the process fun; such unconventional ideas help participants unleash their creativity and build on others' input.

8. An emergency department nursing team found that patients whose discharge instructions were reviewed by a registered nurse had much better understanding of their diagnosis and follow-up than patients whose discharge instructions were not reviewed. The team had evaluated which of the following elements?
  A. A structure element
  B. A process element
  C. An outcome element
  D. A hierarchical element

CORRECT ANSWER—C. *Rationales:* Improved patient understanding of discharge instructions is an outcome and a goal of care. The process element in patient discharge reflects the nature of the action and how discharge teaching is done. For example, the nurse reviews instructions with responsible family members and ascertains by way of return demonstration or verbalization that the instructions are understood. The structure element in patient discharge addresses environment, instrumentation, and qualification of personnel. For example, all patients must have instructions reviewed by a registered nurse, and the patient must sign a written copy of the instructions. Hierarchy refers to the placing of people or things in a rank order according to importance and does not relate to this question.

9. In response to a collective bargaining initiative, a manager is allowed to do which of the following?
  A. Prevent employees from engaging in recruiting activities during nonworking hours
  B. Prevent employees from participating in informal union activities in patient care areas, even during breaks
  C. Withhold desirable assignments from union organizers
  D. Provide wage increases or special considerations to discourage employees from joining the union

CORRECT ANSWER—B. *Rationales:* Federal laws allow management to prevent employees from engaging in collective bargaining in patient care areas. The same laws prohibit managers from preventing union activities during nonworking hours, from withholding desirable assignments from staff engaging in union activities, and from providing special favors to discourage union activity or membership.

10. An emergency nursing staff was struggling to reach a fair distribution of major holidays worked. The manager facilitated meetings in which each staff member agreed to work half of the holidays. Although a couple of members were not completely satisfied with the decision, they said they could "live with it." This type of decision making is known as which of the following?
  A. Consensus
  B. Group vote
  C. Minority poll dissention
  D. Authoritative facilitative coaching

CORRECT ANSWER—A. *Rationales:* The scenario depicts the process of reaching consensus, whereby an agreeable best solution is negotiated in a group. Group vote and minority poll dissention refer to voting and polling (a more informal term) and are limited to merely counting responses: the winning option is the one with the most votes. Neither coaching nor authoritative actions were described.

11. Many emergency departments have customer service committees whose charge is to improve customer relations. Effectiveness is most likely to occur in which of these scenarios?
  A. An all-nurse committee because nurses have the most patient contact
  B. A committee that includes all disciplines and levels of staff and management
  C. A small committee of managers who can respond most effectively to complaints
  D. A multidisciplinary staff-level committee that monitors patient complaints closely and tracks numbers and types of complaints against staff members

CORRECT ANSWER—B. *Rationales:* Optimal customer service includes all staff, at all levels, in all disciplines. The committee works best when the problem is "owned" by those delivering service to customers as well as those in authority. An all-nurse committee places inappropriate emphasis on nursing. It is evident that nurses do have a great deal of patient contact and, therefore, opportunity to set a customer-friendly tone. But there are countless factors that are not directly related to nursing, such as billing, medical diagnosis, and housekeeping. Waiting for complaints is passive, and an after-the-damage-is-done strategy, which is limited to monitoring, does not improve goals.

12. An applicant for an emergency nursing position is qualified, depending on many variables, including personal qualities, education, experience, and credentials. An applicant's ENPC (Emergency Nursing Pediatric Course), TNCC (Trauma Nursing Core Course), ACLS (Advanced Cardiac Life Support), and CEN (Certified Emergency Nurse) certification as well as RN (Registered Nurse) licensure are examples of which qualifications?
  A. Personal qualities
  B. Experience
  C. Educational preparation
  D. Credentials

CORRECT ANSWER—D. *Rationales:* Certifications, courses, and licenses are known as credentials. Experience is an applicant's work history. Educational preparation refers to degrees held as well as academic institutions and programs attended. Personal qualities are subjectively measured and include perceptions of voice, dress, sense of humor, and energy level.

13. A department with a shared governance model would probably have which of these scheduling processes?
A. Self-scheduling of staff
B. Management scheduling of staff
C. Designated staff leader scheduling of staff
D. A centralized system that includes computer-generated scheduling

CORRECT ANSWER—A. *Rationales:* Self-scheduling is the option usually found in shared governance models, which emphasize staff accountability and involvement in operating a unit. Management scheduling, or having a designated staff leader for scheduling, places the work of schedule preparation directly on the manager (or designee); it de-emphasizes staff maturity and responsibility. A centralized system with computer-generated scheduling would provide little opportunity for staff input and is a poor fit with the decentralized approach underlying the shared governance model.

14. The purpose of research in emergency nursing is to do which of the following?
A. To enhance the professional status of emergency nursing
B. To generate a scientific knowledge base for validating and improving practice
C. To evaluate new medical devices and drugs
D. To help nurses identify problems in their clinical setting

CORRECT ANSWER—B. *Rationales:* The purpose of nursing research is to generate a scientific knowledge base for validating and improving practice. Although the professional status of emergency nursing may be incidentally enhanced by research, such enhancement is not the focus or goal. Identification of new problems may be an outcome of nursing research, but most research depends on problem or question identification. Emergency nurses may have opportunities to participate in drug studies and product evaluation programs, but neither represents the purpose of nursing research.

15. Research that aims to examine the feelings and perceptions of emergency nurses working with battered women patients is probably which type of study?
A. Qualitative
B. Quasi-scientific
C. Quantitative
D. Experimental

CORRECT ANSWER—A. *Rationales:* A study that examines thoughts and perceptions is one that lends itself to a qualitative design. Qualitative research is concerned with understanding human beings and the nature of their transactions with themselves and their surroundings. The process is not quasi-scientific but rather a well-accepted mode of rigorous, systematic inquiry used in the social sciences. Quantitative research methods analyze data statistically while striving for precision and control over external variables; context may be overlooked. Experimental research involves doing something to some of the subjects and not doing something to others; in it, subjects are randomly assigned to either group.

SAMPLE TEST

Questions

1. Which is the best unit of measure for identifying early shock in a trauma patient?
   A. Hemoglobin and hematocrit
   B. Central venous pressure
   C. Blood pressure
   D. Heart rate

2. Immediately after delivery of a baby's head, the nurse should do which of the following?
   A. Suction the airway
   B. Feel for the umbilical cord around the baby's neck
   C. Stimulate the baby to cry
   D. Deliver the upper shoulder

3. Which of the following statements is true regarding the outcome of reimplantation?
   A. Reimplantation is less successful in guillotine injuries than in crush injuries.
   B. The more distal the amputation, the more successful the chance of reimplantation.
   C. Amputation reimplantation is more successful in adults than in children.
   D. The outcome of reimplantation is the same whether the injury occurred on an oil-coated machine or a shard of glass.

4. Which of the following is the treatment for a patient who has inhaled cyanide?
   A. Administration of naloxone (Narcan)
   B. Administration of ipecac to perform gastric emptying
   C. Administration of amyl nitrate pearls
   D. Administration of activated charcoal

5. What does the Consolidated Omnibus Budget Reconciliation Act of 1989 (COBRA) mandate for a patient who presents to a hospital that does not offer the services required?
   A. The patient must be medically screened and stabilized before transport to another health care agency.
   B. The patient can be transferred to another facility, regardless of condition before admission to the emergency department.
   C. The COBRA mandate has no requirements regarding this situation.
   D. The emergency department has the right to refuse patients whenever necessary.

6. Hypertensive crisis secondary to monoamine oxidase inhibitor use also results in which of the following?
   A. Hypothermia
   B. Bradycardia
   C. Hyperthermia
   D. Heart block

7. Neuroleptic malignant syndrome is characterized by which of the following signs?
   A. Hypothermia related to dopaminergic hypoactivity in the hypothalamus
   B. Muscle rigidity, akinesia, agitation
   C. Hyperpyrexia, bradycardia, hypotension
   D. Hyperpyrexia, diaphoresis, hypotension

8. Continuous nitroglycerin (Tridil) infusion is indicated for the management of which of the following conditions?
   A. Increased intracranial pressure
   B. Cerebral hemorrhage
   C. Head trauma
   D. Pulmonary edema

9. Which of the following communication techniques is most effective when communicating with an anxious patient?
A. Silence
B. Active listening
C. Questioning
D. Verbalizing support

10. What should the patient who has taken an overdose of a beta blocker receive?
A. Lidocaine (Xylocaine)
B. Glucagon
C. $D_{50}W$
D. Bretylium (Bretylol)

11. Triage is effective when an infant with a glassy stare is classified as which of the following?
A. Acutely ill and categorized emergent
B. Not acutely ill and categorized nonurgent
C. Acutely ill and categorized urgent
D. Acutely ill and categorized nonurgent

12. Which of the following is a priority nursing diagnosis for the brain dead patient who has diabetes insipidus and is awaiting preparation for organ harvest?
A. Altered cerebral tissue perfusion
B. Fluid volume deficit
C. Fluid volume excess
D. Impaired gas exchange

13. Which of the following are the expected compensatory cardiovascular mechanisms in response to shock?
A. Increased pulse rate and increased contractility of the heart
B. Decreased pulse rate and increased contractility of the heart
C. Increased pulse rate and decreased contractility of the heart
D. Decreased pulse rate and decreased contractility of the heart

14. Which is the most commonly reported physical abnormality resulting from critical incident stress?
A. Appetite loss
B. Sleep disturbance
C. Intimacy loss
D. Fatigue

15. Successful fluid replacement in a 2-year-old child is evidenced by which of the following urine level outputs?
A. 1 to 2 ml/kg/hour
B. 3 to 5 ml/kg/hour
C. 0.5 to 1.0 ml/kg/hour
D. 0.75 to 1.5 ml/kg/hour

16. Turner's sign, found on physical assessment, is indicative of which of these conditions?
A. Retroperitoneal hemorrhage
B. Mediastinal bleeding
C. Increased intracranial pressure
D. Splenic injury

17. A brain dead patient with neurogenic diabetes insipidus will develop which of the following?
A. Hypernatremia, hyperkalemia, hyperosmolar serum, hyposmolar urine
B. Hypernatremia, hypokalemia, hyperosmolar serum and urine
C. Hyponatremia, hyperkalemia, hyposmolar serum and urine
D. Hypernatremia, hypokalemia, hyperosmolar serum, hyposmolar urine

18. A 4-year-old child with severe respiratory distress requires intubation and mechanical ventilation. The emergency department nurse anticipates the use of which size endotracheal tube for a child this age?
A. 5 mm
B. 4 mm
C. 3 mm
D. 6 mm

19. Which of the following is the priority nursing diagnosis for a patient who presents with peritonitis?
A. **Pain**
B. Inadequate nutrition
C. Decreased intravascular fluid volume
D. High risk for systemic infection

20. After cardiac transplantation, which is the usual presenting sign or symptom of acute myocardial infarction?
A. Substernal chest pain
B. Congestive heart failure
C. Tachycardia
D. Jaw pain

21. After an industrial accident, a patient with a laceration to the hand and wrist presents to the triage area. Assessment priority should be directed toward which area?
A. Tetanus immunization status
B. Time of last oral intake
C. Presence of industrial contaminants
D. Neurovascular status of injured extremity

22. The doctor orders a continuous infusion of epinephrine (Adrenalin) 1 mg in 250 ml of D_5W by way of infusion pump at 1.25 mcg/minute. What is the infusion rate in milliliters per hour (assuming the use of microdrip 60 gtt/ml tubing)?
A. 34 ml/hour
B. 23 ml/hour
C. 15 ml/hour
D. 19 ml/hour

23. A patient presents to the emergency department complaining of rapid heartbeat, shortness of breath, and syncope. Cardiac monitoring shows supraventricular tachycardia. Vital signs reveal a pulse of 164 beats/minute, blood pressure 80/50 mm Hg, and respirations 28 breaths/minute. I.V. access is established and oxygen is administered. The emergency nurse should anticipate an order for which of the following drugs?
A. Digoxin (Lanoxin)
B. Diltiazem (Cardizem)
C. Bretylium (Bretylol)
D. Adenosine (Adenocard)

24. Classic signs of increased intracranial pressure include all of the following except which?
A. Widening pulse pressure
B. Tachycardia
C. Altered level of consciousness
D. Bradycardia

25. A patient comes to the emergency department complaining of left calf pain that occurs during his morning walk each day. He states that the pain disappears with rest. Which condition should the emergency nurse suspect?
A. Claudication
B. Compartment syndrome
C. Muscle cramps
D. Deep vein thrombosis

26. Which nursing intervention is appropriate for the sudden-cardiac-death survivor?
A. Notifying the patient's support system, including family, friends, and clergy
B. Making decisions for the patient and encouraging the patient to rest
C. Providing the patient with privacy so that he or she can reflect on the situation
D. All of the above

27. Which nursing diagnosis is appropriate for a schizophrenic patient?
A. Personal identity disturbance
B. Altered thought processes
C. Acute confusion
D. Spiritual distress

28. Helicopter transport is arranged. Which device best assures continued correct placement of an endotracheal tube during flight?
A. Cardiac monitor
B. Electronic end-tidal carbon dioxide detector
C. Pulse oximeter
D. Laryngoscope

29. Bradycardia and atrioventricular node conduction disturbances are most often associated with which of the following conditions?
A. Cardiogenic shock
B. Anterior wall infarction
C. Inferior wall infarction
D. Heart failure

30. Which of the following tissue pressure measurements is indicative of compartment syndrome?
  A. 5 to 10 mm Hg
  B. 10 to 20 mm Hg
  C. 20 to 30 mm Hg
  D. 30 to 40 mm Hg

31. Parkinson's disease occurs because of degeneration of which part of the brain?
  A. Temporal lobe
  B. Pituitary gland
  C. Basal ganglia
  D. Medulla

32. The following patients present to the emergency department for treatment after a building explosion and collapse. Which would receive priority care?
  A. A 17-year-old with an open head injury, a Glasgow Coma Scale of 3, fixed and dilated pupils, a pulse rate of 140 beats/minute, and a blood pressure of 60 mm Hg on palpation
  B. A 32-year-old with several facial lacerations who is otherwise stable with a Glasgow Coma Scale of 15
  C. A 43-year-old with a severed left leg, controlled bleeding at the severance site, a pulse rate of 138 beats/minute, a respiratory rate of 32 breaths/minute, and a blood pressure of 88/64 mm Hg
  D. An unresponsive 68-year-old who arrives with third-degree burns over 95% of her body and a blood pressure of 60 mm Hg on palpation

33. A nitroprusside (Nipride) drip is prepared by mixing 50 mg of the drug in 250 ml of D_5W. The nurse is instructed to administer 3 mcg/kg/minute. The patient weighs 89 kg. Which of the following drip rates is correct (the drip factor of the pump tubing is 60 gtt/ml)?
  A. 10 ml/hour
  B. 32 ml/hour
  C. 80 ml/hour
  D. 75 ml/hour

34. Which of the following facts about the principles of disaster documentation is true?
  A. Always use small disaster tags so that they can stay with the patient throughout the emergency department stay.
  B. Have as many carbon copies as possible on the tag so that they can be used to update the command post instead of verbally communicating.
  C. Keep record keeping and charting as close to day-to-day operations as possible.
  D. None of the above is true.

35. Which of the following statements indicates an understanding of genital herpes treatment?
  A. "As long as I am taking the acyclovir (Zovirax) I can continue sexual activity."
  B. "I'll share my prescription for acyclovir with my partner."
  C. "I know that lesions may be getting ready to erupt if I have itching and a tingling sensation in the vaginal area."
  D. "I need to douche twice a day for the next week with Betadine and water."

36. Kawasaki disease is manifested by which of the following signs?
  A. Erythema of the palms and soles
  B. Butterfly rash
  C. Exophthalmos
  D. Koplik's spots

37. Which of the following is the primary nursing diagnosis for a patient with acute congestive heart failure?
  A. Anxiety
  B. Decreased cardiac output
  C. Altered tissue perfusion
  D. Impaired gas exchange

38. Expected outcomes for a family after a sudden infant death syndrome (SIDS) death include all except which of the following?
  A. Verbalizing positive memories of the infant
  B. Accepting a referral for a SIDS support group
  C. Verbalizing concerns about the cause of death
  D. Verbalizing that the baby may have smothered or choked to death

39. Which of the following is not indicative of a positive peritoneal lavage?
    A. Aspiration of 10 ml of gross blood
    B. Presence of intestinal contents
    C. Return of fluid that does not contain blood or white blood cells
    D. Return of cloudy fluid

40. A patient arrives at the emergency department complaining of substernal chest pain. Cardiac monitoring reveals sinus bradycardia with uniform premature ventricular contractions. After a saline lock has been started, the patient becomes unresponsive. The monitor reveals ventricular fibrillation. The emergency nurse defibrillates the patient at 200 joules, 300 joules, and 360 joules. The patient remains in ventricular fibrillation. Cardiopulmonary resuscitation is initiated. The patient is intubated by the doctor. Which is the next action?
    A. Defibrillate at 360 joules.
    B. Administer epinephrine 1 mg I.V.
    C. Administer lidocaine hydrochloride (Xylocaine) 1.5 mg/kg I.V.
    D. Administer sodium bicarbonate 1 mEq/kg I.V.

41. The decision to transfer a patient should be based on all except which of the following?
    A. Written policies of the emergency department
    B. Medical insurance approval
    C. Need for a specialized unit
    D. Need for a specialized procedure

42. A patient who is experiencing a situational crisis presents to the emergency department. The emergency nurse should do which of the following?
    A. Obtain an order to administer antianxiety medication, such as diazepam (Valium)
    B. Encourage verbalization of feelings, give emotional support, and initiate health-related teaching
    C. Orient the patient to reality (person, time, and place) and apply safety restraints
    D. Insist that the patient identify the precipitating factors and his or her emotional response to the event

43. Tetany results when pathogenic organisms are introduced into human tissue. Which bacteria are responsible for this disease?
    A. *Pasteurella multocida*
    B. *Clostridium*
    C. *Enterobacter*
    D. *Streptococcus*

44. When evaluating the care of a patient with bipolar disease in the emergency department, which is the priority determination?
    A. The patient's thought process was organized before discharge.
    B. The patient was safe in the emergency department environment and was able to verbalize the appropriate use of lithium carbonate (Lithonate) on discharge.
    C. The patient's nutritional status was evaluated.
    D. The patient's auditory hallucinations had subsided before discharge.

45. After falling 20 feet from a platform, a patient is admitted to the emergency department. He is complaining of chest pain that radiates to the back. Chest X-rays show widening of the mediastinum. What do these symptoms probably represent?
    A. Ruptured hemidiaphragm
    B. Pneumothorax
    C. Ruptured trachea
    D. Ruptured aorta

46. Which is the nursing priority when caring for a suspected schizophrenic patient who is delusional?
    A. Obtain a psychiatric consult as soon as possible.
    B. Assist with the medical workup because the behavior could be organic and medical causes need to be ruled out.
    C. Anticipate an order for lithium carbonate (Lithonate).
    D. Insist that the delusions are not real.

47. A patient arrives in the emergency department and is placed on the monitor. Identify the rhythm.

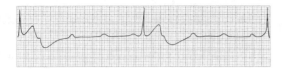

A. Idioventricular
B. Third-degree heart block
C. Sinus bradycardia
D. Wenkebach

48. Which of the following may cause children to become fatigued during increased work of breathing?
A. Increased residual capacity
B. Increased tidal volumes
C. Lower glucose stores than adults
D. Decreased metabolic demands

49. Which is the most common cause of retinal detachment?
A. Degenerative changes in the elderly
B. Direct trauma associated with sports activities
C. Blunt trauma from assault to eye
D. Hereditary factors

50. A patient with known bipolar disorder (manic-depressive illness) is brought to the emergency department by friends who state that he has not been taking his medicine. The emergency department nurse should expect to find which of the following?
A. Labile emotions, hyperactivity or hypoactivity, poor social judgment, and grandiose context to speech
B. An increase in heart rate, respiratory rate, and blood pressure
C. Normal thought process
D. All of the above

51. Which is the correct intervention for a patient with a positive halo sign?
A. Instructing the patient to perform the Valsalva's maneuver as an attempt to open the ear canal
B. Suctioning the fluid from the ear canal
C. Applying a loose sterile dressing over the ear or nose
D. Inserting packing to absorb the fluid

52. Which of the following equipment will be prepared for use before the transport of a conscious burn patient?
A. An ice container for irrigation saline
B. A cooling blanket
C. An end-tidal carbon dioxide detector
D. I.V. infusion pump

53. Which of the following distinguishes myocardial contusion from angina?
A. Chest pain that is not affected by coronary vasodilators
B. Arrhythmias
C. Hypotension, distended neck veins, and muffled heart sounds
D. ECG changes

54. A dystonic reaction can be caused by which of the following medications?
A. Diazepam (Valium)
B. Haloperidol (Haldol)
C. Amitriptyline (Elavil)
D. Clonazepam (Klonopin)

55. A 3-year-old child weighing 15 kg is brought to the emergency department after being found floating in a pond. Initially, the child's rhythm is ventricular fibrillation. Which is the appropriate initial energy level for defibrillation of this patient?
A. 15 joules
B. 30 joules
C. 100 joules
D. 200 joules

56. Before administering a chelating drug to a patient with heavy metal poisoning, the nurse should include which priority nursing assessment?
   A. Level of consciousness
   B. Respiratory status
   C. Urine output
   D. Blood pressure

57. Diazoxide (Hyperstat) is often used in the treatment of hypertensive crisis. Which is the usual method of administration?
   A. Continuous I.V. infusion 200 mg/L
   B. 10 to 50 mg I.M.
   C. 50 to 100 mg I.V. bolus every 5 to 10 minutes
   D. Continuous I.V. infusion 5 g/minute

58. During an unusually busy day in the emergency department, the following patients present themselves to the triage nurse within a 6-minute period. One bed is available for examinations. Which patient should take priority?
   A. A 13-year-old male with groin pain that was more severe 1½ hours ago
   B. A 58-year-old male with urgency and hesitancy to urinate. Onset was 6 hours ago
   C. A 27-year-old female with severe bilateral lower abdominal pain
   D. A 42-year-old female with flank pain, fever, nausea, and vomiting

59. A patient presents to the emergency department complaining of a sudden onset of chest pain that increases with deep breathing and lying flat. The pain decreases somewhat with sitting up and leaning forward. Vital signs are blood pressure 100/60 mm Hg, pulse 100 beats/minute, respirations 22 breaths/minute, and temperature 103.4° F (39.7° C). Which of the following conditions should the emergency nurse suspect?
   A. Myocardial infarction
   B. Pleurisy
   C. Pericarditis
   D. Endocarditis

60. Why should Allen's test be performed before the insertion of an arterial line?
   A. To ensure that the monitor has been zeroed correctly
   B. To ensure that collateral circulation to the hand is adequate
   C. To ensure that no phlebitis is present in the radial artery
   D. To ensure that the transducer is at the level of the right atrium

61. An 80-kg hypertensive patient is ordered nitroprusside (Nipride) to infuse at 5 mcg/kg/minute by way of an infusion pump. The concentration is 100 mg in 250 ml of D_5W. What is the infusion rate in milliliters per hour (assuming the use of microdrip 60 gtt/ml tubing)?
   A. 60 ml/hour
   B. 53 ml/hour
   C. 56 ml/hour
   D. 70 ml/hour

62. Prolonged seizure activity can result in which of the following conditions?
   A. Hyperglycemia
   B. Alkalosis
   C. Hypothermia
   D. Acidosis

63. A patient with an insect in the left ear arrives in the emergency department. Which is the most effective way to remove the insect?
   A. Irrigate the ear with copious amounts of water.
   B. Using an ear speculum to visualize the insect, gently grasp and remove it using forceps.
   C. Instill mineral oil into the ear canal.
   D. All of the actions above are appropriate.

64. Which of the following is the primary side effect of thrombolytic therapy?
   A. Reperfusion arrhythmias
   B. Bleeding
   C. Release of oxygen-free radicals
   D. Hypotension

65. Cocaine-induced myocardial ischemia may be related to which of the following conditions?
A. Coronary artery vasoconstriction
B. Coronary thrombosis
C. Increased myocardial oxygen consumption
D. All of the above

66. At which point is the patient owed a duty of care?
A. At the time of arrival at the emergency department
B. After admission to the emergency department
C. Once the doctor has examined the patient and found an emergent condition
D. At the time a treatment plan has been established

67. Which are the most frequent early systemic signs of septic shock?
A. Hyperthermia, tachycardia, wide pulse pressure, tachypnea, respiratory alkalosis, and mental obtundation
B. Hypothermia, bradycardia, narrow pulse pressure, tachypnea, respiratory acidosis, and coma
C. Hypothermia, tachycardia, narrow pulse pressure, tachypnea, respiratory alkalosis, and confusion
D. Hyperthermia, bradycardia, wide pulse pressure, tachypnea, respiratory acidosis, and mental obtundation

68. The pumping ability of the heart depends on which of the following four factors?
A. Contractility, preload, heart rate, afterload
B. Contractility, heart rate, cardiac output, cardiac index
C. Heart rate, cardiac output, left ventricular hypertrophy, pulmonary venous congestion
D. None of the above

69. Which nursing diagnosis is most appropriate for a suicidal patient being cared for in the emergency department?
A. Risk for injury
B. Spiritual distress
C. Ineffective coping
D. Social isolation

70. Hyperflexion of the upper extremities and hyperextension of the lower extremities are described as which of the following?
A. Decortication
B. Hypotonia
C. Spasticity
D. Decerebration

71. Which of the following injuries is most consistent with shaken baby syndrome?
A. Bilateral arm fractures
B. Basilar skull fractures
C. Retinal hemorrhages
D. Petechiae on the trunk

72. Achieving which prothrombin time is the goal of warfarin sodium (Coumadin) therapy?
A. Equal to that of the control
B. Less than that of the control
C. One and one half times that of the control
D. Three times that of the control

73. Which of the following is an appropriate treatment for a patient with a diagnosis of herpes?
A. Decrease fluid intake.
B. Insert an indwelling urinary catheter.
C. Keep lesions moist.
D. Apply tight-fitting Dacron undergarments.

74. Irritation of the vagal centers in the medulla produces which of the following symptoms?
A. Vomiting
B. Headache
C. Papilledema
D. Restlessness and irritability

75. When an error in documentation is made in the medical record, how should the error be corrected?
    A. Tear out the sheet with the error and recopy all the information on a new sheet, make the correct entry, and initial the sheet to indicate that it is a copy.
    B. Apply correction fluid over the error and record the correct information over it.
    C. Draw a single line through the incorrect entry. Date the error and initial it, and give the reason for the error.
    D. Scribble through the incorrect information as well as possible and then make the correct entry.

76. Triage has been effective when the patient presenting with congestive heart failure is classified as which of the following?
    A. Urgent
    B. Acute
    C. Nonacute
    D. Referable

77. Which is the priority nursing diagnosis for a patient with an open, depressed skull fracture?
    A. Pain related to fracture
    B. Risk for infection related to trauma
    C. Body image disturbance related to trauma
    D. Acute confusion related to head trauma

78. Which of the following is the antidote for heparin sodium overdose?
    A. Vitamin K (AquaMEPHYTON)
    B. Dimercaprol (BAL in Oil)
    C. Naloxone (Narcan)
    D. Protamine sulfate

79. Which is the priority nursing diagnosis for a patient with endocarditis?
    A. Altered cardiopulmonary tissue perfusion
    B. Impaired gas exchange
    C. Pain
    D. Fluid volume deficit

80. Which is the primary treatment for a patient who complains of back pain?
    A. Rest
    B. Cold applications
    C. Weight loss
    D. Stretching exercises

81. Which of the following diagnostic findings indicate the need for mechanical ventilation?
    A. A PaO_2 of 80 mm Hg on room air
    B. A vital capacity less than 10 ml/kg
    C. A normal work of breathing
    D. A $PaCO_2$ of 42 mm Hg

82. The lowest level of electrical energy required to initiate consistent capture with a pacemaker is referred to as which of the following?
    A. Underdrive pacing
    B. Pacing threshold
    C. Sensing threshold
    D. Demand pacing

83. Which of the following is an essential part of the emergency department record for the patient discharged home?
    A. Remarks of other personnel caring for the patient
    B. Discharge instructions and follow-up instructions
    C. The patient's comments regarding the care received
    D. The apparent intellectual level of the patient

84. Which of the following nursing diagnoses is of concern for a patient with a mandibular fracture?
    A. Fluid volume deficit
    B. Altered cerebral tissue perfusion
    C. Ineffective airway clearance
    D. Decreased cardiac output

85. Which of the following is a true statement about the responsibilities of the disaster committee?
A. The committee should review the disaster plan only after a disaster occurs.
B. The committee may disband once the disaster plan is developed or revised.
C. The committee needs to continually reevaluate and revise the disaster plan.
D. The committee should plan disaster exercises at times of low census to ensure maximum staff attendance.

86. After a motor vehicle crash, a patient presents to the emergency department with an injury to the right leg. On physical assessment, the nurse notices that the patient is unable to raise his leg when it is straightened and lacks sensation to the anterior thigh. Assessment of the left leg is normal. What is the possible cause of this finding?
A. Damage to the median nerve
B. Damage to the femoral nerve
C. Damage to the tibial nerve
D. Damage to the peroneal nerve

87. Which of the following is the earliest and most common respiratory alteration in patients with intracranial injury?
A. Apneustic breathing
B. Biot's respirations
C. Cheyne-Stokes respirations
D. Cluster breathing

88. When assessing a patient with moderate to severe anxiety, the emergency nurse should expect which of the following objective findings?
A. Rapid, pressured speech; restlessness; and tachycardia
B. Exaggerated startle response, hyperactivity, and warm, dry skin
C. Dry mouth, clammy skin, and constricted pupils
D. Irritability, bradycardia, and dilated pupils

89. Which is the most common underlying cause of pediatric cardiopulmonary arrest?
A. Genetic cardiac abnormalities
B. Electrolyte disturbances
C. Hypoxemia
D. Primary cardiac arrhythmias

90. Preoperative antibiotic therapy in a patient with an open fracture to the distal tibia will do which of the following?
A. Allow systemic prophylaxis in the event the wound is deeper than initially believed
B. Not do any good because the open wound is easily cleaned and debrided during surgery
C. Reach an effective blood concentration before or at the time of wound closure and, thus, limit the threat of infection
D. Work equally effectively if administered by mouth or I.V.

91. Which of the following is an acceptable reason to transfer a patient?
A. Lack of necessary resources
B. Delay in mobilizing resources
C. Inability to stabilize the patient
D. All of the above

92. A patient's ECG reveals ST-segment changes in leads II, III, and aVF. The emergency nurse suspects damage to which wall of the myocardium?
A. Inferior
B. Lateral
C. Anterior
D. Apical

93. Which of the following statements indicates successful education of the patient with migraine headaches who is taking ergotamine tartrate (Cafergot)?
A. "I need to pick up my oral contraceptives after I leave here today."
B. "I have enrolled in biofeedback therapy."
C. "For lunch I am having a hot dog with a chocolate milk shake."
D. "I should take propranolol only when I have a full-blown migraine."

94. During a physical examination, which is the most characteristic finding in diagnosing asthma?
A. Dark circles under the eyes
B. Bluish, boggy nasal turbinates
C. Expiratory wheezing
D. Moist crackles

95. Initial treatment for the adult patient with a severe anaphylactic reaction includes which of the following drugs?
A. Administration of diphenhydramine (Benadryl) 25 mg I.M.
B. Administration of epinephrine 0.1 to 0.5 mg of a 1:1,000 solution
C. Administration of epinephrine 0.1 to 0.25 mg of a 1:10,000 solution
D. Cimetidine (Tagamet) 300 mg I.V.

96. The nurse should seek clarification of which of the following orders for a 5-year-old child who has ingested a large amount of paint thinner?
A. Ipecac
B. Activated charcoal
C. Gastric lavage
D. Oxygen delivered at 2 L/minute

97. An understanding of discharge instructions is demonstrated if the patient states which of the following after having a hand sutured?
A. "I must return to the emergency department in 3 days for suture removal."
B. "I can shower in 8 hours."
C. "I must elevate the injured area above the level of my heart."
D. "I can expect redness at the site for the first week."

98. It is important to assess which of the following in the patient receiving magnesium sulfate?
A. Urine output, respirations, reflexes
B. Urine output, reflexes, vaginal bleeding
C. Urine output, reflexes
D. All of the above

99. A patient presents to the emergency department after being attacked and sexually assaulted. Which is the most accurate nursing diagnosis for this patient?
A. Rape-trauma syndrome
B. Fear
C. Anxiety
D. Hopelessness

100. Honeybees and bumblebees cause a painful wound with swelling and intense itching. Which of the following is true about the treatment of these stings?
A. Heat should be applied to the sting area.
B. Removal of the stinger is done by scraping the area with a dull object.
C. Removal of the stinger is accomplished by grasping the stinger and pulling it away from the skin.
D. Ice should be applied and the extremity lowered below the heart.

101. During patient assessment, the nurse finds the patient's pupils to be pinpoint. What might this indicate?
A. Opioid overdose
B. Midbrain damage
C. Severe anoxia
D. Previous cataract surgery

102. Symptoms suggesting a scabies infestation include which of the following?
A. Raised, scaly, round patches with relatively flat centers on the hands, feet, trunk, and groin
B. Pink macular rash over palms, soles, hands, feet, wrists, and ankles
C. Pruritus that intensifies at night
D. Generalized urticaria

103. Which of the following statements indicates a lack of understanding of long leg cast and extremity care?
A. "I will keep the cast dry."
B. "If a foreign object drops into the cast, I will attempt to retrieve it before calling my follow-up care provider."
C. "I will wiggle my toes at least once each hour."
D. "I will keep my leg elevated above the level of my heart for the next 24 hours."

104. A patient with heavy vaginal bleeding after a spontaneous abortion is started on an oxytocin (Pitocin) infusion. Which of the following would indicate that the medication was effective?
A. Increased urine output
B. Cessation of bleeding
C. Increased abdominal cramping
D. Increased heart rate

105. Which of the following is the initial biologic response to new wounds?
A. Inflammation
B. Hemostasis
C. Cell proliferation
D. Scar formation

106. Which nursing diagnosis is most appropriate for a patient with esophageal varices?
A. Anxiety
B. Altered gastrointestinal tissue perfusion
C. Impaired gas exchange
D. Fluid volume deficit

107. Which document outlines a patient's wishes regarding emergency treatment if the patient is unable to speak for himself or herself?
A. Durable power of attorney for health care
B. Last will and testament
C. Advanced directive
D. Instructions for care after death

108. Which type of learning is demonstrated when the nurse teaches a parent to change the sterile dressing on a child's arm?
A. Cognitive
B. Affective
C. Social
D. Psychomotor

109. Priority treatment for a patient with suspected blunt abdominal trauma includes which of the following?
A. Inserting two large-bore I.V. lines, administering 2 units of blood, and inserting an indwelling urinary catheter
B. Securing the airway, obtaining a toxicologic screen, and administering tetanus toxoid
C. Obtaining chest and cervical spine X-rays and inserting two large-bore I.V. lines
D. Securing the airway, inserting two large-bore I.V. lines, and obtaining a type and crossmatch for 6 units of blood

110. Which of the following is a priority nursing intervention in a patient presenting with a suspected pelvic fracture?
A. Placing and inflating the pneumatic antishock garment
B. Administering pain medication
C. Preparing for an X-ray
D. Administering high-flow oxygen

111. A patient receiving beta blockers shows which response to a shock state?
A. Increased pulse rate and hypotension
B. Bradycardia, hypotension, and decreased renin secretion
C. Increased pulse rate and hypertension
D. Bradycardia and hypertension

112. A patient is admitted to the emergency department complaining of blurred vision and moderate left eye pain. Physical exam reveals a hazy cornea and small, irregular pupil with sluggish reaction on the left. Which ocular impairment is the most likely?
A. Conjunctivitis
B. Glaucoma
C. Iritis
D. Central retinal artery occlusion

113. A patient presents to the emergency department after slicing his wrist on a piece of steel while at work. How is extensor tendon function assessed?
A. Instructing the patient to push downward and upward against resistance with all five digits
B. Instructing the patient to abduct and adduct his fingers without finger flexion
C. Instructing the patient to oppose his thumb to his little finger
D. Testing sensation over the dorsal surface of the thumb and index, second, and middle fingers

114. The patient is provided discharge instructions regarding corneal abrasions. Which of the following statements would assure the nurse that the patient understands the instructions?
A. "I should be able to remove the eye patch after 1 hour."
B. "I should return to be checked in 1 week."
C. "The pain should be relieved within a few hours without medications."
D. "I will need to see a doctor tomorrow."

115. Which nursing diagnosis is most appropriate for a patient with myasthenia gravis?
A. Fluid volume excess related to hypervolemic therapy
B. Ineffective breathing pattern related to weakness of respiratory muscles
C. Impaired physical mobility related to paralysis and spasticity
D. Pain related to tissue trauma secondary to spinal fractures

116. Which of the following is the minimum acceptable oxygen delivery mode for an unconscious multisystem trauma patient under the influence of alcohol?
A. Simple face mask delivering 50% oxygen at 8 to 10 L/minute
B. Nasal cannula delivering 44% oxygen at 6 L/minute
C. Endotracheal intubation with bag-valve-mask device delivering oxygen at 100%
D. Nonrebreather mask delivering 90% oxygen at 15 L/minute

117. A patient is diagnosed with acute pancreatitis. Which of the following drugs can be used to treat the severe pain?
A. Meperidine (Demerol)
B. Codeine
C. Morphine
D. Hydromorphone hydrochloride (Dilaudid)

118. Which nursing diagnosis is the highest priority for a patient with injuries from sea urchins?
A. Risk for poisoning related to injection of neurotoxins
B. Impaired skin integrity related to foreign-body irritants
C. Anxiety related to perceived threat of death
D. Pain related to soft tissue injury

119. Which of the following conditions can mimic brain death and must be corrected before the diagnosis of brain death?
A. Hyperphosphatemia
B. Alcohol intoxication
C. Hypertension
D. Hyperthermia

120. Which of the following is the strongest clue that a patient may be violent?
A. An 18-year-old man with a history of violence
B. Rapid, loud speech and heavy alcohol consumption
C. Clenched fists, pacing, and tense posture
D. The patient complains of extreme pain and has had to wait several hours

121. A patient involved in a motor vehicle accident complains of right shoulder pain when lying flat. Examination reveals right upper quadrant guarding. Vital signs are blood pressure 90/50 mm Hg, pulse 130 beats/minute, respirations 26 breaths/minute, and temperature 98.4° F (36.9° C). Chest X-ray reveals rib fractures in the lower right chest. The nurse should suspect injury to which of the following organs?
A. Spleen
B. Colon
C. Pancreas
D. Liver

122. Discharge instructions to the family of a patient with a concussion from a head injury should include which of the following?
A. Aspirin (acetylsalicylic acid) 650 mg every 4 hours for complaints of mild discomfort
B. Propoxyphene hydrochloride (Darvon) 65 mg every 4 hours for severe pain
C. Return immediately if the patient behaves in a way that is not normal for the patient
D. Neurologic symptoms shall subside in 4 to 8 hours

123. Which of the following is not a physical finding consistent with acute cholecystitis?
A. Fever
B. Right upper quadrant tenderness
C. Positive Murphy's sign
D. Kehr's sign

124. Which nursing diagnosis is most appropriate for a patient with an eyelid laceration?
A. Fluid volume deficit related to excessive blood loss
B. Altered cerebral tissue perfusion related to injury
C. Risk for infection related to break in skin integrity
D. Body image disturbance related to swelling

125. Which of the following is the initial intervention in caring for a child with pertussis?
A. Control fever with antipyretics
B. Institute isolation measures
C. Administer antibiotics
D. Initiate seizure precautions

126. A woman in her 30th week of pregnancy is brought to the emergency department after a motor vehicle accident. She is complaining of constant, severe abdominal pain. Examination reveals a rigid uterus and no vaginal bleeding. Vital signs are blood pressure 90/58 mm Hg, pulse 140 beats/minute, respirations 32 breaths/minute, temperature 99.2° F (37.3° C), and fetal heart tones 190 beats/minute. The nurse should suspect which of the following?
A. Placenta previa
B. Abruptio placentae
C. Premature labor
D. Ruptured uterus

127. Ventricular shunts are used to treat which of the following conditions?
A. Pneumocephalus
B. Encephalopathy
C. Subdural empyema
D. Hydrocephalus

128. Which of the following is a function of the disaster communications center?
A. Commanding and controlling the incident
B. Coordinating with local emergency medical services and community resources
C. Gathering internal information
D. Supervising the care of incoming casualties

129. A teenager is brought to the emergency department by his parents, who state that he has been smoking ice (the smokable form of methamphetamine). Which of the following assessment findings indicates recent ingestion of an amphetamine?
A. Extreme self-confidence
B. Hypotension
C. Flushed skin
D. Fatigue

130. A patient with acute closed-angle glaucoma is admitted to the emergency department. Signs and symptoms include severe eye pain, a fixed and slightly dilated pupil, a hard globe, a foggy-appearing cornea, nausea, vomiting, severe headache, halos around lights, and diminished peripheral vision. Which therapy is most appropriate for this patient?
A. Instillation of pilocarpine (Pilocar) eyedrops every 15 minutes
B. Systemic administration of analgesia
C. Administration of acetazolamide (Diamox)
D. All of the above

131. The nurse should prepare to administer which of the following cofactors to a patient with methanol poisoning?
A. Folic acid
B. Thiamine
C. Pyridoxine
D. Calcium

132. A young adult presents to the emergency department triage desk complaining of blurred vision. Lid ptosis is present, and the nurse notes that ocular movement is limited. The patient also complains of having some difficulty swallowing. Based on these findings, the nurse should specifically question the patient about which of the following?
A. Recent viral illnesses
B. Use of home canned foods
C. Presence of numbness or tingling
D. Recent travel

133. A patient with a history of alcohol abuse and cirrhosis presents to the emergency department. The patient is vomiting large amounts of bright red blood and is poorly responsive. Vital signs are blood pressure 80/50 mm Hg, pulse 140 beats/minute, respirations 36 breaths/minute, and temperature 99.8° F (37.7° C). The emergency nurse should do which of the following first?
A. Suction blood from airway
B. Insert two large-bore I.V. lines
C. Insert a nasogastric tube
D. Administer I.V. vitamin K (AquaMEPHYTON)

134. Labetalol (Normodyne) is ordered for a patient with acute cocaine overdose. The nurse should evaluate the patient's response to the drug by observing for which of the following?
A. Normalization of temperature
B. Lowering of blood pressure
C. Absence of seizures
D. Increase in pupil size

135. A patient with multiple facial injuries and suspected cervical spine injuries develops severe respiratory distress. Jaw-thrust maneuvers are unsuccessful in improving the patient's respiratory effort. Which is the least desirable method for establishing an airway in this patient?
A. Orotracheal intubation
B. Nasotracheal intubation
C. Needle cricothyrotomy
D. Surgical cricothyrotomy

136. Which of the following is the most serious side effect of vasopressin (Pitressin) I.V. therapy in the patient with bleeding esophageal varices?
A. Coronary vasoconstriction
B. Abdominal cramping
C. Water intoxication
D. Tissue damage due to infiltration

137. The nurse should prepare to administer which of the following drugs to a patient who has overdosed on fentanyl (Sublimaze)?
A. Physostigmine (Antilirium)
B. Flumazenil (Romazicon)
C. Atropine
D. Naloxone (Narcan)

138. A woman is admitted to the emergency department with a 2-hour history of right lower quadrant pain, which is increasing in severity. She is nauseated and has been vomiting. She also has a 7-day history of moderate vaginal bleeding. Which of the following indicates a strong suspicion for an ovarian cyst?
A. Elevated white blood cell count
B. Decreased hemoglobin
C. Elevated human chorionic gonadotropin levels
D. Decreased calcium level

139. Which is the main priority in the care of the patient with acute pancreatitis?
A. Pain control
B. Nutritional support
C. Causal correction
D. Fluid resuscitation

140. Six hours after eating dinner at a friend's house, a patient is admitted to the emergency department. The patient has signs of staphylococcal food poisoning. The friend was recently treated for a staphylococcal infection on his hand. Which is the highest priority nursing diagnosis for this patient?
A. Altered nutrition: less than body requirements
B. Fluid volume deficit
C. Diarrhea
D. Risk for infection

141. Which of the following diagnoses is most important in a patient with a pulmonary contusion?
A. Ineffective airway clearance related to effects of injury
B. Impaired gas exchange related to blood extravasation into lung
C. Pain related to injury and chest movement with breathing
D. Anxiety related to pain and hospitalization

142. The emergency department nurse knows that the most important principle in patient education is which of the following?
A. Providing the most up-to-date information available
B. Alleviating the patient's guilt associated with not knowing appropriate self-care
C. Determining patient readiness to learn new information
D. Building on previous information

143. Which of the following nursing diagnoses would be a priority for a patient with compartment syndrome?
A. Anxiety related to a crisis event
B. Pain related to ischemic injury secondary to compartment pressure increase
C. Altered peripheral tissue perfusion related to increased compartment pressure
D. Risk for impaired skin integrity related to decreased blood supply

144. A 12-year-old child is brought to the emergency department by his mother. The child has had a rash over his entire body and inside his mouth for 1 day. The patient also has a sore throat, headache, cough, and a low-grade fever of 100.8° F (38.2° C). Based on these findings, the doctor makes a preliminary diagnosis of which of the following diseases?
A. Scarlet fever
B. Fifth disease
C. Rubella
D. Roseola infantum

145. Which treatment is appropriate for a patient with central retinal artery occlusion?
A. Surgical decompression
B. Anticoagulant therapy
C. Gentle ocular massage
D. All of the above

146. Which lung sound requires immediate nursing intervention?
A. Crackles
B. Rhonchi
C. Stridor
D. Wheezing

147. A patient involved in a motor vehicle accident arrives in the emergency department complaining of severe abdominal pain. Vital signs are blood pressure 100/50 mm Hg, pulse 120 beats/minute, respirations 28 breaths/minute, and temperature 98.9° F (37.2° C). Chest X-ray reveals right rib fractures. The nurse should most strongly suspect which of the following?
A. Splenic injury
B. Perforated stomach
C. Pancreatic injury
D. Lacerated liver

148. Abrupt withdrawal of corticosteroid therapy puts a patient at risk for which of the following?
A. Glaucoma
B. Adrenal crisis
C. Psychic disturbances
D. Tardive dyskinesia

149. Hyperosmolar hyperglycemic nonketotic syndrome can be identified by which of the following laboratory values?
A. Blood glucose levels between 300 and 500 mg/dl
B. Plasma osmolality greater than 350 mOsm/kg
C. Normal blood urea nitrogen level
D. Arterial blood gases: pH 7.12; PaO_2 94 mm Hg; $PaCO_2$ 38 mm Hg; and HCO_3- 18 mEq/L

150. When evaluating the ECG of a patient with a potassium deficit, the nurse should expect which of the following changes?
A. Shortened QT interval
B. Tall, peaked T waves
C. Widened QRS complex
D. Inverted or flattened T waves

151. Chemical burns constitute a true ocular emergency. Which assessment finding is consistent with a chemical burn?
A. Corneal whitening
B. Dilated, nonreactive pupils
C. Redness with purulent discharge
D. Corneal irregularity with luster

152. A gardener is brought to the emergency department by his family. After spilling insecticide on himself as he filled a sprayer, he developed these symptoms, including headache, ataxia, and difficulty breathing. Before assessing this patient, the nurse should do which of the following?
A. Double glove
B. Identify the type of insecticide
C. Determine how much insecticide was spilled
D. Apply respiratory protection

153. On arrival in the emergency department, a multitrauma patient had a hematocrit (HCT) of 42%. Serial HCT reveal drops that do not correlate with the amount of I.V. fluid received. After 1 liter of fluid, the HCT was 35%; after 2 liters, the HCT is 29.5%. The nurse notices that the urinary catheter drainage is now hematuric and the patient is bleeding from the nasogastric and endotracheal tube sites. The doctor makes a diagnosis of disseminated intravascular coagulation. Based on this diagnosis, the nurse can expect to do which of the following?
A. Administer heparin
B. Administer fresh frozen plasma
C. Administer cryoprecipitate
D. All of the above

154. Which is the priority nursing diagnosis for a semiresponsive patient with ethanol intoxication?
A. Ineffective airway clearance related to alcohol intoxication
B. Risk for injury related to alcohol intoxication
C. Acute confusion related to alcohol intoxication
D. Altered nutrition: less than body requirements related to alcohol intoxication

155. Herpes zoster is an inflammatory condition with localized burning and shearing pain. Which type of lesion best fits the diagnosed rash?
A. Papule
B. Vesicle
C. Bulla
D. Pustule

156. Which of the following nursing diagnoses is appropriate for a patient diagnosed with pyelonephritis?
A. Risk for fluid volume deficit
B. Impaired tissue integrity
C. Altered renal tissue perfusion
D. Decreased cardiac output

157. Septic shock frequently causes which condition in children?
A. Hyperglycemia
B. Metabolic alkalosis
C. Hypoglycemia
D. Hypercalcemia

158. A woman arrives in the emergency department complaining of a 2-week history of lower abdominal–pelvic pain and a yellowish, foul-smelling vaginal discharge. Her pain is increasing. Vital signs are blood pressure 94/60 mm Hg, pulse 120 beats/minute, respirations 28 breaths/minute, temperature 101° F (38.3° C), pulse oximetry 94% (room air). Her white blood cell count is 16×10^3 µl, hemoglobin is 12.2 g/dl, and hematocrit is 38%. Which of the following procedures should not be performed?
A. Nasogastric tube insertion
B. Pelvic exam
C. Culdocentesis
D. Administration of I.V. fluids

159. Which of the following X-ray findings is evident in a patient with pancreatitis?
A. Free air under the diaphragm
B. Dilated loops of bowel
C. Sentinel loops of bowel
D. Abnormal air-fluid levels in the bowel

160. Which of the following does treatment for hyperkalemia include?
A. Administration of 10% glucose infusion with regular insulin
B. Administration of stored blood
C. Administration of calcium gluconate
D. None of the above

161. Successful repair of a renal pedicle injury should be evaluated by which of the following?
A. No extravasation of contrast on cystography
B. Visualization of kidney on excretory urography
C. Patency on retrograde urethrography
D. Normal kidney-ureter-bladder X-ray

162. A patient with sexually transmitted disease may have pain related to all except which of the following?
A. Dysuria
B. Discharge
C. Lesions
D. Pruritus

163. Which of the following is associated with intestinal obstruction?
A. Distention, vomiting, and visible peristalsis
B. Right upper quadrant tenderness, fever, and jaundice
C. Abdominal free air, distention, and rebound tenderness
D. Nausea, abdominal mass, and bruit

164. Cellular function is abnormal during a shock state and results in which type of metabolism?
A. Aerobic metabolism
B. Metabolic alkalosis
C. Anaerobic metabolism
D. None of the above

165. A trauma patient who is in shock and has been diagnosed with a fractured pelvis and a lacerated spleen requires immediate blood replacement. Which type of blood should be administered?
A. O-positive packed red blood cells
B. O-negative packed red blood cells
C. Type-specific, uncrossmatched packed red blood cells
D. Typed and crossmatched packed red blood cells

166. Which of the following is a contraindication for lumbar puncture?
A. Increased intracranial pressure
B. Warfarin sodium (Coumadin) therapy
C. Infection of the cutaneous or osseous areas at the lumbar puncture site
D. All of the above

167. Arterial blood gas measurements for a trauma patient consist of pH 7.48, $PaCO_2$ 30 mm Hg, PaO_2 84 mm Hg, HCO_3- 22 mEq/L. The patient is in which metabolic state?
A. Metabolic acidosis
B. Respiratory alkalosis
C. Respiratory acidosis
D. Metabolic alkalosis

168. Which patient has the highest risk for developing cardiogenic shock?
A. An elderly nursing home patient with pneumonia
B. A patient with acute anterolateral wall infarction
C. A restrained front-seat automobile passenger involved in a rear end crash
D. A patient who underwent cardiac surgery 4 weeks ago and who now presents with abdominal pain

169. Which of the following is the primary nursing diagnosis for an acutely burned patient in the emergency department?
A. Pain
B. Fluid volume deficit
C. Impaired skin integrity
D. Ineffective thermoregulation

170. When evaluating patient teaching, the nurse knows that the hypercalcemic patient has good understanding of the condition if the patient states which of the following?
A. "Exercise will help release calcium from my bones."
B. "Decreasing my intake of milk will prevent excessive intake of calcium."
C. "By increasing my fluid intake to 3 liters a day, I will eliminate more calcium from my system."
D. All of the above

171. Which of the following determines whether or not reimplantation can occur?
A. Availability of a reimplantation team
B. Whether the amputated part is an upper or a lower extremity
C. Occupation of the patient
D. Patient's insurance status

172. Which nursing diagnosis best explains the effect of cyanide poisoning?
A. Altered cardiopulmonary tissue perfusion
B. Ineffective airway clearance
C. Ineffective breathing pattern
D. Impaired gas exchange

173. The treatment plan for a patient in cardiogenic shock should have which of the following outcomes?
A. Increased left ventricular end-diastolic pressure
B. Increased systemic vascular resistance
C. Decreased cardiac output
D. Decreased left ventricular end-diastolic pressure

174. The patient receiving I.V. immune globulin therapy suddenly develops chest tightness, dyspnea, back pain, and chills. Which intervention is a priority for this patient?
A. Assess vital signs
B. Stop the infusion
C. Administer epinephrine (Adrenalin) 0.01 mg/kg S.C.
D. Administer diphenhydramine (Benadryl)

175. Which drug should be administered when a patient in septic shock develops bilateral pulmonary crackles and an S_3 heart sound?
A. Nitroprusside sodium (Nipride)
B. Nitroglycerin (Nitro-Bid)
C. Dopamine hydrochloride (Intropin)
D. Dobutamine hydrochloride (Dobutrex)

176. Which of the following fractures leads to severe complications in the pediatric patient?
A. Open fractures
B. Closed fractures
C. Dislocation fractures
D. Epiphyseal growth plate fractures

177. An important intervention in treating open pneumothorax is covering the wound. This is accomplished with which of the following?
A. Sterile saline–moistened gauze
B. Porous dressing taped on all four sides
C. Transparent nonporous dressing
D. Nonporous dressing taped on three sides

178. The nurse has administered nalbuphine hydrochloride (Nubain), a known opioid antagonist, for pain control. The nurse knows that the patient needs assessment for opioid dependence after which of the following outcomes?
A. Respiratory depression
B. Nausea and vomiting
C. Gooseflesh and diarrhea
D. Seizures

179. A patient is admitted to the emergency department. He has a stab wound to the heart, and the knife is still impaled in his chest. The patient's vital signs are blood pressure 70/40 mm Hg, pulse rate 132 beats/minute, respirations 28 breaths/minute and shallow, and oral temperature 98.4° F (36.9° C). Which nursing diagnosis best describes this patient's condition?
A. Impaired gas exchange
B. Decreased cardiac output
C. Risk for fluid volume deficit
D. Ineffective airway clearance

180. Which of the following is associated with hepatitis A?
A. Left upper quadrant pain
B. Right upper quadrant pain
C. Dark, tarry stools
D. Hematuria

181. An emergency department nurse has made a serious medication error on a pediatric patient. The nurse manager spoke promptly with the nurse privately, asked for her version of the story, reviewed medication error prevention strategies, and helped the nurse inform peers of the problem that led to the error. The nurse manager has provided which of the following?
A. Constructive feedback
B. Emotional support
C. Recognition
D. Goal setting

182. Autotransfusion can be performed on a patient with major blood loss from the chest. How many hours before the transfusion can the loss occur?
A. 4 hours
B. 10 hours
C. 8 hours
D. 5 hours

183. A patient is being treated with I.V. epinephrine and antihistamines after an anaphylactic reaction. Which evaluation finding suggests effective treatment?
A. Blood pressure 86/62 mm Hg
B. pH 7.45, PaO_2 86 mm Hg, $PaCO_2$ 30 mm Hg
C. Patent airway, no pulmonary basilar wheezes
D. Pulmonary basilar wheezes

184. A multitrauma patient has just arrived in the emergency department. Nasotracheal intubation was initiated at the scene by an emergency medical service unit. Which intervention must be done first?
A. Connect the nasotracheal tube to a volume ventilator.
B. Obtain arterial blood gas measurements to determine acid-base status.
C. Verify nasotracheal tube placement.
D. Attach the patient to a cardiac monitor and pulse oximeter.

185. A patient develops anaphylactic shock after receiving radiopaque dye and is on atenolol (Tenormin) 100 mg P.O. daily for hypertension. Which intervention should be implemented?
   A. Do not administer glucocorticoids.
   B. Administer high doses of epinephrine and Glucagon 5 to 15 mcg/minute I.V.
   C. Do not administer diphenhydramine (Benadryl).
   D. Administer high doses of inhaled bronchodilators.

186. Which nursing diagnosis is most appropriate for a patient with an intestinal obstruction?
   A. Fluid volume excess
   B. Impaired gas exchange
   C. Hypothermia
   D. Fluid volume deficit

187. A patient admitted to the emergency department has many learning needs in relation to an immediate problem. How does the nurse determine what these learning needs may be?
   A. Interview the patient or significant other to determine the extent of the patient's knowledge concerning the immediate complaint.
   B. Explain what the patient needs to know, and ask if the patient or significant other is aware of this information.
   C. Give the patient or significant other a handout of the health care organization's patient education offerings, and ask if any of the classes listed are of interest.
   D. Enroll the patient in patient education classes, and tell the patient or significant other when and where the classes will be held.

188. Which of the following statements from a patient discharged from the emergency department with acute otitis externa indicates an understanding of instructions?
   A. "I should wear earplugs when swimming."
   B. "I should make position changes slowly."
   C. "I need to keep my home uncluttered."
   D. "I should contact my doctor if my ear aches and the pain increases when I lay down."

189. Which of the following is the purpose of corticosteroids in a patient diagnosed with a brain tumor?
   A. Control absence seizures
   B. Provide symptomatic relief of agitation
   C. Reduce cerebral edema
   D. Reduce pain

190. Which of the following is a true definition of a disaster?
   A. A situation that results in more than three injured at a single location
   B. A natural occurrence, such as an earthquake or a tornado
   C. A situation that produces an immediate patient load greater than the normal emergency medical system and health care facilities can handle
   D. A situation in which many people are killed at once

191. Which is the most effective treatment of intrapulmonary shunt in the adult respiratory distress syndrome patient?
   A. Administer a diuretic
   B. Increase the FIO_2
   C. Implement positive end-expiratory pressure
   D. Decrease fluid intake

192. Which nursing diagnosis is most appropriate for a patient with eclampsia?
   A. Risk for injury
   B. Anxiety
   C. Decreased cardiac output
   D. Fluid volume deficit

193. Which acid-base imbalance is most likely seen in a patient with chronic obstructive pulmonary disease?
   A. Metabolic acidosis
   B. Respiratory acidosis
   C. Metabolic alkalosis
   D. Respiratory alkalosis

194. After a motor vehicle accident, a patient arrives in the emergency department complaining of dyspnea and sharp shoulder pain. Objective data reveal decreased breath sounds on the left, heart sounds shifted to the right, and bowel sounds in the middle chest. Which diagnosis is the most likely?
A. Hemothorax
B. Ruptured diaphragm
C. Aortic dissection
D. Tracheobronchial disruption

195. Which of the following statements about applying a splint is true?
A. The splint must immobilize the joint above and below the injury.
B. A traction splint is used only for femur fractures.
C. The extremity must be readjusted so that it is in a neutral position before applying the splint.
D. Air splints are ideal for patients being transported by air because they cushion the patient during the bumpy air ride.

196. When giving a patient discharge instructions about reducing the incidence of emboli, which action by the patient indicates the need for further teaching?
A. Leaning over to tie shoelaces
B. Moving the legs from side to side
C. Sitting with the legs crossed
D. Walking in and out of the room

197. Which of the following products is indicated for posterior epistaxis?
A. Merocel nasal tampon
B. 16-g indwelling urinary catheter
C. Nasostat nasal balloon
D. Gelfoam hemostatic agent

198. A 3-year-old child in respiratory distress is admitted to the emergency department. Vital signs are respiratory rate 44 breaths/minute, pulse 160 beats/minute, and temperature 99.8° F (38.2° C). Nasal mucous membranes are pale, bluish gray, and boggy with clear mucoid discharge. There is a high-pitched wheeze on expiration throughout the chest. Chest X-ray shows overdistended lungs. Which diagnosis is the most probable?
A. Bronchiolitis
B. Foreign-body obstruction
C. Asthma
D. Hypersensitivity pneumonitis

199. Which of the following is a true statement about epididymitis?
A. Elevation of the testis increases pain.
B. A child with epididymitis should be screened for possible molestation.
C. It is not necessary to examine and treat sexual partners.
D. Fertility is not affected in a patient with epididymitis.

200. Which of the following is the primary nursing diagnosis for a patient with angina?
A. Fluid volume excess
B. Decreased cardiac output
C. Pain
D. Altered cardiopulmonary tissue perfusion

201. The emergency department nurse should expect a patient with severe burn injuries to have which of the following electrolyte abnormalities in the immediate postburn phase?
A. Increased potassium, decreased sodium
B. Increased potassium, increased sodium
C. Decreased potassium, decreased sodium
D. Decreased potassium, increased sodium

202. A 4-year-old child presents with abrupt onset of high fever, stridor, drooling, tachypnea, and severe throat pain. Which diagnosis is the most likely?
A. Epiglottitis
B. Retropharyngeal abscess
C. Bacterial tracheitis
D. Viral croup syndrome

203. Which is the least effective intervention for a patient with flail chest?
   A. Apply a sandbag to the flail area of the chest.
   B. Intubate and ventilate the patient.
   C. Control pain to allow full lung expansion.
   D. Limit fluids unless hypovolemic shock is present.

204. Which of the following is a true statement about pelvic fractures?
   A. Pelvic fractures usually involve only one fracture site.
   B. Pelvic fractures are always stable.
   C. Bleeding associated with a pelvic fracture is usually arterial.
   D. Open pelvic fractures are associated with high mortality.

205. Which intervention is most appropriate for a patient with croup?
   A. Administering humidified air (mist therapy)
   B. Administering 100% oxygen by way of a face mask
   C. Administering corticosteroids
   D. Administering nebulized racemic epinephrine

206. After ruling out medical causes, which intervention is most appropriate for hyperventilation?
   A. Place a paper bag over the patient's nose and mouth.
   B. Place the patient in a position to facilitate breathing.
   C. Talk with the patient, providing reassurance.
   D. Monitor arterial blood gases.

207. When introducing change to an emergency department, which of the following tactics would increase acceptance?
   A. Do not burden the staff with the responsibility for input in the planning phase.
   B. Make several changes at once followed by a longer quiet phase with no changes.
   C. Always explain the reason for change.
   D. After carefully eliciting input from all staff, be firm and confident in presenting a final plan that should endure for the long term.

208. Which of the following is a common finding in a patient with an open pneumothorax?
   A. A chest wound with sucking sounds
   B. Increased breath sounds over the affected area
   C. Resonance over the affected area
   D. Hemoptysis

209. A patient presents with an ankle injury. The ankle is moderately swollen, ecchymotic, and painful to palpation over the lateral and medial malleolus. Which of the following is a nursing priority?
   A. Applying ice and elevating the ankle
   B. Teaching the principles of crutch walking
   C. Getting an order for pain medication
   D. Applying a traction splint with 15 lb of traction

210. Which nursing diagnosis is appropriate for a patient with a suspected esophageal rupture?
   A. Fluid volume excess
   B. Risk for infection
   C. Decreased cardiac output
   D. Impaired gas exchange

211. Which of the following injuries should result in radiographic assessment by arteriography?
   A. An injury to a long bone
   B. A penetrating injury with the possibility of a fracture
   C. An open fracture
   D. An injury with suspected vascular damage

212. An elderly patient is brought to the emergency department by his neighbor, who states that he found the patient in his unheated home. The outdoor temperature is 27° F (2.8° C). The patient is lethargic and confused. Vital signs are blood pressure 90/46 mm Hg, pulse 50 beats/minute, respirations 14 breaths/minute, and temperature 89.6° F (32° C). Which of the following statements about the treatment of patients with severe hypothermia is true?
A. The application of warm blankets is sufficient to prevent further heat loss.
B. Active and rapid external warming is the treatment of choice for this patient.
C. Complications of rewarming include metabolic acidosis and cardiac arrhythmias.
D. After the temperature returns to normal, the patient may be safely discharged.

213. Adenosine (Adenocard) is administered to a patient with paroxysmal supraventricular tachycardia. The patient complains of faintness and becomes pale. The monitor shows asystole. The emergency nurse should do which of the following?
A. Begin cardiopulmonary resuscitation
B. Administer 1 mg of atropine sulfate by I.V. push
C. Observe the patient for several seconds
D. Administer epinephrine (Adrenalin) by I.V. push

214. A repeat clean-catch urine specimen (or a catheterized specimen) may need to be collected if which of the following is reported in the urinalysis?
A. Presence of bacteria
B. Presence of increased epithelial cells
C. Presence of increased white blood cells
D. Presence of pus

215. Which nursing diagnosis best describes the effect of rapid infusion of room temperature crystalloids and stored refrigerated blood to a trauma patient in shock?
A. Decreased cardiac output
B. Altered renal, cardiac, and GI tissue perfusion
C. Hypothermia
D. Risk for altered body temperature

216. Which of the following is the purpose of patient classification systems in emergency departments?
A. To assist in the assignment of appropriate triage categories
B. To group patients according to the amount and complexity of their nursing care requirements so that staffing can be appropriated judiciously
C. To provide a system for prediction of census data
D. To validate the accuracy of diagnosis-related groups in fixing prospective payment for different groups of patients

217. An adult is brought to the emergency department with a burn injury. He has partial-thickness burns to his entire chest, right arm, and right thigh. Which of the following is a fairly accurate estimate of the body surface area that has been burned?
A. 45%
B. 27%
C. 18%
D. 36%

218. A patient is given instructions after treatment for heat cramps. Which of the following statements indicates that the patient understands the discharge instructions?
A. "I will take salt tablets while working outside."
B. "I will drink plenty of fluids and rest during the middle of the day."
C. "I will do most of my outside work between 11 a.m. and 2 p.m."
D. "If I experience these symptoms again, I will drink more fluids and continue working."

219. A patient presents to the emergency department complaining of shortness of breath, dizziness, and chest pain after a diving trip with friends. Which condition should the emergency nurse suspect?
A. Decompression sickness
B. Air embolism
C. Nitrogen narcosis
D. Spontaneous pneumothorax

220. When treating a patient involved in a radiation accident, the emergency nurse should do which of the following?
A. Treat life-threatening problems only after decontaminating the victim
B. Wear protective clothing
C. Wear a radiation meter
D. All of the above

221. A patient with a LeFort II fracture is transferred to the emergency department. The nurse looks for free-floating movement of which of the following?
A. Unilateral periorbital area
B. Nose and dental arch
C. Teeth and lower maxilla
D. All facial bones

222. Learning occurs best when there is two-way interaction. Which of the following methods allows for this?
A. A list of do's and don'ts written at the sixth-grade level
B. A short videotape that provides useful information and demonstration
C. An audiotaped discussion of the do's and don'ts
D. A discussion and demonstration involving the nurse and patient

223. A 5-year-old patient with a pea in his ear is admitted to the emergency department. The nurse needs which of the following to remove the pea?
A. Alligator forceps
B. 30-ml syringe
C. Lidocaine
D. Triethanolamine polypeptide oleate-condensate (Cerumenex)

224. A patient presents to the triage desk and complains of feeling like he is hungover. The symptoms have occurred for several mornings and go away as the day progresses. The patient also states that other family members have similar symptoms. Which of the following assessment questions is most appropriate for the triage nurse to ask?
A. Has anyone at work had similar symptoms?
B. Do you own a car?
C. Do you use gas heat or appliances?
D. Have you had any numbness or tingling?

225. A patient is admitted to the emergency department complaining of a sudden onset of right-sided facial weakness, drooling, and inability to close the right eyelid. The patient is alert and oriented. Slight speech impairment is noted. When the patient attempts to close the right eyelid, the eyeball moves upward. All other assessment findings are negative. Which of the following nursing diagnoses is most appropriate for this patient?
A. Risk for injury
B. Ineffective airway clearance
C. Impaired gas exchange
D. Pain

226. After ingesting a bottle of aspirin in a suicide attempt, a patient with severe salicylate poisoning has been admitted to the emergency department. The nurse should prepare to add which of the following medications to the patient's I.V. fluids?
A. Calcium gluconate
B. Folic acid
C. Sodium bicarbonate
D. Magnesium

227. Which of the following statements indicates that a patient with Ménière's disease understands the discharge instructions?
A. "I will put these eyedrops in my right eye every 6 hours."
B. "I'm going to send my daughter home tonight; she doesn't need to stay."
C. "I need to sit up slowly when I get out of bed."
D. "I'll put an ice pack on my ear to help the pain."

228. A patient is admitted to the emergency department after sustaining injuries in an explosion. The patient was near the area of explosion and was thrown to the ground. The patient has a fractured right humerus, a concussion, tinnitus, and a sanguineous discharge from a painful right ear. Which of the following is an appropriate intervention for this patient regarding her painful right ear?

A. Instruct the patient on the importance of following the prescribed antibiotic regimen.

B. Irrigate the right ear with warm normal saline.

C. Instill Auralgan eardrops for pain relief.

D. Investigate for evidence of cerebrospinal fluid.

229. A patient is admitted to the emergency department complaining of right ear pain. A diagnosis of acute external otitis, or swimmer's ear, is made. All except which of the following are signs and symptoms to expect?

A. Tender ear

B. Swollen canal

C. Bulging tympanic membrane

D. Redness to pinna

230. A patient with a severe posterior epistaxis of short duration is admitted to the emergency department. The patient is pale, weak, and slightly dizzy and complains of a headache. Vital signs are blood pressure 200/110 mm Hg, pulse 104 beats/minute, respirations 28 breaths/minute, and temperature 98° F (36.7° C). Which of the following laboratory test results is possible?

A. Markedly decreased hemoglobin

B. Decreased platelet count

C. Diminished prothrombin time

D. Increased creatinine level

231. All emergency nurses are compelled to treat with dignity the homeless patient with multiple minor complaints by which directive?

A. Personal or religious beliefs

B. Code of Ethics for Emergency Nurses

C. Clinical expertise

D. State and federal laws

232. Which of the following amputations is not favorable for successful reimplantation?

A. Multiple digits

B. Thumb

C. Pediatric extremity

D. Injuries at multiple levels on the same extremity

233. Which is the treatment of choice for a patient with an esophageal rupture?

A. Immediate intubation

B. Insertion of a nasogastric tube

C. Antibiotic administration

D. Chest tube insertion

234. Increasingly, health care agencies use a planning program style of budgeting in which the manager must justify all budget items each year. The manager must also detail cost-effectiveness for each expenditure. What is the name for this type of budgeting?

A. Zero-base budgeting

B. Cost-benefit budgeting

C. Fixed-ceiling budgeting

D. Flexible budgeting

235. When does intussusception occur in an infant?

A. The proximal bowel invaginates into the distal bowel.

B. Hypertrophy and hyperplasia of the circular antral and pyloric musculature result in gastric outlet obstruction.

C. A section of intestine twists on its own axis.

D. Solidified feces cause a mechanical obstruction.

236. Which type of injury is characterized by a pulling or stressing of a muscle or tendon beyond normal limits and results in damage to the fibers without bleeding?

A. Sprain

B. Abrasion

C. Strain

D. Contusion

237. Which of the following findings indicates worsening pulmonary function in a patient with flail chest?
   A. Accessory muscle use
   B. Increased pain with movement
   C. Increased blood pressure
   D. Shallow respirations

238. Which of the following is a symptom of radial head dislocation (nursemaid's elbow) in a pediatric patient?
   A. Ligamentous instability
   B. Excessive swelling
   C. Refusal to use arm
   D. Loss of arm length

239. The release of histamine in the antigen-antibody reaction during anaphylactic shock results in which condition?
   A. Vasodilation
   B. Vasoconstriction
   C. Increased myocardial contractility
   D. Decreased vascular permeability

240. About 16 hours after a fall, a patient is transferred to an emergency department from a nursing home. The fall resulted in a comminuted fracture of the left hip. About 1 hour after arrival in the emergency department, the patient begins to complain of chills and difficulty breathing. On auscultation of the patient's chest, the emergency nurse notes petechiae over the patient's anterior chest and neck. Which of the following is the likely cause of the patient's symptoms?
   A. Compartment syndrome
   B. Pulmonary embolus
   C. Fat embolus
   D. Myocardial infarction

241. Five days after a colon resection, a diabetic patient presents to the emergency department. This morning during a bout of coughing he felt a "pop." The incision is open and intestines are protruding from the wound. Which intervention is most appropriate for the emergency nurse?
   A. Gently push the intestines back into the abdomen.
   B. Cover the intestines with saline-moistened gauze.
   C. Apply and inflate all sections of a pneumatic antishock garment.
   D. Allow the intestines to be exposed to air.

242. Which of the following fractures has the highest potential for hemorrhage leading to hypovolemia?
   A. **Femur fracture**
   B. Forearm fracture
   C. Pelvic fracture
   D. Ankle fracture

243. Which records should accompany a patient being transferred to a trauma center?
   A. Chest X-ray
   B. Laboratory results
   C. Emergency department chart
   D. All of the above

244. Which of the following is the earliest indicator of a change in a patient's neurologic status?
   A. Pupillary reaction
   B. Motor response
   C. Capillary refill
   D. Level of consciousness

245. A patient with a hemothorax from blunt chest trauma is admitted to the emergency department. Three hours after receiving a blood transfusion, the patient begins to lose 200 ml of blood each hour from the chest tube. Which of the following is the most likely explanation for this finding?
   A. A vessel has been disrupted and requires surgical repair.
   B. This is the expected rate of chest tube drainage.
   C. The patient is having a transfusion reaction.
   D. A second chest tube should have been inserted to manage the loss.

246. Which of the following is the definitive therapy for a patient with pneumothorax?
A. Administer analgesics.
B. Insert two I.V. lines with large-bore needles.
C. Administer supplemental oxygen.
D. Perform tube thoracotomy.

247. Which of the following is an appropriate intervention for a trauma patient with hypovolemic shock and a urine specific gravity of 1.050?
A. Hold all I.V. fluids.
B. Administer a bolus of 40 ml/kg of crystalloid.
C. Insert an indwelling urinary catheter.
D. Administer furosemide (Lasix) 40 mg I.V.

248. The best way to evaluate a patient's integration of new information provided by the nurse is which of the following?
A. Using a pretest and posttest
B. Analyzing the content of the questions the patient asks
C. Asking the patient to explain how the information can be incorporated into the patient's lifestyle
D. Providing the patient with information about how to incorporate the information into the patient's lifestyle

249. Which of the following is the initial treatment for a patient with a tracheobronchial injury?
A. Suctioning to maintain airway patency
B. Preparing for chest tube insertion
C. Providing intubation and mechanical ventilation
D. Preparing for surgical intervention

250. A patient arrives in the emergency department complaining of joint pain, low-grade fever, and pruritus. The patient reports that his urine is dark colored. Which of the following is the most likely diagnosis for this patient?
A. Lyme disease
B. Hepatitis
C. Diphtheria
D. Human immunodeficiency virus

Answer Sheet

	A B C D		A B C D		A B C D		A B C D
1.	○ ○ ○ ○	26.	○ ○ ○ ○	51.	○ ○ ○ ○	76.	○ ○ ○ ○
2.	○ ○ ○ ○	27.	○ ○ ○ ○	52.	○ ○ ○ ○	77.	○ ○ ○ ○
3.	○ ○ ○ ○	28.	○ ○ ○ ○	53.	○ ○ ○ ○	78.	○ ○ ○ ○
4.	○ ○ ○ ○	29.	○ ○ ○ ○	54.	○ ○ ○ ○	79.	○ ○ ○ ○
5.	○ ○ ○ ○	30.	○ ○ ○ ○	55.	○ ○ ○ ○	80.	○ ○ ○ ○
6.	○ ○ ○ ○	31.	○ ○ ○ ○	56.	○ ○ ○ ○	81.	○ ○ ○ ○
7.	○ ○ ○ ○	32.	○ ○ ○ ○	57.	○ ○ ○ ○	82.	○ ○ ○ ○
8.	○ ○ ○ ○	33.	○ ○ ○ ○	58.	○ ○ ○ ○	83.	○ ○ ○ ○
9.	○ ○ ○ ○	34.	○ ○ ○ ○	59.	○ ○ ○ ○	84.	○ ○ ○ ○
10.	○ ○ ○ ○	35.	○ ○ ○ ○	60.	○ ○ ○ ○	85.	○ ○ ○ ○
11.	○ ○ ○ ○	36.	○ ○ ○ ○	61.	○ ○ ○ ○	86.	○ ○ ○ ○
12.	○ ○ ○ ○	37.	○ ○ ○ ○	62.	○ ○ ○ ○	87.	○ ○ ○ ○
13.	○ ○ ○ ○	38.	○ ○ ○ ○	63.	○ ○ ○ ○	88.	○ ○ ○ ○
14.	○ ○ ○ ○	39.	○ ○ ○ ○	64.	○ ○ ○ ○	89.	○ ○ ○ ○
15.	○ ○ ○ ○	40.	○ ○ ○ ○	65.	○ ○ ○ ○	90.	○ ○ ○ ○
16.	○ ○ ○ ○	41.	○ ○ ○ ○	66.	○ ○ ○ ○	91.	○ ○ ○ ○
17.	○ ○ ○ ○	42.	○ ○ ○ ○	67.	○ ○ ○ ○	92.	○ ○ ○ ○
18.	○ ○ ○ ○	43.	○ ○ ○ ○	68.	○ ○ ○ ○	93.	○ ○ ○ ○
19.	○ ○ ○ ○	44.	○ ○ ○ ○	69.	○ ○ ○ ○	94.	○ ○ ○ ○
20.	○ ○ ○ ○	45.	○ ○ ○ ○	70.	○ ○ ○ ○	95.	○ ○ ○ ○
21.	○ ○ ○ ○	46.	○ ○ ○ ○	71.	○ ○ ○ ○	96.	○ ○ ○ ○
22.	○ ○ ○ ○	47.	○ ○ ○ ○	72.	○ ○ ○ ○	97.	○ ○ ○ ○
23.	○ ○ ○ ○	48.	○ ○ ○ ○	73.	○ ○ ○ ○	98.	○ ○ ○ ○
24.	○ ○ ○ ○	49.	○ ○ ○ ○	74.	○ ○ ○ ○	99.	○ ○ ○ ○
25.	○ ○ ○ ○	50.	○ ○ ○ ○	75.	○ ○ ○ ○	100.	○ ○ ○ ○

	A	B	C	D		A	B	C	D		A	B	C	D		A	B	C	D
101.	○	○	○	○	126.	○	○	○	○	151.	○	○	○	○	176.	○	○	○	○
102.	○	○	○	○	127.	○	○	○	○	152.	○	○	○	○	177.	○	○	○	○
103.	○	○	○	○	128.	○	○	○	○	153.	○	○	○	○	178.	○	○	○	○
104.	○	○	○	○	129.	○	○	○	○	154.	○	○	○	○	179.	○	○	○	○
105.	○	○	○	○	130.	○	○	○	○	155.	○	○	○	○	180.	○	○	○	○
106.	○	○	○	○	131.	○	○	○	○	156.	○	○	○	○	181.	○	○	○	○
107.	○	○	○	○	132.	○	○	○	○	157.	○	○	○	○	182.	○	○	○	○
108.	○	○	○	○	133.	○	○	○	○	158.	○	○	○	○	183.	○	○	○	○
109.	○	○	○	○	134.	○	○	○	○	159.	○	○	○	○	184.	○	○	○	○
110.	○	○	○	○	135.	○	○	○	○	160.	○	○	○	○	185.	○	○	○	○
111.	○	○	○	○	136.	○	○	○	○	161.	○	○	○	○	186.	○	○	○	○
112.	○	○	○	○	137.	○	○	○	○	162.	○	○	○	○	187.	○	○	○	○
113.	○	○	○	○	138.	○	○	○	○	163.	○	○	○	○	188.	○	○	○	○
114.	○	○	○	○	139.	○	○	○	○	164.	○	○	○	○	189.	○	○	○	○
115.	○	○	○	○	140.	○	○	○	○	165.	○	○	○	○	190.	○	○	○	○
116.	○	○	○	○	141.	○	○	○	○	166.	○	○	○	○	191.	○	○	○	○
117.	○	○	○	○	142.	○	○	○	○	167.	○	○	○	○	192.	○	○	○	○
118.	○	○	○	○	143.	○	○	○	○	168.	○	○	○	○	193.	○	○	○	○
119.	○	○	○	○	144.	○	○	○	○	169.	○	○	○	○	194.	○	○	○	○
120.	○	○	○	○	145.	○	○	○	○	170.	○	○	○	○	195.	○	○	○	○
121.	○	○	○	○	146.	○	○	○	○	171.	○	○	○	○	196.	○	○	○	○
122.	○	○	○	○	147.	○	○	○	○	172.	○	○	○	○	197.	○	○	○	○
123.	○	○	○	○	148.	○	○	○	○	173.	○	○	○	○	198.	○	○	○	○
124.	○	○	○	○	149.	○	○	○	○	174.	○	○	○	○	199.	○	○	○	○
125.	○	○	○	○	150.	○	○	○	○	175.	○	○	○	○	200.	○	○	○	○

	A	B	C	D			A	B	C	D
201.	○	○	○	○		226.	○	○	○	○
202.	○	○	○	○		227.	○	○	○	○
203.	○	○	○	○		228.	○	○	○	○
204.	○	○	○	○		229.	○	○	○	○
205.	○	○	○	○		230.	○	○	○	○
206.	○	○	○	○		231.	○	○	○	○
207.	○	○	○	○		232.	○	○	○	○
208.	○	○	○	○		233.	○	○	○	○
209.	○	○	○	○		234.	○	○	○	○
210.	○	○	○	○		235.	○	○	○	○
211.	○	○	○	○		236.	○	○	○	○
212.	○	○	○	○		237.	○	○	○	○
213.	○	○	○	○		238.	○	○	○	○
214.	○	○	○	○		239.	○	○	○	○
215.	○	○	○	○		240.	○	○	○	○
216.	○	○	○	○		241.	○	○	○	○
217.	○	○	○	○		242.	○	○	○	○
218.	○	○	○	○		243.	○	○	○	○
219.	○	○	○	○		244.	○	○	○	○
220.	○	○	○	○		245.	○	○	○	○
221.	○	○	○	○		246.	○	○	○	○
222.	○	○	○	○		247.	○	○	○	○
223.	○	○	○	○		248.	○	○	○	○
224.	○	○	○	○		249.	○	○	○	○
225.	○	○	○	○		250.	○	○	○	○

Answers and Rationales

1. CORRECT ANSWER—**B.** *Rationales:* Central venous pressure (CVP) is the best unit of measure for identifying shock in a trauma patient. CVP measures right-sided heart pressure, which reflects blood and fluid status. A normal CVP measurement is 4 to 10 cm H_2O pressure. A value less than 4 cm may indicate hypovolemia or vasodilation. Hemoglobin and hematocrit are not the best indicators of early shock in a trauma patient because they may be normal in the early phase of shock unless there has been massive blood loss. It normally takes 4 to 6 hours for the actual blood loss to be reflected in the hemoglobin and hematocrit levels.
Nursing process step: Assessment

2. CORRECT ANSWER—**B.** *Rationales:* The umbilical cord may be wrapped around the baby's neck. The nurse should look and feel around the neck. If the umbilical cord is present, the nurse should attempt to slip it over the baby's head. If the cord is too tight, the nurse should clamp it in two places and cut between the clamps. Then, the airway may be suctioned. The baby may need to be stimulated to cry after delivery. The shoulders are not delivered until the nurse has checked for the umbilical cord.
Nursing process step: Intervention

3. CORRECT ANSWER—**B.** *Rationales:* Parts that are distally positioned, such as fingers and toes, have less muscle tissue involvement and, therefore, have a good reimplantation rate. Because of extensive damage to blood vessels and the increased risk of debris-contaminated tissue, crush injuries have a less successful reimplantation rate than guillotine injuries (those that are severed with an extremely sharp cutting edge rather than a twisting or tearing type of injury). Contaminated versus clean injury: Injuries caused by sharp glass or a sharp knife have less need for debridement than injuries sustained in a crush injury from a surface that is coated with soil, rust, or oil. Other factors that affect reimplantation success include the age of the patient (children have more successful implantations because of generally healthier vascular systems) and care of the amputated part before reattachment (amputated parts should be kept cool and reattached within 6 hours of the injury).
Nursing process step: Analysis

4. CORRECT ANSWER—**C.** *Rationales:* Ingestion or inhalation of cyanide produces an intracellular anoxic poisoning by preventing oxidative phosphorylation; the result is anaerobic metabolism, lactic acidosis, and decreased adenosine triphosphate production. Cyanide ingestion quickly results in apnea, seizures, and coma. Gastric emptying, therefore, may be a treatment option but only through lavage. The use of oral agents such as ipecac may result in aspiration. Naloxone is used in the treatment of narcotic analgesic overdose. Activated charcoal is used in a variety of toxic poisonings, although it is not commonly used in patients who have ingested ethanol, hydrocarbon, or cyanide.
Nursing process step: Intervention

5. CORRECT ANSWER—**A.** *Rationales:* This rule prohibits unstable, critical patients from being diverted to hospitals farther away rather than being transported to the closest emergency department. Even though the hospital may not offer the needed services, the patient must be medically stable before transport to another facility. This is a specific mandate in the 1989 COBRA. The emergency department cannot refuse critical or unstable patients for any reason.

6. CORRECT ANSWER—**C.** *Rationales:* Hypertensive crisis secondary to psychotropic drug therapy is characterized by hyperthermia, chest pain, tachycardia, and palpitations.
Nursing process step: Assessment

7. CORRECT ANSWER—**B.** *Rationales:* Neuroleptic malignant syndrome is thought to occur as a result of dopaminergic blockade at receptor sites secondary to administration of neuroleptic agents. Classic signs include hyperthermia, muscle rigidity, diaphoresis, tachycardia, hypertension, and akinesia.
Nursing process step: Assessment

8. CORRECT ANSWER—**D.** *Rationales:* Nitroglycerin reduces preload and is, therefore, beneficial in the management of acute pulmonary edema. Nitroglycerin's vasodilator properties prevent its use in the management of cerebral hemorrhage, head trauma, and increased intracranial pressure.
Nursing process step: Intervention

9. CORRECT ANSWER—**B.** *Rationales:* Communicating with an anxious patient requires that the nurse be an active listener and provide an environment in which the patient can maintain self-control. Questioning an anxious person tends to increase the patient's anxiety and verbalizing support takes away the patient's self-control. Silence may imply doubt on the part of the listener.
Nursing process step: Intervention

10. CORRECT ANSWER—**B.** *Rationales:* After a beta-adrenergic blocker or calcium channel blocker overdose, glucagon is administered in a dose of 50 to 150 mcg/kg to reverse the effects of beta blockade. Glucagon enhances myocardial contractility and increases heart rate and atrioventricular conduction in a separate cellular pathway distinct from the adrenergic receptor pathway. Therefore, it is able to stimulate the myocardium in the presence of beta-adrenergic blockade. Lidocaine and bretylium are used in the treatment of ventricular tachyarrhythmias. $D_{50}W$ is used in the treatment of hypoglycemia.
Nursing process step: Intervention

11. CORRECT ANSWER—**A.** *Rationales:* The ability to respond and focus in children is synonymous with an adult being oriented to person, place, and time. An infant who has a glassy stare (indicating an inability to focus) may suggest serious central nervous system derangement, necessitating emergent treatment.
Nursing process step: Evaluation

12. CORRECT ANSWER—**B.** *Rationales:* The brain dead patient with diabetes insipidus has lost the ability to produce antidiuretic hormone. The result is a high urine output that, if left untreated, can be as high as 24 L/24 hours. This can result in a fluid volume deficit. The high urine output can be managed with fluid resuscitation and vasopressin (Pitressin) until the patient can be prepared for organ harvest. The patient's oxygenation is being managed with mechanical ventilation, so there should not be impaired gas exchange. The brain dead patient has had an alteration in cerebral tissue perfusion, but it is no longer of concern.
Nursing process step: Analysis/Nursing diagnosis

13. CORRECT ANSWER—A. *Rationales:* Initial response to low perfusion states result in increased secretion of catecholamines (epinephrine and norepinephrine). Vasoconstriction of the peripheral vessels shunts blood to the vital organs (heart and brain). The heart rate and contractility increase in an effort to increase preload. When compensatory mechanisms fail, peripheral vessels dilate and peripheral and splanchnic pooling occur.
Nursing process step: Evaluation

14. CORRECT ANSWER—B. *Rationales:* Sleep disturbances (nightmares, insomnia) are the earliest and most frequently reported physical symptom after critical incident stress. Loss of appetite, loss of intimacy, and fatigue may also be seen but are less common.
Nursing process step: Assessment

15. CORRECT ANSWER—A. *Rationales:* A 2-year-old child receiving adequate fluid replacement has a normal urine output of 1 to 2 ml/kg/hour.
Nursing process step: Evaluation

16. CORRECT ANSWER—A. *Rationales:* Turner's sign is a discoloration of the flank area as a result of a retroperitoneal bleed. Blood in the mediastinum is indicative of an aortic disruption and is seen best on an upright chest X-ray. Increased intracranial pressure is exhibited by alterations in mental status, blood pressure, heart rate, and respirations. Splenic injury produces referred pain to the left shoulder and neck and is known as Kehr's sign.
Nursing process step: Assessment

17. CORRECT ANSWER—D. *Rationales:* Neurogenic diabetes insipidus occurs after insult to the hypothalamus or the posterior pituitary gland, resulting in an alteration in antidiuretic hormone (ADH) secretion. After traumatic injury to the brain, ADH levels can decrease, resulting in high urine output. Classic signs include high serum sodium and osmolality, hypokalemia, and low urine osmolality due to excessive urine output.
Nursing process step: Assessment

18. CORRECT ANSWER—A. *Rationales:* The nurse should anticipate the use of a 5-mm endotracheal tube (ETT). ETT size is estimated using the following formula:

(16 + age in years) ÷ 4 = ETT size in millimeters

In the given scenario, the equation would be:

(16 + 4) ÷ 4 = 5 mm

Nursing process step: Intervention

19. CORRECT ANSWER—C. *Rationales:* The patient with peritonitis may experience decreased intravascular fluid volume related to a fluid shift in the peritoneal space, vomiting, and decreased oral intake. Pain is also a factor and should be addressed as appropriate. The patient with peritonitis has inadequate nutrition, but nutrition is not a priority concern in the emergency department. The patient with peritonitis is at risk for systemic infection and should receive I.V. antibiotics.
Nursing process step: Analysis

20. CORRECT ANSWER—B. *Rationales:* Congestive heart failure is the most common presenting symptom after cardiac transplantation. Because of the lack of vagal innervation of the transplanted heart, tachycardia, chest pain, and jaw pain related to ischemia are not possible.
Nursing process step: Assessment

21. CORRECT ANSWER—D. *Rationales:* Of primary importance in patients with orthopedic injury is the determination of neurovascular status. Impaired neurovascular status may be limb-threatening or life-threatening. Tetanus immunization, last oral intake, and the presence of contaminants are secondary concerns.
Nursing process step: Assessment

22. CORRECT ANSWER—**D.** *Rationales:* The concentration of epinephrine is 1 mg divided by 250 ml = 0.004 mg/ml or 4 mcg/ml. To infuse 1.25 mcg/minute, the nurse should infuse 19 ml/hour. Use the following formula: Dosage in micrograms per minute multiplied by 60 minutes divided by the concentration of drug = pump setting: 1.25 mcg/minute × 60 minutes = (75) divided by 4 mcg/ml = 18.75, or 19 ml/hour.
Nursing process step: Intervention

23. CORRECT ANSWER—**D.** *Rationales:* Adenosine is the drug of choice for paroxysmal supraventricular tachycardia; 6 mg is given rapid I.V. push over 1 to 3 seconds. If there's no response in 1 to 2 minutes, 12 mg may be given. Bretylium is used to treat refractory ventricular fibrillation. Digoxin and diltiazem are considered third-line drugs in the treatment of supraventricular tachycardia.
Nursing process step: Intervention

24. CORRECT ANSWER—**B.** *Rationales:* Tachycardia is not an indicator of increased intracranial pressure. The earliest and most sensitive indicator of increased intracranial pressure is a change in the level of consciousness. A compensatory mechanism that attempts to provide adequate cerebral perfusion pressure as intracranial pressure increases is Cushing's triad. Signs of the triad include widening pulse pressure, bradycardia, and increased systolic blood pressure.
Nursing process step: Assessment

25. CORRECT ANSWER—**A.** *Rationales:* Extremity pain that is regularly produced by the same degree of exercise and is relieved by rest is probably claudication. The other conditions are not immediately relieved by rest and are not consistent in presentation.
Nursing process step: Assessment

26. CORRECT ANSWER—**A.** *Rationales:* Survivors of sudden death need the support of loved ones. Therefore, the emergency department nurse should ensure that the family has been notified. The survivor needs to participate in decision making regarding the treatment plan. Providing opportunities for decision making decreases the patient's feelings of powerlessness. When possible, have someone stay with the patient to promote security.
Nursing process step: Intervention

27. CORRECT ANSWER—**B.** *Rationales:* Alteration in thought processes (disorganized thinking) is one of the hallmark signs of psychosis. The psychotic patient has difficulty recognizing reality. The patient does not have a personal identity disturbance and is not confused or in spiritual distress.
Nursing process step: Analysis

28. CORRECT ANSWER—**B.** *Rationales:* During helicopter transfer, assessment of breath sounds is difficult. An electronic end-tidal carbon dioxide detector best assures that the patient is ventilating. Cardiac monitors show rate changes, but a rate change is a nonspecific finding. Pulse oximetry is not accurate in the presence of vibrations such as those experienced during transfer. A laryngoscope allows visual assessment of tube placement but is not useful for constant monitoring.
Nursing process step: Evaluation

29. CORRECT ANSWER—**C.** *Rationales:* Patients with inferior wall infarction may experience bradycardia and atrioventricular conduction disturbances. Anterior wall infarction may lead to tachycardia and heart block. Tachycardia is also a sign of heart failure and cardiogenic shock, both complications of myocardial infarction.
Nursing process step: Assessment

30. CORRECT ANSWER—**D.** *Rationales:* Normal tissue pressure is less than 20 mm Hg. Tissue pressures in excess of 30 mm Hg with suspicious clinical findings are usually indicative of compartment syndrome and require further intervention.
Nursing process step: Intervention

31. CORRECT ANSWER—**C.** *Rationales:* Parkinson's disease is a degenerative condition of the basal ganglia. It can also be induced as a result of drug therapy. Such drugs include neuroleptics, antihypertensives, and antiemetics.
Nursing process step: Assessment

32. CORRECT ANSWER—**C.** *Rationales:* The patient with a severed leg has a serious injury that requires immediate attention and is amenable to medical intervention. Therefore, that patient would receive priority in this scenario. The patient with an open head injury and the patient with severe burns are hemodynamically compromised and have a grave prognosis. In addition, the resources to treat them during a disaster are inappropriate. The patient with facial lacerations is stable and the injuries are relatively minor; therefore, that patient's care can be delayed.
Nursing process step: Assessment

33. CORRECT ANSWER—**C.** *Rationales:* First determine the concentration:

$$\frac{50 \text{ mg}}{250 \text{ ml}} = 0.2 \text{ mg/ml}$$

then, because the dose is ordered mcg/kg/min convert to mcg/ml:

$$0.2 \times 1,000 = 200 \text{ mcg/ml}$$

Then set up the following equation:

$$\frac{\text{Dosage} \times \text{patient's weight (in kg)} \times 60}{\text{Infusion concentration}}$$

$$\frac{3 \text{ mcg/kg/min} \times 89 \text{ kg} \times 60}{200 \text{ mcg/ml}} = 80.1$$

Round off to 80 ml/hr.

Nursing process step: Intervention

34. CORRECT ANSWER—**C.** *Rationales:* During times of increased stress, confusion, and overwhelming patient volumes, the use of familiar forms and medical records increases compliance with documentation of patient care. Disaster tags can minimize and standardize documentation. They are most useful if they have multiple copies, and these copies are distributed to the command post, public relations, or admissions.
Nursing process step: Planning/Intervention

35. CORRECT ANSWER—**C.** *Rationales:* Prodromal symptoms, which include itching, tingling, and paresthesia, may occur a few hours to 2 days before actual eruption of herpes lesions. Acyclovir reduces the duration of viral shedding, which begins just before lesion appearance and continues for about 12 days, but sexual activity should cease until lesions are healed or a posttreatment examination is done. All partners should have their own examination and treatment regimen. Douching is not recommended because it disturbs the normal flora that assists with preventing infection.
Nursing process step: Evaluation

36. CORRECT ANSWER—**A.** *Rationales:* Kawasaki disease is a form of vasculitis that attacks multiple body systems. Signs and symptoms include elevated temperature, conjunctivitis, "strawberry" tongue and lips, cervical lymphadenopathy, erythema of the palms and soles, and periungual desquamation. A butterfly rash (malar erythema) is associated with lupus erythematosus. Exophthalmos is associated with Graves' disease, a thyroid disorder. Koplik's spots, which are associated with rubeola, are reddened areas with gray-blue centers on the buccal mucosa.
Nursing process step: Assessment

37. **CORRECT ANSWER—B.** *Rationales:* Decreased cardiac output is the most common characteristic of congestive heart failure. Although all the listed nursing diagnoses are applicable to the patient with congestive heart failure, decreased cardiac output is the distinguishing factor. Decreased cardiac output can lead to decreased tissue perfusion. Impaired gas exchange may result from fluid overload and pulmonary edema. Subsequent hypoxia can lead to anxiety in the patient with acute congestive heart failure.
Nursing process step: Analysis

38. **CORRECT ANSWER—D.** *Rationales:* The family members should indicate a basic understanding of SIDS. Verbalizing that the baby may have smothered or choked demonstrates that they are not well informed or do not comprehend what they have been told about SIDS. It is normal for family members to be concerned about the cause of death and to verbalize positive memories about the child. Accepting a referral for a SIDS support group demonstrates that they are ready to move on.
Nursing process step: Evaluation

39. **CORRECT ANSWER—C.** *Rationales:* The return of cloudy fluid or the aspiration of gross blood or intestinal contents represents a positive peritoneal tap. The return of clear fluid would indicate a negative tap.
Nursing process step: Evaluation

40. **CORRECT ANSWER—B.** *Rationales:* Following the advanced cardiac life support guidelines for ventricular fibrillation, the appropriate action is to administer epinephrine 1 mg I.V. The patient may be defibrillated at 360 joules within 30 to 60 seconds. Lidocaine may then be administered in persistent ventricular fibrillation. Sodium bicarbonate is not indicated at this point, and its use should be guided by arterial blood gas levels.
Nursing process step: Intervention

41. **CORRECT ANSWER—B.** *Rationales:* Decisions regarding patient transfer must be based on need for additional or specialized care. "Dumping" uninsured or underinsured patients is not an acceptable reason for transfer. Lack of insurance is not a reason to prevent transfer of a patient to a specialized facility.
Nursing process step: Assessment

42. **CORRECT ANSWER—B.** *Rationales:* Immediate psychosocial interventions should focus on getting the patient to identify the cause of the distress and to identify coping behaviors successfully used in the past. The emergency nurse must support the patient and initiate health-related teaching. Giving antianxiety medications will not address the underlying problem. These patients are not disoriented and do not require restraints. Denial may be used as a coping mechanism before the patient is ready to face the situation. The patient should not be pressured to talk about the crisis.
Nursing process step: Intervention

43. **CORRECT ANSWER—B.** *Rationales: Clostridium tetani* is a gram-positive anaerobic spore that produces bacteria that inhabit the intestinal tracts of humans and animals. The bacterium enters the bloodstream and travels to the central nervous system. *Clostridium* can survive in soil for years. *Pasteurella multocida, Enterobacter,* and *Streptococcus* are commonly associated with dog bites.
Nursing process step: Analysis

44. **CORRECT ANSWER—B.** *Rationales:* The patient's safety is the first priority in the emergency department. Psychiatric patients should be told how to take their medications, and they should be able to verbalize an understanding of the instructions. It is unrealistic to expect the patient's thought process to be organized or the patient's auditory hallucinations to subside completely before discharge. The emergency department is not the place for a complete nutritional evaluation.
Nursing process step: Evaluation

45. CORRECT ANSWER—**D.** *Rationales:* The widened mediastinum along with clinical correlation represents a ruptured aorta. Blood leaking into the mediastinum increases intrathoracic pressure, resulting in pain and increased respiratory rate. A ruptured hemidiaphragm or pneumothorax is evident on chest X-ray and does not involve a widening of the mediastinum. A ruptured trachea could produce a pneumomediastinum on chest X-ray.
Nursing process step: Assessment

46. CORRECT ANSWER—**B.** *Rationales:* Organic reasons for delusional behavior must be ruled out before the patient is considered a psychiatric emergency. A psychiatric consult can be obtained once the patient is cleared medically. Lithium carbonate is not the drug of choice for this patient. Lithium is used for bipolar disease, not schizophrenia. Insisting that the delusions are not real will only antagonize the patient.
Nursing process step: Intervention

47. CORRECT ANSWER—**B.** *Rationales:* In third-degree heart block, there is no relation between P waves and QRS complexes. The atria and ventricles beat independent of one another. Idioventricular rhythms are wide complex and are usually slower and without P waves. Sinus bradycardia has a P wave for each QRS complex. Wenkebach has progressively longer PR intervals until a QRS complex is dropped. It has a regularly irregular rhythm.
Nursing process step: Assessment

48. CORRECT ANSWER—**C.** *Rationales:* Glucose is needed to sustain the work of the diaphragm in breathing. Because children have small stores of glucose, they are likely to suffer respiratory distress more quickly than adults. Decreased metabolic demands do not cause fatigue. Increased vital capacity and tidal volumes improve oxygenation and decrease the work of breathing.
Nursing process step: Analysis

49. CORRECT ANSWER—**A.** *Rationales:* Degenerative changes in the elderly, direct trauma, blunt trauma, and hereditary factors can all lead to retinal detachment. The most common cause is degenerative changes in the elderly. Minimal to moderate trauma to the eye may cause retinal detachment, but in such cases, predisposing factors play an important role. Severe trauma may cause retinal tears and detachment, even if there are no predisposing factors.
Nursing process step: Assessment

50. CORRECT ANSWER—**A.** *Rationales:* Labile emotions, hyperactivity or hypoactivity, poor social judgment, and grandiose context to speech are classic signs of bipolar disease. Vital signs are usually normal, unless other contributing factors are present. Patients with bipolar disease may have impaired thinking related to rapid progression of thoughts, flight of ideas, and grandiosity.
Nursing process step: Assessment

51. CORRECT ANSWER—**C.** *Rationales:* A positive halo sign indicates leaking of cerebrospinal fluid, usually from the ears or nose. Performing the Valsalva's maneuver, coughing, suctioning, and blowing of the nose increases intracranial pressure. Additional pressure will in turn increase the risk of further tearing of the dura mater and increase the release of cerebrospinal fluid. To reduce the risk of increased intracranial pressure or the introduction of infection, the fluid should be allowed to flow freely with minimal intervention.
Nursing process step: Intervention

52. CORRECT ANSWER—**D.** *Rationales:* Monitoring I.V. infusion rates is often difficult in transport; therefore, an I.V. infusion regulating pump is helpful. Iced saline is important for initial burn cooling, but it could precipitate hypothermia during transport. Cooling blankets are similarly not warranted. Pain should be controlled with analgesics. An end-tidal carbon dioxide monitor is of no value unless the patient is intubated.
Nursing process step: Analysis

53. CORRECT ANSWER—**A.** *Rationales:* The pain associated with myocardial contusion is not affected by coronary vasodilators. Both myocardial contusion and angina may result in arrhythmias and ECG changes. Hypotension, distended neck veins, and muffled heart sounds represent findings of cardiac tamponade.
Nursing process step: Assessment

54. CORRECT ANSWER—**B.** *Rationales:* Haloperidol is a phenothiazine and is capable of causing dystonic reactions. Diazepam and clonazepam are both benzodiazepines, and amitriptyline is a tricyclic antidepressant. Benzodiazepines and tricyclic antidepressants do not cause dystonic reactions. Benzodiazepines can cause drowsiness, lethargy, and hypotension. Tricyclic antidepressants can cause a decreased level of consciousness, tachycardia, dry mouth, and dilated pupils.
Nursing process step: Intervention

55. CORRECT ANSWER—**B.** *Rationales:* The initial defibrillation attempt would be 2 joules/kg. If unsuccessful, double the energy level for the second and third attempts.
Nursing process step: Intervention

56. CORRECT ANSWER—**C.** *Rationales:* Chelating agents bind with a heavy metal and the compound formed is primarily excreted in the urine. The patient should have adequate urine output before administration of chelating agents. The nurse should monitor renal function and urine output during and after therapy. Level of consciousness, respiratory status, and blood pressure should be monitored, but they are not specific to chelation therapy.
Nursing process step: Assessment

57. CORRECT ANSWER—**C.** *Rationales:* Diazoxide has a rapid onset of action and may be given 50 to 100 mg I.V. bolus every 5 to 10 minutes until blood pressure is lowered. A dose of 300 mg should not be exceeded. The sustained effect may be 4 to 12 hours.
Nursing process step: Intervention

58. CORRECT ANSWER—**A.** *Rationales:* Testicular torsion occurs as a sudden onset of testicular pain and, possibly, nausea, vomiting, and swelling of testes. Pain that significantly decreases may be a detrimental sign pointing to testicular ischemia, which may occur from 2 to 4 hours past initial onset. The patients with urinary retention, pelvic inflammatory disease, and pyelonephritis are in pain and moderate distress, but they can wait, if necessary.
Nursing process step: Assessment

59. CORRECT ANSWER—**C.** *Rationales:* Pericarditis is an inflammation of the pericardium. The symptoms described are indicative of pericarditis. The pain of myocardial infarction generally does not change with deep breathing or a change in position. Pleurisy and endocarditis are usually gradual in onset.
Nursing process step: Assessment

60. CORRECT ANSWER—**B.** *Rationales:* Allen's test is performed to ensure that collateral circulation to the hand is adequate. The radial and ulnar arteries are compressed simultaneously. The patient is then instructed to open and close a fist several times. The hand will become blanched. The radial artery is released, and the hand is observed for hyperemia. The procedure is repeated with the ulnar artery.
Nursing process step: Intervention

61. CORRECT ANSWER—**A.** *Rationales:* The concentration of nitroprusside is 0.4 mg/ml, or 400 mcg/ml (100 mg divided by 250 ml). To infuse 5 mcg/kg/minute, the nurse needs to infuse 60 ml/hour and should use this formula: Dosage in micrograms per kilogram per minute multiplied by the patient's weight in kilograms multiplied by 60 minutes divided by the concentration of the drug in micrograms per milliliter.
5 mcg/kg/minute × 80 kg = (400) × 60 minutes = (24,000) divided by 400 mcg/ml = 60 ml/hour
Nursing process step: Intervention

62. CORRECT ANSWER—**D.** *Rationales:* Status epilepticus is seizure activity that exceeds 30 minutes' duration or is a series of seizures that do not allow for full recovery between events. Prolonged seizure activity can result in loss of base reserve that will lead to metabolic acidosis. Other complications associated with status epilepticus include hyperthermia, hypoglycemia, cardiac arrhythmias, hypoxia, increased intracranial pressure, and airway obstruction.
Nursing process step: Evaluation

63. CORRECT ANSWER—**C.** *Rationales:* Insects are the most common foreign materials in the ears of adults. To remove an insect from a patient's ear, the nurse should instill mineral oil to fill the ear canal and then direct a light at the canal opening. The insect will crawl toward the light and out of the canal. Instilling water will cause the insect to swell and make removing it more difficult. Using forceps may cause the insect to break into pieces and necessitate further intervention.
Nursing process step: Intervention

64. CORRECT ANSWER—**B.** *Rationales:* Bleeding is the primary side effect of thrombolytic therapy. The nurse should establish three I.V. sites before administering therapy and should avoid giving the patient I.M. injections and drawing arterial blood gases. The patient should be monitored for bleeding. Reperfusion arrhythmias and hypotension may occur with thrombolytic therapy and are treated symptomatically.
Nursing process step: Evaluation

65. CORRECT ANSWER—**D.** *Rationales:* Cocaine-induced myocardial ischemia has been associated with coronary artery vasoconstriction, coronary thrombosis, and increased myocardial oxygen consumption. In addition, these patients often suffer from tachyarrhythmias.
Nursing process step: Evaluation

66. CORRECT ANSWER—**A.** *Rationales:* On arrival at the emergency department, the patient is owed a duty of care by the doctor and hospital staff.

67. CORRECT ANSWER—**A.** *Rationales:* The early clinical indicators for septic shock include hyperthermia, tachycardia, wide pulse pressure, tachypnea (resulting in respiratory alkalosis), and mental obtundation ranging from mild disorientation to confusion, lethargy, agitation, and coma. While alive in the body, bacteria and other microorganisms release endotoxins. Endotoxins activate the mediators — tumor necrosis factor, interleukin-1, and interferon-γ — which elicit a febrile response, resulting in hyperthermia. (Note that patients who are elderly, very young, or immunocompromised may be unable to elicit a febrile response to the chemical mediators and may develop hypothermia). Tachycardia is initiated by the sympathetic response to the increase in body temperature and the decrease in cardiovascular insufficiency from the dilation of the ventricles and vasodilation of the vasculature. Tachypnea is from the direct effects of endotoxins or secondary to kallikreins, bradykinin, prostaglandins, or complement activation. The wide pulse pressure comes from decreases in systemic vascular resistance and vasodilation of the vasculature. The altered mental state is thought to be from an altered state of amino acid metabolism or a disruption of the blood-brain barrier.
Nursing process step: Assessment

68. CORRECT ANSWER—**A.** *Rationales:* The pumping ability of the heart depends on contractility (force of ventricular contraction), preload (ventricular filling, end-diastolic volume), heart rate, and afterload (pressure against which the ventricle pumps). Cardiac output and index are the result of the pumping ability of the heart.
Nursing process step: Evaluation

69. CORRECT ANSWER—**A.** *Rationales:* The suicidal patient is at risk for injury, and nursing interventions should be directed at keeping the patient from harming himself. Suicidal patients may also suffer from spiritual distress, social isolation, and ineffective coping, but these involve long-term interventions and are not the priority while the patient is in the emergency department.
Nursing process step: Analysis

70. CORRECT ANSWER—**A.** *Rationales:* Decorticate and decerebrate posturing are indicative of cerebral damage. In decortication, the upper extremities are abducted with obvious flexion of the arms, wrists, and fingers; the lower extremities are hyperextended with plantar flexion. Hypotonia (flaccidity) presents with decreased muscle tone and weakness. Spasticity is an increase in muscle resistance to passive movement and is followed by a sudden decrease in resistance. Decerebration presents as hyperextension of the upper and lower extremities.
Nursing process step: Analysis

71. CORRECT ANSWER—**C.** *Rationales:* Retinal hemorrhages result from a temporary obstruction of venous return and are consistent with being shaken. Bilateral arm fractures, basilar skull fractures, and petechiae on the trunk may result from other forms of child abuse.
Nursing process step: Assessment

72. CORRECT ANSWER—**C.** *Rationales:* The recommended therapeutic range is 1.5 to 2.5 times the control time. Prothrombin times equal to or less than the control are of no therapeutic value. Prothrombin times greater than 3 times the control have no added benefit and may be associated with a higher risk of bleeding.
Nursing process step: Evaluation

73. CORRECT ANSWER—**B.** *Rationales:* Many women present with distended bladders because of the intense, scalding pain from urine touching the lesions. These women can benefit from the use of an indwelling urinary catheter for bladder relief and continuous urine drainage. Fluid intake should be increased rather than decreased to dilute the acid urine and to correct or prevent dehydration. Lesions should be kept dry, and loose-fitting cotton underwear is recommended. Other treatment regimens include the use of sitz baths and anesthetic ointments as well as acyclovir ointment for pain control.
Nursing process step: Planning/Intervention

74. CORRECT ANSWER—**A.** *Rationales:* Vomiting occurs secondary to increased intracranial pressure as the vagal centers of the medulla become irritated. Headache is usually in response to increased intracranial pressure, localized swelling, and distortion of blood vessels. Papilledema occurs as the result of edema of the optic nerve. Restlessness and irritability (altered level of consciousness) are signs of increased intracranial pressure.
Nursing process step: Assessment

75. CORRECT ANSWER—**C.** *Rationales:* Anything other than a single line, date, initials, and reason is suspect to legal counsel, insurance examiners, and other responsible authorities.

76. CORRECT ANSWER—**B.** *Rationales:* A patient presenting with congestive heart failure is classified as acute, which means that the patient must be seen within 30 to 60 minutes of arrival at the emergency department. A patient classified as urgent must be seen immediately. A nonacute patient can wait in turn to be seen, and a referable patient can be seen at the doctor's discretion and may be referred to another doctor at another time.
Nursing process step: Evaluation

77. CORRECT ANSWER—**B.** *Rationales:* All the diagnoses are appropriate for the patient with an open, depressed skull fracture. The problem that requires the most immediate attention is risk for infection related to trauma. If the fracture line is open even a few millimeters at the time of impact, it can allow dirt, hair, and glass to enter the cranial vault. Complications of infection include encephalopathy and meningitis.
Nursing process step: Analysis/Nursing diagnosis

78. CORRECT ANSWER—D. *Rationales:* Protamine sulfate, when given alone, acts as an anticoagulant. When given in the presence of heparin sodium, a stable salt is formed and the anticoagulant ability of both medications is lost. Vitamin K is the antidote for warfarin sodium (Coumadin) ingestion. Dimercaprol is used to promote the excretion of arsenic, gold, and mercury. Naloxone is effective in reversing the effects of opioid narcotics.
Nursing process step: Intervention

79. CORRECT ANSWER—A. *Rationales:* The patient with endocarditis may experience a decrease in cardiac output due to valvular dysfunction from vegetation. The vegetation causes emboli to form, which travel through the bloodstream to other organs, causing infarctions in the major organs. These infarctions lead to decreased tissue perfusion. Pain may be present at the left upper area of the stomach, radiating to the left shoulder. The patient may also complain of shortness of breath and a productive cough. Therefore, pain and impaired gas exchange are appropriate for this patient, but the priority diagnosis is altered tissue perfusion, which is also the cause of the other diagnoses.
Nursing process step: Analysis/Nursing diagnosis

80. CORRECT ANSWER—A. *Rationales:* The primary treatment for a patient with back pain is rest. Anti-inflammatory and antispasmodic medications will help the patient rest. Applying heat, not cold, is recommended. Weight loss and stretching exercises are interventions that should be initiated after acute pain subsides.
Nursing process step: Intervention

81. CORRECT ANSWER—B. *Rationales:* The key rationale for initiation of mechanical ventilation is apnea, $PaCO_2$ greater than 50 mm Hg, PaO_2 less than 50 mm Hg, pH less than 7.25, A-a gradient greater than 350 mm Hg, increased work of breathing, and a vital capacity of less than 10 ml/kg.
Nursing process step: Assessment

82. CORRECT ANSWER—B. *Rationales:* The lowest level of electrical energy required to initiate consistent capture with a pacemaker is referred to as pacing threshold. It is determined by achieving pacing at a high level and then gradually decreasing the energy level until capture ceases. For successful capture, the energy is then set a few milliamperes above the threshold. Underdrive pacing is used to interrupt tachyarrhythmias. Demand pacers fire only when the heart rate drops below a set rate.
Nursing process step: Evaluation

83. CORRECT ANSWER—B. *Rationales:* Discharge and follow-up instructions can serve as a defense in litigation if it can be demonstrated that the patient was nonadherent to instructions and, therefore, furthered his or her own injury. The patient's remarks, the remarks of other personnel, and the patient's intellectual level should be included in the record only if the discharging nurse believes that the comments illustrate the patient's ability or willingness to adhere to instructions.

84. CORRECT ANSWER—C. *Rationales:* A mandibular fracture can predispose the patient to an ineffective airway because associated bleeding, edema, or tongue displacement can obstruct the airway. A nasopharyngeal or an oropharyngeal airway may be needed. Fluid volume deficit, altered tissue perfusion, and decreased cardiac output do not present problems related to a singular mandibular injury.
Nursing process step: Analysis/Nursing diagnosis

85. CORRECT ANSWER—C. *Rationales:* Disaster preparedness planning is an ongoing process and should not end with the revision or development of a plan. Plan revision may occur after a disaster, but this is not the only time to make changes. Census fluctuations are too unpredictable to adequately plan a disaster exercise.
Nursing process step: Evaluation

86. CORRECT ANSWER—**B.** *Rationales:* Damage to the femoral nerve results in the patient's inability to raise the affected leg when it is straight, extend the knee, or sense stimulus to the anterior thigh. Median nerve injuries are evidenced by inability to dorsiflex the affected wrist or extend the metacarpophalangeal joints. Sensory deviation with median nerve injury results in altered sensation to the dorsal web space between the thumb and index finger. Tibial nerve injuries result in altered plantar flexion of the foot and sensory changes to the sole. Peroneal nerve damage results in altered dorsiflexion of the foot and sensory changes to the web space between the great and second toes.
Nursing process step: Assessment

87. CORRECT ANSWER—**C.** *Rationales:* Cheyne-Stokes respirations are characterized by respirations of increasing depth and frequency followed by a period of apnea lasting for 10 to 60 seconds. The changes in rate and depth are in response to levels of carbon dioxide. Periods of apnea occur when the stimulation to respiratory centers diminishes. Apneustic breathing is characterized by a pause of 2 to 3 seconds after a full or prolonged inspiration. Biot's respirations are irregular and unpredictable with deep and shallow random breaths and pauses. Cluster breathing appears as a group of irregular breaths with periods of apnea at irregular intervals.
Nursing process step: Assessment

88. CORRECT ANSWER—**A.** *Rationales:* The sympathetic nervous system responds to a perceived threat by releasing epinephrine, which causes vasoconstriction. This vasoconstriction results in tachycardia, cold and clammy skin, dry mouth, and dilated pupils. Warm and dry skin, constricted pupils, and bradycardia would not occur.
Nursing process step: Assessment

89. CORRECT ANSWER—**C.** *Rationales:* Hypoxemia is the most common underlying cause of pediatric cardiopulmonary arrest. It leads to marked bradycardia and, eventually, asystole in the pediatric patient. Ensuring optimum oxygenation is the most important intervention in this patient population. The other options may lead to cardiopulmonary arrest in the pediatric patient, but they are much less common.
Nursing process step: Analysis

90. CORRECT ANSWER—**C.** *Rationales:* Antibiotic therapy should be administered as soon as possible after traumatic injury. Research indicates that antibiotics given preoperatively are most effective because the bacterial count is low and the bacteria are most amenable to antibiotics. The goal of early antibiotic therapy is to reach an effective blood concentration before or at the time of wound closure and, thus, limit the threat of infection. I.V. administration of antibiotics results in higher concentrations than oral dosing.
Nursing process step: Evaluation

91. CORRECT ANSWER—**D.** *Rationales:* The lack of necessary resources, a delay in mobilizing resources, and the inability to stabilize the patient are all acceptable reasons for transferring a patient.
Nursing process step: Assessment

92. CORRECT ANSWER—**A.** *Rationales:* Changes in leads II, III, and aVF are indicative of damage to the inferior wall of the heart. The lateral wall shows changes in leads I, II, III, aVL, V_5, and V_6. Anterior changes are shown in leads V_1 through V_4, I, and aVL. Apical damage is shown in leads II, aVF, V_5, and V_6.
Nursing process step: Assessment

93. CORRECT ANSWER—**B.** *Rationales:* Preventive measures are an important part of migraine headache management. Biofeedback therapy, relaxation tapes, and assertiveness training can reduce stressors that may precipitate an event. A patient who is taking ergotamine tartrate should avoid using oral contraceptives during pharmacologic management of the migraine. The patient should be instructed to avoid excessive caffeine, nitrates, alcohol, wheat, and chocolate; ingesting these foods may precipitate an attack. Propranolol (Inderal) should be taken as a prophylactic measure against migraine headaches. It is a beta blocker that acts by inhibiting vasodilation.
Nursing process step: Evaluation

94. CORRECT ANSWER—**C.** *Rationales:* The most characteristic finding of asthma is expiratory wheezing; however, absence of wheezing could indicate increased severity of the attack. The nurse should remember that not all wheezing signals asthma. Dark circles under the eyes, also known as allergic shiners, and bluish, boggy nasal turbinates are seen in patients with allergies as well as asthma. Therefore, these are not significant findings for diagnosing asthma. Moist crackles indicate the presence of fluid in the lungs' small airways and are heard in patients with pneumonia and early stages of pulmonary edema.
Nursing process step: Assessment

95. CORRECT ANSWER—**C.** *Rationales:* The initial pharmacologic treatment for an anaphylaxis-allergic reaction is epinephrine. Epinephrine slows the release of cellular chemical mediators and causes vasoconstriction. This vasoconstriction improves hypotensive states and decreases edematous tissue. In severe anaphylaxis, a 1:10,000 epinephrine solution should be administered I.V. slowly in a 0.1- to 0.25-mg dose. The administration of 0.1 to 0.5 mg of 1:1,000 S.C. epinephrine is an appropriate intervention as treatment for allergic reactions that are not true anaphylaxis. Diphenhydramine, a histamine receptor antagonist, can be administered in doses of 25 to 50 mg by way of oral, I.V., or I.M. routes. Cimetadine, also a histamine receptor antagonist, is not a first-line drug in the treatment of anaphylactic reactions.
Nursing process step: Intervention

96. CORRECT ANSWER—**A.** *Rationales:* Ipecac is contraindicated in the ingestion of most petroleum distillates, such as paint thinner, because of the potential for aspiration. The risk for aspiration must be weighed against the toxicity of the petroleum product ingested. Activated charcoal may be ordered to absorb toxins in the petroleum product. Gastric lavage may be ordered to remove toxins if the airway is protected by endotracheal intubation. Oxygen may be ordered if aspiration has occurred.
Nursing process step: Intervention

97. CORRECT ANSWER—**C.** *Rationales:* Elevating the area above the heart reduces swelling and pain. It is recommended that sutures to a hand be left intact until day 8 to 10. For improved cosmetic results, sutures involving the forehead, nose, and eyelid may be removed in 3 to 5 days. Patients should be advised to keep the area clean and dry for the first 24 hours. Showers may be taken after that, but the patient should avoid prolonged soaking of the site. Redness is a sign of infection, and the patient should consult a doctor if redness appears. Other signs of infection include red streaks, purulent drainage, fever, lymph node enlargement, and swelling.
Nursing process step: Evaluation

98. **CORRECT ANSWER—A.** *Rationales:* Magnesium sulfate is used to control seizures in pregnancy-induced hypertension. Urine output of less than 30 ml/hour should be reported. The drug should be withheld if respirations are fewer than 16 breaths/minute; magnesium sulfate may cause respiratory depression. Hypermagnesemia may result in depressed patellar reflexes. Vaginal bleeding is not associated with magnesium sulfate administration.
Nursing process step: Assessment

99. **CORRECT ANSWER—A.** *Rationales:* The nursing diagnosis of rape-trauma syndrome refers to both the acute and the long-term phases experienced by the victim of sexual assault. Specific nursing interventions can be planned based on this diagnosis. The rape victim may also experience fear, anxiety, and hopelessness; however, these diagnoses are not specific.
Nursing processes step: Analysis/Nursing diagnosis

100. **CORRECT ANSWER—B.** *Rationales:* Removal of the stinger is best done by using a dull object to scrape the stinger from the surface of the skin. Cold packs, not heat, should be applied to the site. Grasping and pulling the stinger are not recommended because those actions may release more venom from the sac. The area should be cleaned and cold packs applied to the site. Elevating the extremity reduces accompanying edema.
Nursing process step: Intervention

101. **CORRECT ANSWER—A.** *Rationales:* An opioid overdose or pontine hemorrhage produces pupils that can be described as "barely visible" or pinpoint. The patient with midbrain damage has pupils that are nonreactive and midposition. Severe anoxia results in bilateral fixed and dilated pupils. Previous cataract surgery should be suspected in the patient with keyhole-shaped pupils.
Nursing process step: Assessment

102. **CORRECT ANSWER—C.** *Rationales:* Symptoms associated with scabies infestation include red-brown linear markings on the wrists, between the fingers, at the belt and nipple line, and in the genital area. Pruritus is present and is accentuated at night when the activity of the mites increases. Raised, scaly, round patches with relatively flat centers on the hands, feet, trunk, and groin are associated with ringworm. A pink macular rash over the palms, soles, hands, feet, wrists, and ankles is associated with Rocky Mountain spotted fever. The rash later becomes petechial and mimics meningococcemia. Urticaria is rapidly appearing wheals or papules that are the result of a vascular allergic reaction. It is often accompanied by severe itching.
Nursing process step: Assessment

103. **CORRECT ANSWER—B.** *Rationales:* A foreign object dropped into the cast may result in a wound or pressure sore to the skin. If a wound occurs, the risk for infection is great. Therefore, the patient must be instructed not to attempt to retrieve the object and to call the follow-up care provider instead. Keeping the cast dry will maintain cast stability and prevent premature degradation. Having the patient wiggle the toes at least once every hour assists with circulation and assures distal neuromotor function. Elevating the extremity above the level of the heart promotes venous drainage and decreased extremity swelling and pain.
Nursing process step: Evaluation

104. **CORRECT ANSWER—C.** *Rationales:* Oxytocin causes uterine smooth muscle to contract and, therefore, increases abdominal cramping. It does not increase urine output or heart rate. Vaginal bleeding should slow down but does not cease completely.
Nursing process step: Evaluation

105. CORRECT ANSWER—**B.** *Rationales:* Normal healing consists of a series of steps: The first is hemostasis. In this step, vasoconstriction, coagulation, and platelet aggregation occur. The second step in wound healing is inflammation. This is caused by capillary dilation, which allows increased blood flow to the site of injury. During this stage, granulocytes, lymphocytes, neutrophils, and macrophages migrate to the injury. As the products of injury are removed, reconstructive cells proliferate and lead to scar formation.
Nursing process step: Assessment

106. CORRECT ANSWER—**D.** *Rationales:* Massive hemorrhage can occur with bleeding esophageal varices and lead to a severe fluid volume deficit. Treatment is aimed at stabilization by replacing volume and tamponading the bleeding. The patient also experiences anxiety related to hemorrhage and fear of death as well as anxiety related to hypoxia. If bleeding is not controlled, the patient will develop altered tissue perfusion. Impaired gas exchange may occur if inadequate tissue perfusion persists.
Nursing process step: Analysis

107. CORRECT ANSWER—**C.** *Rationales:* The advanced directive is a legal document outlining a person's wishes regarding health care if the person is unable to speak for himself or herself. The durable power of attorney for health care gives another person the power to make health care decisions for the patient when and if the patient is unable to make decisions for himself or herself. The last will and testament and instructions for care after death are not read until after the patient's death.

108. CORRECT ANSWER—**D.** *Rationales:* Psychomotor learning requires the coordination of the brain and extremities to complete a task. Cognitive learning is a mental process that does not involve the extremities. Affective learning involves feelings and attitudes rather than cognitive or psychomotor skills. Social is not a type of learning.
Nursing process step: Analysis

109. CORRECT ANSWER—**D.** *Rationales:* All the interventions may be appropriate for the patient with suspected blunt abdominal trauma. However, the priority of care should always be airway stabilization and then I.V. access. Fluid resuscitation is begun as needed. A nasogastric tube and an indwelling urinary catheter should be inserted. Additional diagnostic tests are performed based on patient stability.
Nursing process step: Intervention

110. CORRECT ANSWER—**D.** *Rationales:* The number one intervention for a trauma patient is the administration of high-flow oxygen. The application of a pneumatic antishock garment, radiologic evaluation, and analgesic administration can occur once the priorities of airway, breathing, and circulation are complete.
Nursing process step: Intervention

111. CORRECT ANSWER—**B.** *Rationales:* Beta blockers may mask the signs of shock. The sympathetic stimulation causing an increase in heart rate is blocked by beta blockers. The patient may present with bradycardia, hypotension, and decreased renin secretion.
Nursing process step: Intervention

112. CORRECT ANSWER—**C.** *Rationales:* Iritis produces blurred vision and unilateral pain that is moderate to severe. The cornea appears clear to hazy and pupils are irregular and small with sluggish reaction. Conjunctivitis results in no change in vision, has a clear cornea, normal pupil size, and purulent or mucopurulent discharge. Glaucoma is marked by severe, sudden onset pain; decreased visual acuity; hazy, lusterless cornea; and a semidilated, nonreactive pupil on the affected side. Central retinal artery occlusion is painless and causes a sudden unilateral loss of vision. The pupil in the affected eye is dilated and nonreactive.
Nursing process step: Assessment

113. CORRECT ANSWER—**A.** *Rationales:* Extensor tendons are prone to injury. The nurse should look for strength along with motor response when the patient extends and flexes against resistance. Tendon lacerations that go unrecognized and, thus, untreated can lead to permanent deformity. The remaining tests are used to determine peripheral nerve damage.
Nursing process step: Assessment

114. CORRECT ANSWER—**D.** *Rationales:* A patient with a corneal abrasion must receive daily outpatient follow-up care. If the injury is bilateral, the patient is generally admitted to the hospital. Ophthalmologic consultation should be made if the corneal abrasion fails to resolve in 48 to 72 hours. The eye patch should be left in place until the eye is seen by a doctor the next day. The pain is often severe and requires medication for relief.
Nursing process step: Evaluation

115. CORRECT ANSWER—**B.** *Rationales:* With myasthenia gravis, various muscle groups become fatigued. When the diaphragm or the intercostal muscles become involved, the patient is at risk for ineffective breathing. One appropriate treatment is plasmapheresis, which can create a fluid volume deficit, not excess. Myasthenia gravis is a chronic and progressive weakness of voluntary muscle groups, not the paralysis of them. Therefore, impaired physical mobility related to paralysis and spasticity is not appropriate. Myasthenia gravis involves the muscular, not the skeletal, system; therefore, pain related to tissue trauma secondary to spinal fractures is not an appropriate diagnosis.
Nursing process step: Analysis / Nursing diagnosis

116. CORRECT ANSWER—**C.** *Rationales:* A patient with alcohol intoxication is often unable to maintain an airway. The safest airway for this patient is intubation. A patient sustaining multisystem trauma should receive high concentrations of oxygen to maintain adequate cellular oxygenation. The nasal cannula is a passive device that requires the patient to perform adequate minute ventilations (tidal volume × respiratory rate). The nasal cannula can deliver a maximum oxygen of 44%. The simple face mask can deliver up to 60% oxygen, but it often results in carbon dioxide accumulation and respiratory acidosis. The nonrebreather mask can deliver adequate oxygenation to patients who can protect their airway.
Nursing process step: Intervention

117. CORRECT ANSWER—**A.** *Rationales:* Meperidine, a nonopioid analgesic, is the drug of choice for pain control in pancreatitis. Opioids can cause spasms of the sphincter of Oddi and exacerbate pain. The spasms block the normal flow of pancreatic enzymes and raise the levels of the enzymes in the pancreas. The increased enzyme levels worsen autodigestion in the pancreas and exacerbate pain.
Nursing process step: Intervention

118. CORRECT ANSWER—**A.** *Rationales:* Stings from sea urchins can rapidly lead to respiratory arrest in a patient with multiple wounds. Priority treatments should be made based on the assessment of airway, breathing, and circulation. Until embedded spines are removed, the patient remains at risk for developing systemic reactions. Impaired skin integrity related to foreign-body irritants, anxiety related to perceived threat of death, and pain related to soft tissue injury are appropriate diagnoses for the patient with sea urchin injuries, but they are not the priority problem.
Nursing process step: Analysis/Nursing diagnosis

119. CORRECT ANSWER—**B.** *Rationales:* Agents that cause severe depression of the central nervous system, such as alcohol, can mimic brain death. Hypophosphatemia, not hyperphosphatemia, severely impairs neuronal functioning. Hyperthermia and hypertension do not result in brain death–like syndromes. Instead, patients who are hypothermic or hypotensive need to have the parameters corrected before initiation of brain death protocols.
Nursing process step: Analysis

120. CORRECT ANSWER—**C.** *Rationales:* Clenched fists, pacing, and tense posture demonstrate escalation of violent behavior. The emergency department nurse needs to recognize this behavior early so that appropriate intervention can occur. An 18-year-old man who has a history of violence and rapid, loud speech and who has consumed large amounts of alcohol may be violent, especially if he has been waiting several hours and is in extreme pain.
Nursing process step: Assessment

121. CORRECT ANSWER—**D.** *Rationales:* Lower right rib fractures are often associated with liver injury. The nurse may also find decreased hematocrit from bleeding. Kehr's sign (pain in the left shoulder secondary to diaphragmatic irritation by blood) and Ballance's sign (fixed dullness to percussion in the left flank and dullness in the right flank that disappears with a change in position) may also be present. Injury to the spleen is associated with left upper quadrant pain and lower left rib fractures. Colon injuries are often associated with rectal bleeding and free air, which is detected by X-ray, under the diaphragm. Pancreatic injuries are associated with left upper quadrant or epigastric pain and Turner's sign (ecchymosis in the flank area suggesting retroperitoneal bleeding).
Nursing process step: Assessment

122. CORRECT ANSWER—**C.** *Rationales:* A change in the patient's behavior or mental status may indicate increased intracranial pressure. The family should be advised to return with the patient immediately if the patient's behavior becomes abnormal. Aspirin should be avoided by a patient with a head injury because it may increase bleeding. The use of narcotics is not recommended because these drugs may mask signs associated with increased intracranial pressure (increased drowsiness, confusion, and lack of coordination). Symptoms of a concussion should subside within 24 to 48 hours. The patient should be reevaluated if the symptoms exceed this length of time.
Nursing process step: Intervention

123. CORRECT ANSWER—**D.** *Rationales:* A patient with acute cholecystitis presents with fever, right upper quadrant tenderness, and a positive Murphy's sign. Murphy's sign is pain in the right upper quadrant on inspiration; the pain prevents the patient from taking a deep breath. Kehr's sign, which is associated with abdominal bleeding, is referred pain in the left shoulder and is caused by diaphragmatic irritation from blood.
Nursing process step: Assessment

124. CORRECT ANSWER—**C.** *Rationales:* In a trauma situation, an open wound has a great potential for infection. Fluid volume deficit and a decrease in cerebral tissue perfusion will probably not occur with an isolated eye laceration. Swelling will occur after an eye laceration, but it is generally short term.
Nursing process step: Analysis/Nursing diagnosis

125. CORRECT ANSWER—**B.** *Rationales:* To prevent the possible spread of infection, respiratory isolation should be initiated when pertussis is suspected. Isolation is recommended to prevent the transmission of airborne infectious diseases. With respiratory isolation, gowns and gloves are not indicated. Masks, however, are to be worn by any staff member who comes within arm's length of the patient. Additional interventions should focus on the patient's symptoms: control fever with antipyretics, administer antibiotics, and initiate seizure precautions as necessary.
Nursing process step: Intervention

126. CORRECT ANSWER—**B.** *Rationales:* The symptoms described are typical in a patient with abruptio placentae, which is the separation of the placenta from the uterus before delivery. It is also often associated with blunt abdominal trauma. If the outer edges of the placenta remain attached, bleeding may be concealed. In placenta previa, the placenta develops in the lower part of the uterus, and it may cover the opening. The patient presents with painless vaginal bleeding. The patient in premature labor does not have a rigid uterus. A patient with a ruptured uterus shows signs of shock and does not have fetal heart tones.
Nursing process step: Assessment

127. CORRECT ANSWER—**D.** *Rationales:* Hydrocephalus is treated with ventricular shunts, which are surgically implanted to augment drainage of cerebrospinal fluid from the brain. Pneumocephalus is treated by evacuation of air through the use of subarachnoid screws. Encephalopathy is treated with drugs: anticonvulsants, steroids, and antibiotics. Subdural empyema is a collection of material between the dura and arachnoid layers; it is treated with antimicrobial therapy and surgical drainage.
Nursing process step: Intervention

128. CORRECT ANSWER—**D.** *Rationales:* Coordinating agency (and multiagency) response and using and coordinating community resources are crucial functions of the communications center. Incident command and supervising care during a disaster are accomplished by designated medical team members who are on-scene or in the hospital treatment areas. The communications center gathers information from internal and external sources.
Nursing process step: Analysis

129. CORRECT ANSWER—**A.** *Rationales:* Amphetamines are stimulants. They cause increased energy, decreased appetite, extreme self-confidence, tachycardia, arrhythmias, hypertension, vasoconstriction, and insomnia. Fatigue is a sign of amphetamine withdrawal.
Nursing process step: Assessment

130. CORRECT ANSWER—**D.** *Rationales:* Miotic drops are given to decrease the pupil size and allow for aqueous humor drainage. Morphine is given to reduce pain, and acetazolamide or osmotic diuretics are given to reduce intraocular pressure. Surgery may be indicated if pharmacologic intervention is unsuccessful.
Nursing process step: Intervention

131. CORRECT ANSWER—**A.** *Rationales:* Folic acid is the cofactor necessary for metabolizing toxic metabolites of methanol to nontoxic metabolites in the liver. Thiamine and pyridoxine are the cofactors administered for ethylene glycol ingestion. Calcium may be administered if hypocalcemia occurs in ethylene glycol ingestion.
Nursing process step: Intervention

132. CORRECT ANSWER—B. *Rationales:* This patient presents with classic signs of botulism poisoning. This toxin causes descending paralysis. The earliest signs are visual, followed by dysphagia and, later, respiratory paralysis. Improperly canned foods are the primary source of this toxin. A form of this toxin is found in honey and may cause signs of botulism poisoning in infants. It is not a problem for adults. A history of recent viral infection and the presence of numbness or tingling are signs of Guillain-Barré syndrome. Recent travel is not specific to the symptoms mentioned.
Nursing process step: Assessment

133. CORRECT ANSWER—A. *Rationales:* Establishing a clear airway is the first priority of care. Airway, breathing, and circulation are always included in the primary assessment and take precedence over other problems. The other interventions are a high priority after establishment of an airway.
Nursing process step: Intervention

134. CORRECT ANSWER—B. *Rationales:* Cocaine is a stimulant drug. It causes hyperthermia, tachycardia, hypertension, and seizures. Labetalol is an alpha- and beta-adrenergic blocking agent. Its effect is to slow tachycardia and lower blood pressure. It does not have a direct affect on temperature or pupils. The drug used for seizures is a benzodiazepine.
Nursing process step: Evaluation

135. CORRECT ANSWER—B. *Rationales:* Contraindications to nasotracheal intubation include suspected basilar skull fractures and nasal fractures. Nasotracheal intubation may also put the patient at risk for developing encephalitis or meningitis. Orotracheal intubation is the most common method for establishing an airway. It is not the method of choice in obvious cervical spine injuries, but 96% of patients with cervical spine injuries can be intubated safely. Cricothyrotomy is a surgical procedure used to establish an airway. Needle cricothyrotomy is generally performed on children younger than age 12 when an airway cannot be obtained by other means. Surgical cricothyrotomy is not recommended for children younger than age 12 because damage to the cricoid cartilage could harm the only structure supporting the larynx and the upper trachea.
Nursing process step: Intervention

136. CORRECT ANSWER—A. *Rationales:* Coronary vasoconstriction, abdominal cramping, water intoxication, and tissue damage from infiltration are all side effects of vasopressin therapy. The most serious side effect is coronary vasoconstriction, which can cause arrhythmias, ischemia, and decreased cardiac output.
Nursing process step: Evaluation

137. CORRECT ANSWER—D. *Rationales:* Fentanyl is an opioid. The antidote for opioids is naloxone. Physostigmine is the antidote for anticholinergics except cyclic antidepressants. Flumazenil is the antidote for benzodiazepines. Atropine is the antidote for organophosphates.
Nursing process step: Intervention

138. CORRECT ANSWER—B. *Rationales:* Ovarian cysts, if they rupture, can cause hemorrhage and hypovolemic shock. Serial hematocrits and hemoglobin levels are helpful in the evaluation process. The white blood cell count is not significantly elevated unless peritonitis has occurred. This patient's pain is only 2 hours old; therefore, the likelihood of peritonitis is low. An elevated human chorionic gonadotropin level indicates a possible ectopic pregnancy. A decreased calcium level is not important to this diagnosis.
Nursing process step: Assessment

139. CORRECT ANSWER—**D.** *Rationales:* Although controlling pain, supporting nutrition, and treating the underlying cause are important aspects of care, fluid resuscitation is the priority. Severe hypovolemic shock may result in acute pancreatitis, and it must be treated with judicious fluid and electrolyte replacement.
Nursing process step: Intervention

140. CORRECT ANSWER—**B.** *Rationales:* Staphylococcal food poisoning results from a bacterial toxin formed in food. Patients present with severe abdominal pain, cramps, vomiting, diarrhea, perspiration, and fever. In some cases, the patient is in shock. Symptoms appear 1 to 6 hours after eating. The cause is usually food that has been contaminated by a preparer with a staphylococcal infection on the hand. Although altered nutrition: less than body requirements; diarrhea; and risk for infection are of concern, the highest priority is replacing lost fluid.
Nursing process step: Analysis/Nursing diagnosis

141. CORRECT ANSWER—**B.** *Rationales:* Pulmonary contusion is a potentially life-threatening injury. The most serious problems occur from blood extravasation into the alveoli. This condition leads to hypoxia that often becomes refractory to increases in FIO_2. Fluid resuscitation in the initial treatment also impacts the severity of extravasation. Ineffective airway clearance, pain, and anxiety are significant problems in the patient with pulmonary contusion. Often, each of these consequences can be effectively managed with pain control alone.
Nursing process step: Analysis/Nursing diagnosis

142. CORRECT ANSWER—**C.** *Rationales:* Unless the patient is ready to accept new information, building on previous knowledge is useless. The readiness factor is critical to acceptance and integration of new information. Patient guilt can not be alleviated until the patient understands the intricacies of the condition and the physiologic response to the disease.
Nursing process step: Assessment

143. CORRECT ANSWER—**C.** *Rationales:* Altered peripheral tissue perfusion is the primary nursing diagnosis associated with compartment syndrome. Tissue perfusion to an extremity with increased compartment pressure is diminished as the pressures within the tissue exceed the peripheral blood pressure. This results in compromised tissue perfusion and leads to ischemia and cell death. Anxiety related to a crisis event, pain related to ischemic injury secondary to compartment pressure increase, and risk for impaired skin integrity related to decreased blood supply are all appropriate nursing diagnoses for a patient with compartment syndrome; however, they do not receive the same priority attention as altered tissue perfusion.
Nursing process step: Analysis/Nursing diagnosis

144. CORRECT ANSWER—**C.** *Rationales:* The symptoms are consistent with rubella, a childhood disease that is transmitted through droplets or direct contact with infected people. Scarlet fever is identified by a fine rash that is primarily found on the chest, neck, axillae, and inner thighs. The rash does not effect the face and is usually accompanied by high fever and vomiting. Fifth disease is distinguished by an intensely red rash that begins on the face and then develops on the trunk and extremities. The rash clears centrally, leaving a lacy appearance that can last for weeks. There is no accompanying fever. Roseola infantum is identified by a high fever (104° F [30° C]) that abruptly stops and is followed by a rash that fades on pressure.
Nursing process step: Analysis

145. CORRECT ANSWER—**D.** *Rationales:* Within 30 to 60 minutes after onset, an anterior chamber paracentesis should be performed by an ophthalmologist. Some centers have used tissue plasminogen activator and heparin for partial retinal artery occlusions with success. Gentle ocular massage may be performed by a doctor before the arrival of an ophthalmologist. Breathing into a paper bag to increase carbon dioxide causes retinal arteriole vasodilation until definitive therapy can be performed.
Nursing process step: Intervention

146. CORRECT ANSWER—C. *Rationales:* Stridor is a loud, musical noise that can be heard without a stethoscope. It most often is the result of partial upper airway obstruction and is common in croup and epiglottitis. It requires immediate intervention. Crackles are popping noises heard most often during inspiration, and they indicate the presence of fluid, pus, or mucus in the smaller airways. When the nurse hears crackles, the patient should be instructed to cough and breathe deeply. Then the nurse should auscultate again; the crackles may have cleared. Rhonchi are snoring, low-pitched sounds produced by air passing through narrowed air passages. Wheezing is a high-pitched, musical sound that can be heard during inspiration and expiration. It usually accompanies an asthma attack or bronchospasm.
Nursing process step: Assessment

147. CORRECT ANSWER—D. *Rationales:* Liver injuries are often associated with lower right rib fractures. Lacerations of the liver may cause profuse bleeding and lead to hypovolemia. The patient with blunt abdominal trauma should be evaluated for other abdominal injuries. Injuries to the spleen are more often associated with left rib fractures. Perforations of the stomach and pancreatic injury are less common.
Nursing process step: Analysis

148. CORRECT ANSWER—B. *Rationales:* Adrenal crisis may occur as the result of sudden withdrawal from corticosteroid therapy. Symptoms of adrenal crisis include fever, myalgia, arthralgia, and malaise. An increased risk for developing glaucoma and subcapsular cataracts can be the result of prolonged use of corticosteroids. Psychic disturbances may present as adverse side effects during use, and they may include euphoria, insomnia, mood swings, and extreme depression. Tardive dyskinesia consists of irreversible, involuntary movements that may develop in people being treated with neuroleptics, such as chlorpromazine (Thorazine).
Nursing process step: Analysis

149. CORRECT ANSWER—B. *Rationales:* Hyperosmolality is the result of accompanying hyperglycemia and hypernatremia. Hyperosmolality causes insulin levels to be reduced, preventing the movement of glucose into the cells and allowing glucose to accumulate in the plasma. Hyperosmolar hyperglycemic nonketotic syndrome is characterized by extremely elevated blood glucose levels, which range from 600 mg/dl to 2,800 mg/dl. The blood urea nitrogen level is normally elevated from severe dehydration. Fluid volume deficit is more severe than in diabetic ketoacidosis; up to 12 liters of fluid must be replaced. Mild metabolic acidosis is reflected in arterial blood gas results from poor perfusion and anaerobic metabolism.
Nursing process step: Assessment

150. CORRECT ANSWER—D. *Rationales:* In addition to flattened or inverted T waves, the ECG may show prolonged QT interval and a prominent U wave. Patients with hypokalemia are also more predisposed to developing ventricular ectopy. A shortened QT interval may be evidenced in hypercalcemia. Tall, peaked T waves with a short QT interval are indicative of hyperkalemia. A widened QRS complex may be observed with hyperkalemia.
Nursing process step: Evaluation

151. CORRECT ANSWER—A. *Rationales:* The most significant assessment finding in a chemical burn to the eye, especially an alkaline burn, is corneal whitening. There is pain and variable visual loss. It is also difficult to define specific eye structures. There may be redness but no purulent discharge. A corneal abrasion presents with corneal irregularity without luster.
Nursing process step: Assessment

152. CORRECT ANSWER—A. *Rationales:* Most insecticides are carbamates or organophosphates. They are highly lipid soluble and are well absorbed through the skin. If protection is not worn, the insecticide may be absorbed through the skin of the health care worker. The type and amount of insecticide spilled can be determined during the assessment. Respiratory protection is necessary if the insecticide is in a vapor or aerosol form. **Nursing process step:** Analysis

153. CORRECT ANSWER—D. *Rationales:* Disseminated intravascular coagulation (DIC) is a condition of excessive coagulation that eventually leads to inadequate homeostasis. The activation of the coagulation system leads to the formation of fibrin that binds with blood to form a clot. In DIC, the clots are deposited in the microvasculature of various organs. Excessive bleeding in DIC results from the consumption of all clotting factors. Fibrin degradation products further aggravate this situation because they act as powerful anticoagulants. Heparin is most effective when administered soon after recognition of symptoms. Fresh frozen plasma and cryoprecipitate are administered to replace clotting factors. **Nursing process step:** Intervention

154. CORRECT ANSWER—A. *Rationales:* Airway is the first priority for all medical situations. The intoxicated patient should be placed in a side-lying position to prevent aspiration in the event of vomiting. An airway adjunct (oropharyngeal or nasopharyngeal airway) will help keep the airway open and prevent the tongue from obstructing it. Because hypoventilation is present in the acutely intoxicated patient, it may become necessary to intubate and ventilate. All the other diagnoses are also applicable but should not be initiated until the airway can be maintained. **Nursing process step:** Analysis/Nursing diagnosis

155. CORRECT ANSWER—B. *Rationales:* Herpes zoster (shingles) is characterized by clusters of vesicles that form in a line along nerve pathways. Vesicles are fluid-filled lesions less than 1 cm in size; the fluid is clear. Papules are solid masses of cellular growth usually less than 5 mm in size. Bulla are fluid-filled lesions larger than 1 cm. Pustules are fluid-filled lesions; unlike a vesicle, the fluid is yellowish. **Nursing process step:** Assessment

156. CORRECT ANSWER—A. *Rationales:* The nausea and vomiting that accompany pyelonephritis can predispose the patient to fluid volume deficit. Nausea and vomiting symptomatology should be treated to avoid this complication. Treatment is especially important in children, who are prone to dehydration. Tissue integrity is not impaired and perfusion to the kidneys is not interrupted. Decreased cardiac output is not a problem for this patient. **Nursing process step:** Analysis

157. CORRECT ANSWER—C. *Rationales:* Septic shock frequently causes hypoglycemia in pediatric patients. Infants have limited glycogen stores that are rapidly depleted during stress. During the resuscitative stage, all pediatric patients should have serum glucose levels monitored. Hypoglycemia should be treated with 2 to 4 ml/kg of 25% dextrose solution I.V. Septic shock results in a metabolic acidosis state from decreased cellular perfusion. Hypercalcemia does not occur. Hypocalcemia results from impaired tissue perfusion during septic shock and should be treated with calcium chloride 10% solution 10 to 20 mg/kg I.V. administered slowly. **Nursing process step:** Assessment

158. CORRECT ANSWER—**C.** *Rationales:* Untreated pelvic inflammatory disease can create a tubo-ovarian cyst. If it ruptures, the patient can develop peritonitis and become septic. Before any invasive procedure, such as a culdocentesis, the infection should be treated with I.V. antibiotics. Therefore, an I.V. line is necessary for antibiotics and for fluid resuscitation. A nasogastric tube is inserted because of decreased peristalsis, which can occur with peritonitis or sepsis. A pelvic exam is performed to obtain cultures and assess the patient.
Nursing process step: Planning/Intervention

159. CORRECT ANSWER—**C.** *Rationales:* In inflammatory conditions, such as pancreatitis, a loop of bowel adjacent to the inflammation may become distended with gas. This is known as a sentinel loop of bowel. Free air under the diaphragm is indicative of perforation. Dilated loops of bowel and abnormal air-fluid levels in the bowel may be indicative of bowel obstruction.
Nursing process step: Assessment

160. CORRECT ANSWER—**A.** *Rationales:* An infusion of 10% glucose and regular insulin is administered to induce the transfer of potassium from the serum to the intracellular fluid. Patients with a potassium excess should receive only fresh blood because the cells in stored blood release potassium during storage. Calcium gluconate is used to reverse magnesium intoxication.
Nursing process step: Intervention

161. CORRECT ANSWER—**B.** *Rationales:* Excretory urography is the test of choice for renal pedicle repair. Dye injected into the venous system should enter the kidney and provide visualization if the renovascular system is intact. Cystography is a diagnostic tool for the bladder, and retrograde urethrography is performed for a urethral injury. A kidney-ureter-bladder X-ray shows the shape, location, and size of these organs. It helps to identify masses or radiopaque calculi.
Nursing process step: Evaluation

162. CORRECT ANSWER—**B.** *Rationales:* A patient with a sexually transmitted disease may complain of painful urination. The pain may be from an associated urinary tract infection or from urine passing over lesions. The lesions themselves may also be painful, and itching can be so severe that it elicits pain (either from the desire to scratch or from actual scratching). A discharge does not produce pain.
Nursing process step: Analysis

163. CORRECT ANSWER—**A.** *Rationales:* Intestinal obstruction may be associated with distention, vomiting, visible peristalsis, localized tenderness, and altered bowel sounds. Right upper quadrant tenderness, fever, and jaundice are related to cholecystitis. Abdominal free air, distention, and rebound tenderness are found with a perforated viscous. Nausea, abdominal mass, and bruit are found in patients with a leaking abdominal aneurysm.
Nursing process step: Assessment

164. CORRECT ANSWER—**C.** *Rationales:* During normal cellular function, an aerobic environment exists. Adequate cellular perfusion of glucose and oxygen occurs, and waste products are removed. When cellular perfusion is reduced, tissue hypoxia ensues and results in an abnormal cellular metabolism, creating an anaerobic environment. A by-product of anaerobic metabolism is lactic acid. Decreased tissue perfusion does not remove the by-product, and metabolic acidosis occurs.
Nursing process step: Assessment

165. CORRECT ANSWER—**B.** *Rationales:* O-negative packed red blood cells are recommended when blood replacement must occur immediately. In some institutions, O-positive packed red blood cells are being administered to male patients without complications. The gender of the patient was not mentioned in the scenario. Type-specific uncrossmatched packed red blood cells take 15 to 20 minutes to process. Typed and cross-matched packed red blood cells require 30 to 60 minutes to process. To prevent transfusion reactions, type-specific or typed and crossmatched blood should be administered as soon as possible.
Nursing process step: Intervention

166. CORRECT ANSWER—**D.** *Rationales:* Increased intracranial pressure, warfarin therapy, and infection of the cutaneous or osseous areas at the lumbar puncture site are contraindications to performing a lumbar puncture, unless the benefits outweigh the risks. Performing a lumbar puncture on a patient with increased intracranial pressure may result in brain stem compression or herniation. Patients on anticoagulation therapy are at increased risk for hemorrhage. Performing a lumbar puncture at the site of infection increases the chance of introducing bacteria into the cerebrospinal fluid.
Nursing process step: Assessment

167. CORRECT ANSWER—**B.** *Rationales:* During the initial phase of shock, respiratory alkalosis occurs as the body attempts to rid itself of the carbonic acid that accumulates as a result of inadequate tissue perfusion. Respiratory acidosis and metabolic acidosis result when fluid or blood loss continues and compensatory mechanisms fail to restore normal cellular function. Metabolic alkalosis occurs in patients who have lost hydrogen ions or have an accumulation of bicarbonate.
Nursing process step: Assessment

168. CORRECT ANSWER—**B.** *Rationales:* Cardiogenic shock is characterized by impaired ability of the heart to pump and decreased contractility of the myocardium. Stroke volume and cardiac output decline and result in increased left ventricular end-diastolic pressure. Myocardial infarction resulting in damage to greater than 40% of the left ventricular myocardium is the most common cause of cardiogenic shock. Other causes of cardiogenic shock are cardiomyopathies, valvular dysfunction, and rupture of papillary muscle. Pericardial tamponade, tension pneumothorax, and pulmonary embolus result in obstructive or restrictive cardiogenic shock. Pneumonia is an inflammation of the lung parenchyma and is the leading cause of death in the geriatric population. Cardiogenic shock is not a complication of pneumonia. Restrained passengers hit from the back are at low risk for developing cardiogenic shock unless they have sustained a myocardial contusion.
Nursing process step: Assessment

169. CORRECT ANSWER—**B.** *Rationales:* After establishing an airway, the immediate concern in the burn patient is fluid resuscitation. Hypovolemia is a result of increased capillary permeability. Pain should be addressed when the patient's condition warrants. If the patient is suffering from full-thickness burns, sensory receptors have been destroyed, and the patient does not feel pain in the area. The patient's impaired skin integrity requires diligent wound care. Rapid fluid loss and disruption in skin integrity also cause difficulty in thermoregulation and may result in hypothermia. Because of problems in thermoregulation, the patient with an infection may not develop a fever.
Nursing process step: Analysis

170. CORRECT ANSWER—**D.** *Rationales:* When a person is immobilized for extended periods, calcium leaves the bones and becomes concentrated in the extracellular fluid. From there, it passes through the kidneys and precipitates to form stones. Milk is high in calcium and should be restricted in patients with hypercalcemia. Increased fluid intake facilitates increased kidney excretion of calcium.
Nursing process step: Evaluation

171. CORRECT ANSWER—**A.** *Rationales:* Having a reimplantation team available is an important factor. Others include the amount of damage to the attachment area or amputated part, length of time since amputation occurred, predicted outcome of reimplantation, and the general physical condition of the patient. It makes no difference whether the amputated part is an upper or a lower extremity. The patient's occupation, although important to consider, should not determine whether or not attempts at reimplantation occur. The insurance status of the patient should never be a factor in the provision of life- and limb-threatening interventions.
Nursing process step: Intervention

172. CORRECT ANSWER—**D.** *Rationales:* Cyanide attaches to the respiratory enzyme cytochrome-*c* oxidase and forms a stable complex, preventing gas exchange at the cellular level. Therapy for cyanide poisoning is aimed at breaking this bond and restoring respiration at the cellular level. Altered tissue perfusion, ineffective airway clearance, and ineffective breathing pattern also occur, but they are a result of the impaired gas exchange.
Nursing process step: Analysis/Nursing diagnosis

173. CORRECT ANSWER—**D.** *Rationales:* The treatment plan for a patient in cardiogenic shock includes administering medications that decrease preload and afterload and increase contractility. As a result of this therapy, left ventricular end-diastolic (LVED) pressure as well as demands on the heart should be reduced. Vasodilators reduce total peripheral resistance and decrease LVED pressure. Catecholamines increase heart rate, heart contractility, and vasodilatation in the postcapillary sphincters and pulmonary system. All other options are clinical manifestations of cardiogenic shock.
Nursing process step: Evaluation

174. CORRECT ANSWER—**B.** *Rationales:* The patient described is having a hemolytic reaction to transfusion therapy. The transfusion should be stopped immediately. The nurse should then initiate infusion of 0.9% normal saline at a keep-vein-open rate. After contacting a doctor, the nurse should be prepared to administer antihistamines and epinephrine. The patient's vital signs should be reassessed frequently, as indicated by hospital policy.
Nursing process step: Intervention

175. CORRECT ANSWER—C. *Rationales:* This patient has pulmonary edema as a result of heart failure. In doses of 5 to 20 g/kg/minute, dopamine hydrochloride stimulates the beta-adrenergic and alpha-adrenergic receptors of the sympathetic nervous system and results in vasoconstriction of peripheral blood vessels, increased heart rate, increased contractility, and enhanced conduction through the atria and ventricles. Dobutamine hydrochloride stimulates the beta receptors of the heart to increase myocardial contractility and stroke volume and results in increased cardiac output. Patients in septic shock also suffer from peripheral vasodilation. Dobutamine hydrochloride does not act on the peripheral vascular beds and is used in conjunction with dopamine hydrochloride. Nitroprusside and nitroglycerin are vasodilators and have the ability to enhance perfusion through vasoconstricted vessels. The pharmacologic activity of vasodilation on the systemic vessels is unpredictable; therefore, the patient should have a thermodilution catheter inserted for measuring systemic vascular resistance. Vasodilators are seldom used in the emergency department.
Nursing process step: Intervention

176. CORRECT ANSWER—D. *Rationales:* Fractures to the epiphyseal growth plate may result in early closure. As the child continues to grow, there may be no growth in the affected bone. If the growth plate fracture is partial, angulated growth may subsequently occur, leading to deformity. Open fractures, closed fractures, and dislocation fractures usually do not result in long-term problems, provided initial orthopedic care is appropriate.
Nursing process step: Analysis

177. CORRECT ANSWER—D. *Rationales:* The dressing of choice for a patient with an open pneumothorax is a nonporous dressing taped on three sides. The dressing should be placed over the wound at the end of expiration. The patient should be monitored closely for worsening of condition. Saline-moistened gauze would increase the potential for infection. When a porous dressing is used, pieces of gauze can move into the chest. If the dressing is taped on all four sides, it predisposes the patient to the development of a tension pneumothorax.
Nursing process step: Intervention

178. CORRECT ANSWER—C. *Rationales:* Administering a drug with opioid antagonist properties may precipitate drug withdrawal in an opioid-dependent patient. Signs of opioid withdrawal include chills, diaphoresis, gooseflesh, abdominal pain, muscle cramps, diarrhea, tearfulness, and irritability. Respiratory depression, nausea, and vomiting are side effects of opioids. Seizures can occur as a result of sedative, hypnotic, or anxiolytic withdrawal.
Nursing process step: Evaluation

179. CORRECT ANSWER—B. *Rationales:* The nursing diagnosis that best describes this patient's condition is decreased cardiac output. The patient has cardiac tamponade that causes blood to collect in the pericardial sac. The pooling blood prevents the atria from filling during diastole. The decrease in atrial filling results in decreased stroke volume and cardiac output. If pump failure is not corrected, the patient will develop impaired gas exchange as a result of impaired cardiac function. Patients with cardiac tamponade do not generally experience a risk for fluid volume deficit; instead, they experience decreased cardiac output related to the heart's inability to pump. Ineffective airway clearance is not an appropriate diagnosis at this time.
Nursing process step: Analysis/Nursing diagnosis

180. CORRECT ANSWER—**B.** *Rationales:* The symptoms associated with hepatitis A include fever, anorexia, malaise, vomiting, nausea, light-colored stools, and dark-colored urine. Hepatitis is also associated with liver inflammation, which causes pain in the right upper quadrant. The spleen, not the liver, is located in the left upper quadrant. Dark, tarry stools are associated with GI bleeding. Hematuria is associated with trauma, anticoagulant therapy, renal tumors, and renal calculi.
Nursing process step: Assessment

181. CORRECT ANSWER—**A.** *Rationales:* The scenario describes constructive feedback because the manager immediately responded respectfully to the staff nurse by speaking with the nurse promptly and privately. The manager also implemented a positive approach to preventing future errors. The scenario doesn't refer to emotional support or goal setting. Recognition is feedback for a positive contribution, not an error.

182. CORRECT ANSWER—**A.** *Rationales:* Autotransfusion should be completed within 4 hours of the injury. Autologous blood is collected from the pleural cavity or mediastinal area and transfused to the patient.
Nursing process step: Intervention

183. CORRECT ANSWER—**C.** *Rationales:* A patent airway without pulmonary basilar wheezes is an indicator that the treatment plan for this patient is correct and that the patient's condition is stabilizing. Blood pressure 86/62 mm Hg, pH 7.45, PaO_2 86 mm Hg, $PaCO_2$ 30 mm Hg, and pulmonary basilar wheezes do not indicate that this patient's condition is improving.
Nursing process step: Evaluation

184. CORRECT ANSWER—**C.** *Rationales:* The priority for an intubated trauma patient is to assess patency of airway. Tubes can become displaced during transport from the emergency medical service unit to the trauma room. To confirm nasotracheal tube placement, the nurse should first listen for air sounds over the epigastric area. If none are present, the nurse should listen over both lung bases during ventilation. All other interventions may be implemented after airway, breathing, and circulation have been assessed.
Nursing process step: Intervention

185. CORRECT ANSWER—**B.** *Rationales:* Patients receiving beta blockers require large, repeated doses of epinephrine to counteract the effects of the beta blockers. Glucagon 5 to 15 mcg/minute I.V. may be beneficial for refractory hypotension associated with beta blockers. All other medications should be administered per recommended doses.
Nursing process step: Intervention

186. CORRECT ANSWER—**D.** *Rationales:* A bowel obstruction results in electrolyte and fluid accumulation within the intestinal lumen and leads to dehydration. These patients frequently experience vomiting, which increases fluid loss. The nursing diagnosis most appropriate for this patient is fluid volume deficit.
Nursing process step: Analysis/Nursing diagnosis

187. CORRECT ANSWER—**A.** *Rationales:* The patient must take part in identifying learning and educational needs. Adults resent being told what they need and when to report. A patient must feel in control and feel confident in meeting some or all of his or her own needs. Only through the interview process can the nurse determine the best approach and method for addressing learning needs. If the patient is enrolled for classes without having any input, the patient is not in control and may become resentful.
Nursing process step: Assessment

188. CORRECT ANSWER—A. *Rationales:* After being diagnosed with acute otitis externa, the patient should be instructed to wear earplugs to keep the infected ear dry. Acute otitis externa is an inflammatory condition of the auricle and external auditory canal usually caused by gram-negative organisms. Keeping the ear dry makes it more difficult for these organisms to grow. Because of risks associated with vertigo, a patient with Ménière's disease would be instructed to change position slowly and keep his or her home uncluttered. A patient with otitis media would be instructed to notify the doctor if ear pain increases when lying down. This may indicate that antibiotic therapy is ineffective.
Nursing process step: Evaluation

189. CORRECT ANSWER—C. *Rationales:* Corticosteroids reduce inflammation and cerebral edema and help prevent increased intracranial pressure. Anticonvulsants are used to control absence seizures. Antipsychotics and antianxiety drugs may be used sparingly to control agitation. Preferably, nonnarcotics are used to relieve pain. Narcotics may make it difficult to assess the patient's level of consciousness.
Nursing process step: Intervention

190. CORRECT ANSWER—C. *Rationales:* A disaster is a situation that produces an immediate patient load greater than the normal emergency medical system and available health care facilities can handle. Many incidents occur that result in more than three casualties. Such events usually do not overwhelm the emergency medical system. Both natural and manmade situations can result in disasters. Multiple-death situations, although terrible and a stress to the system, usually do not constitute a true disaster for the medical system when appropriate scene triage occurs.
Nursing process step: Assessment

191. CORRECT ANSWER—C. *Rationales:* The two causes of intrapulmonary shunt seen in the adult respiratory distress syndrome (ARDS) patient are pulmonary edema and atelectasis. Common treatments for hydrostatic pulmonary edema include diuretics and inotropes and decreased fluid intake. They are not effective treatments for the early stages of ARDS. A key finding in ARDS is refractory hypoxemia that is not improved by increasing the FIO_2. In fact, FIO_2 levels greater than 60% for prolonged periods result in atelectasis, worsening ARDS, and hypoxemia. Adding low levels of positive end-expiratory pressure (5 to 10 cm H_2O) will assist in reopening the alveoli and improving tissue oxygenation.
Nursing process step: Intervention

192. CORRECT ANSWER—A. *Rationales:* A patient with eclampsia may suffer from seizures or coma and must be protected from injury. This patient may also experience anxiety related to concern about her and the baby's health. This patient would not necessarily experience decreased cardiac output or fluid volume deficit.
Nursing process step: Analysis

193. CORRECT ANSWER—B. *Rationales:* Carbon dioxide is an acidic compound that is normally excreted by the respiratory system. The patient with chronic obstructive pulmonary disease presents with an elevated $PaCO_2$, resulting in the development of respiratory acidosis. The patient also has hypoxemia. Metabolic acidosis is a common finding in renal failure, dehydration, and shock. Respiratory alkalosis often occurs with anxiety and other states that lead to hyperventilation. Metabolic alkalosis occurs in situations with increased loss of GI fluids.
Nursing process step: Assessment

194. CORRECT ANSWER—**B.** *Rationales:* The key diagnostic finding that suggests a ruptured diaphragm is the presence of bowel sounds in the middle of the chest. The left side of the diaphragm is more likely to be injured than the right side because it is not as well protected. The abdominal contents herniate into the chest, causing compression of the lungs and great vessels. Hemothorax would produce diminished breath sounds but not shoulder pain or bowel sounds in the chest. Aortic dissection may cause a shift of heart sounds; however, the patient decompensates quickly. A tracheobronchial disruption produces signs consistent with pneumothorax.
Nursing process step: Assessment

195. CORRECT ANSWER—**A.** *Rationales:* A traction splint is used for femur fractures as well as fractures of the proximal tibia. The extremity should be splinted in the position found if the neurovascular status is intact. Air splints are contraindicated for air transport of patients because altitude changes result in pressure changes within the splint, which may cause neurovascular compromise.
Nursing process step: Intervention

196. CORRECT ANSWER—**C.** *Rationales:* Because patients with deep vein thrombosis are among those most likely to develop pulmonary emboli, the nurse should encourage walking and active range-of-motion exercises. To keep pressure from building up in the legs, the patient should not cross them at the knees or ankles. To maintain normal plasma volume, which prevents vascular collapse and venous stasis, the patient should consume adequate fluids. Adequate nutrition also helps to maintain integrity of the alveolar and arterial epithelium.
Nursing process step: Evaluation

197. CORRECT ANSWER—**B.** *Rationales:* A 16-g indwelling urinary catheter can be used to control bleeding and provide hemostasis for a posterior nosebleed. It is inserted into the nares and into the posterior nasal passage. It is then inflated and pulled against the nasopharynx. Other choices include gauze packs connected to a string, the Merocel posterior pack, and the Epistat (a double-balloon catheter). The Merocel nasal tampon is inserted into the anterior nares and swells with blood and nasal secretions, which exert gentle pressure on the inside of the nares. The Nasostat nasal balloon is placed into the affected nares and inflated with 15 to 20 cc of air (normal saline is inserted if bleeding stops). Gelfoam is an absorbable hemostatic agent that stimulates coagulation. The Mercocel nasal tampon, the Nasostat nasal balloon, and the Gelfoam hemostatic agent are for anterior bleeds.
Nursing process step: Planning/Intervention

198. CORRECT ANSWER—**C.** *Rationales:* Based on physical findings and chest films, the correct response is asthma. Bronchiolitis occurs primarily in winter and spring during the first 2 years of life with a peak at 2 to 6 months of age. It begins with a cough, rhinorrhea, and nasal congestion. The symptoms of foreign-body obstruction depend on the degree of obstruction; a sudden onset of coughing, choking, gagging, or wheezing is often seen. Bronchial foreign bodies usually cause wheezing or coughing and are frequently misdiagnosed as asthma. The patient with a bronchial foreign body presents with hyperresonant percussion and diminished breath sounds distal to the foreign body. Hypersensitivity pneumonitis produces patchy infiltrates and atelectasis on chest film.
Nursing process step: Analysis/Nursing diagnosis

199. CORRECT ANSWER—B. *Rationales:* It is rare for a child to contract epididymitis, so the possibility of child molestation should be investigated. Causes of epididymitis include prostatitis, cystitis, and urethral instrumentation. Common causative organisms include *Escherichia coli, Neisseria gonorrhoeae, Mycobacterium tuberculosis,* and *Chlamydia.* Elevation of the testis sometimes relieves the pain. A person with epididymitis should be cautioned that all sexual partners should be examined and treated. Infertility can be a problem if epididymitis is untreated or partially treated because it can cause vas deferens scars or antisperm antibody production.
Nursing process step: Assessment

200. CORRECT ANSWER—D. *Rationales:* Altered tissue perfusion to the myocardium is responsible for the pain associated with angina. This may in turn lead to decreased cardiac output.
Nursing process step: Analysis

201. CORRECT ANSWER—A. *Rationales:* Potassium may increase in the early postburn period from hemolysis of red blood cells and loss of intracellular potassium. Sodium may decrease slightly because of extracellular body fluid loss and sodium trapped in the edema surrounding the burn wound.
Nursing process step: Assessment

202. CORRECT ANSWER—A. *Rationales:* A child with epiglottitis has a sudden high fever (usually 102.9° F [39.4° C]), marked drooling, stridor, severe sore throat, and no cough. A child with retropharyngeal abscess has abrupt onset of high fever, stridor, drooling, severe sore throat, hyperextension of the head, and stiff neck. In bacterial tracheitis, the fever is mild followed by an acute increase. There is a barky cough, no drooling, and minimal or no sore throat. Viral croup syndrome causes a variable temperature (100° to 104° F [37.8° to 40° C]), barky cough, no drooling, and mild or no sore throat.
Nursing process step: Analysis

203. CORRECT ANSWER—A. *Rationales:* A sandbag applied to the injured chest area limits lung expansion and predisposes the patient to atelectasis. Therefore, more current theory recommends that all patients with flail chest be immediately intubated and ventilated to manage the underlying pulmonary contusion. Pain must be controlled to facilitate adequate ventilation. Fluids should be limited to reduce the incidence of pulmonary edema.
Nursing process step: Intervention

204. CORRECT ANSWER—D. *Rationales:* Pelvic fractures always involve at least two fracture sites because of the bony ring structure of the pelvis. They can be stable or unstable; however, more than 66% of them are stable. A fracture of the pelvis can produce bleeding, which is usually venous and caused by the disruption of the pelvic veins. Open pelvic fractures are associated with injuries to the perineum, genitourinary structures, or rectum and have a significantly higher mortality rate.
Nursing process step: Assessment

205. CORRECT ANSWER—A. *Rationales:* The cornerstone of treatment for a patient with croup is humidified air. Oxygen should be administered to the patient if hypoxemia is present; however, 100% oxygen is seldom necessary and delivery by way of a mask is nearly impossible for a child. Corticosteroids remain a controversial treatment choice. In severe cases, a patient may require racemic epinephrine to assist with bronchoconstriction.
Nursing process step: Intervention

206. CORRECT ANSWER—A. *Rationales:* After ruling out medical causes for hyperventilation, returning carbon dioxide to more normal levels is the most appropriate intervention. This can be accomplished by placing a bag over the patient's nose and mouth to permit rebreathing of carbon dioxide. Placing the patient in a comfortable position, providing reassurance, and monitoring arterial blood gases are appropriate; however, the solution is rebreathing carbon dioxide.
Nursing process step: Intervention

207. CORRECT ANSWER—C. *Rationales:* Many people find it difficult to adjust to major changes in structure and ways of operating. Explaining reasons for change makes acceptance more likely. A manager's approach should also include the following: obtaining as much input from staff as possible, making no more than one major change at a time, and letting staff know that if the change does not work, adjustments can usually be made. The goal is to find a workable process.

208. CORRECT ANSWER—A. *Rationales:* Common findings in a patient with an open pneumothorax are sucking sounds from the wound on inspiration, penetrating wound to the chest, diminished or absent breath sounds over the affected area, hyperresonance on the affected side, dyspnea, chest pain, and tachypnea. Hemoptysis occurs most commonly with pulmonary contusion or tracheobronchial injury.
Nursing process step: Assessment

209. CORRECT ANSWER—A. *Rationales:* Elevating the extremity and applying ice slow the swelling process and help relieve pain. Teaching the patient how to walk with crutches is not appropriate at this time because the patient is distracted by the pain. If elevating the ankle and applying ice do not decrease the pain, then an order for medication is appropriate. A traction splint is contraindicated for this patient; the traction splint is indicated for fractures of the femur and proximal tibia only.
Nursing process step: Intervention

210. CORRECT ANSWER—B. *Rationales:* The most appropriate nursing diagnosis is risk for infection related to disruption of the esophagus with contents emptied into the thoracic cavity. Risk for fluid volume deficit (not excess) related to fluid shifts could also occur. Decreased cardiac output is unlikely unless concurrent injuries to nearby vessels have occurred. Impaired gas exchange occurs only if the lung is injured along with the esophagus.
Nursing process step: Analysis/Nursing diagnosis

211. CORRECT ANSWER—D. *Rationales:* Arteriography is helpful if diminished or absent pulses indicate that there may be vascular damage. Arteriography is not clinically indicated for long bone injuries if the vascular status is unaffected. It is not usually indicated in open injuries (including penetrating injury) unless the wound is near major vascular structures or the wounding force was a high-velocity one.
Nursing process step: Assessment

212. CORRECT ANSWER—C. *Rationales:* Complications of rewarming include metabolic acidosis, cardiac arrhythmias, pneumonia, renal failure, pancreatitis, sepsis, and adult respiratory distress syndrome. The application of warm blankets is not sufficient with such severe hypothermia. More active rewarming (peritoneal dialysis, warmed fluids, heated humidified oxygen, extracorporeal blood rewarming) may be needed. Rapid rewarming is not advised because such a patient is vulnerable to cardiac arrhythmias. External rewarming causes peripheral vasodilation. This action may divert blood flow to the skin and shunt cooled blood to the central circulation, thereby causing a brief drop in core temperature. It may also predispose the patient to hypovolemia and ventricular fibrillation. Debilitated and elderly patients with core temperatures under 95° F (35° C) should be hospitalized.
Nursing process step: Intervention

213. CORRECT ANSWER—C. *Rationales:* Adenosine may cause momentary high-grade blocks and asystole that are rapidly resolved. If they do not resolve rapidly, the nurse should begin cardiopulmonary resuscitation. There are no documented cases of asystole lasting longer than 30 seconds.
Nursing process step: Intervention

214. CORRECT ANSWER—**B.** *Rationales:* The presence of an increased number of epithelial cells, especially when they exceed the number of white blood cells, is indicative of a contaminated specimen. Proper cleansing and retrieval of the specimen may not have taken place. The presence of bacteria, white blood cells, and pus suggests pyelonephritis or a urinary tract infection. **Nursing process step:** Planning/Intervention

215. CORRECT ANSWER—**C.** *Rationales:* Rapid infusion of room temperature crystalloids and stored refrigerated blood results in hypothermia in a trauma patient with hemorrhagic shock. Trauma patients in shock are predisposed to hypothermia because of altered perfusion to the hypothalamus (which regulates temperature). Hypothermia in trauma patients may cause coagulopathies and increased acidosis. A shock state results in altered renal, cardiac, and GI tissue perfusion from decreased cardiac output; the condition may worsen with hypothermia. **Nursing process step:** Analysis/Nursing diagnosis

216. CORRECT ANSWER—**B.** *Rationales:* Patient classification systems provide methods for grouping patients according to the amount and complexity of nursing care required. The systems are used to determine staffing in terms of numbers and levels of licensure. Triage categories are assigned to determine priority for initial evaluation or intervention. Triage categories can also be an acuity measure, but they do not reflect the necessary amount or type of nursing care. Census data count and sort patient visits according to such variables as time, reasons, and demographics. Diagnosis-related groups were developed for use in prospective payment for Medicare recipients and are not directly related to nursing care.

217. CORRECT ANSWER—**D.** *Rationales:* The nurse can estimate the percentage of body surface area (BSA) burned using the rule of nines. In an adult, the head compromises 9% BSA; the torso, 18% front and 18% back; arms, 9% each; legs, 18% each; and the perineum, 1%. In a child, the head compromises 18% and each leg is 14%; the other percentages are the same as for an adult. **Nursing process step:** Assessment

218. CORRECT ANSWER—**B.** *Rationales:* Increasing fluid intake and decreasing workload during the hottest part of the day reduce the risk for heat-related illnesses. Salt tablets can contribute to volume depletion by causing a hyperosmotic state. If the patient experiences painful cramps in overworked muscles, the patient should cool off and rest. **Nursing process step:** Evaluation

219. CORRECT ANSWER—**B.** *Rationales:* These symptoms suggest air embolism, which is caused by failure to exhale on ascent. Decompression sickness is caused by nitrogen bubbles in the bloodstream and is manifested by rash, fatigue, and dizziness. Nitrogen narcosis results when the patient breathes dissolved nitrogen under pressure. Symptoms include fatigue, weakness, and decreased consciousness; it may result in death. **Nursing process step:** Assessment

220. CORRECT ANSWER—**B.** *Rationales:* The emergency nurse should wear protective clothing, such as boots, gloves, cap, and mask, to prevent contamination from radiation. A radiation meter is not indicated in this situation. Life-threatening problems may be handled after the nurse has donned protective clothing and before the patient is decontaminated. **Nursing process step:** Intervention

221. CORRECT ANSWER—B. *Rationales:* A LeFort II fracture involves a pyramidal fracture that includes the central portion of the maxilla across the superior nasal area. It may also involve the orbit. This produces a free-floating nose and dental arch. Free-floating movement of the unilateral periorbital area does not describe a clinical situation. However, free-floating movement of the teeth and maxilla describes a LeFort I, and free-floating movement of all the facial bones describes a LeFort III fracture.
Nursing process step: Assessment

222. CORRECT ANSWER—D. *Rationales:* Discussion allows for direct contact as well as questions and answers. Personal contact and interest often make learning easier for the patient, and such contact allows the nurse to evaluate the patient's learning.
Nursing process step: Intervention

223. CORRECT ANSWER—A. *Rationales:* Alligator forceps are used to remove vegetable or other foreign bodies from the ear. The nurse also needs a good light source, large ear speculums, ear curette, and ear suction. If the foreign body is not a vegetable, a 30-ml syringe filled with water may be used to irrigate the ear. (Water causes vegetables to swell so they are even more difficult to remove.) Lidocaine is useful in removing live bugs. Cerumenex is useful in removing earwax buildup only.
Nursing process step: Planning/Intervention

224. CORRECT ANSWER—C. *Rationales:* Common signs of early carbon monoxide poisoning are headache and nausea or flulike symptoms. Because the symptoms improve during the day, an environmental cause, such as a faulty gas appliance or heating system, may be responsible. A car can also be a source of carbon monoxide poisoning. But unless the patient leaves the car's motor running in an attached garage, its unlikely the car is the cause. If the patient reported that symptoms occurred at work (rather than reporting that family members shared similar symptoms), then asking the patient if anyone at work had similar symptoms would be appropriate.
Nursing process step: Assessment

225. CORRECT ANSWER—A. *Rationales:* This patient is experiencing symptoms of Bell's palsy. Risk for injury relates to the risk for corneal abrasion caused by the inability to close the right eyelid. Based on assessment of the patient, ineffective airway clearance and impaired gas exchange are inappropriate diagnoses. Respiratory distress or obstruction is not described. Pain is not correct because no mention of pain is made, and Bell's palsy (cranial nerve VII - facial), unlike trigeminal (cranial nerve V) neuralgia, does not cause much pain.
Nursing process step: Analysis/Nursing diagnosis

226. CORRECT ANSWER—C. *Rationales:* Sodium bicarbonate is used in severe salicylate toxicity to alkalinize the urine to a pH of 7.5 and to enhance excretion of salicylates. Calcium gluconate is the antidote for hydrofluoric acid. Folic acid is given in methanol poisoning, and magnesium is used in hydrofluoric acid exposure.
Nursing process step: Intervention

227. CORRECT ANSWER—C. *Rationales:* Ménière's disease causes vertigo, a ringing or roaring noise in the ears, hearing loss, nausea, and vomiting. Slow positional changes can help the patient control vertigo. Eyedrops are not useful, even if there is some blurred vision. Because of the symptoms, the patient may need help until the vertigo subsides; it would be in this patient's best interest to have assistance at home. Hearing loss may not be permanent and hearing may return. No ear pain is associated with Ménière's disease; thus, an ice pack or other analgesic alternative for pain is unnecessary.
Nursing process step: Evaluation

228. CORRECT ANSWER—**D.** *Rationales:* When a significant traumatic event has occurred, the nurse should check for signs of a basilar skull fracture or other serious injuries. A ruptured tympanic membrane that has sanguineous discharge should be checked for the presence of cerebrospinal fluid. When the ruptured tympanic membrane has been caused by a blast or other traumatic occurrence, antibiotics are not usually indicated. Irrigating the ear is contraindicated in ruptured tympanic membrane. Instead, gentle suctioning of any debris is recommended. Nothing should be instilled in the ear until other associated injuries have been ruled out and diagnosis is complete.
Nursing process step: Planning/Intervention

229. CORRECT ANSWER—**C.** *Rationales:* Swimmer's ear refers to a bacterial or fungal infection in the external ear. Symptoms usually include an ear that is tender to the touch, a swollen ear canal, cellulitis of the pinna and surrounding structure and, possibly, purulent drainage. A bulging tympanic membrane is a symptom of acute otitis media.
Nursing process step: Assessment

230. CORRECT ANSWER—**B.** *Rationales:* A decreased platelet count may be present if a blood dyscrasia is the cause of bleeding. After a bleeding episode, decreased hemoglobin may not be immediately apparent because of hemoconcentration. Hence, more time or serial hemoglobin determinations may be necessary to detect a fall in hemoglobin readings. Prothrombin times may be elevated in bleeding patients because of bleeding disorders or anticoagulant therapy. Creatinine is a test of kidney function.
Nursing process step: Assessment

231. CORRECT ANSWER—**B.** *Rationales:* Code #1 in the Code of Ethics for Emergency Nurses states that "the emergency nurse provides services with respect for human dignity and the uniqueness of the patient, unrestricted by considerations of social or economic status, personal attributes, or the nature of health problems." Personal beliefs cannot compel the behavior of an entire profession; emergency nurses may have many different personal or religious beliefs regarding human dignity. The development of clinical expertise should coincide with a deeper understanding of ethical behavior, but clinical expertise cannot guarantee ethical behavior. Ethics deals with values, actions, and choices of right and wrong. Laws are binding rules of conduct enforced by authority. In many situations, laws and ethics overlap. However, the ethical precept of treating other human beings with dignity and respect for their uniqueness cannot be mandated by law.

232. CORRECT ANSWER—**D.** *Rationales:* Injuries at multiple levels on the same extremity make it unlikely that reimplantation will be successful. Loss of several digits seriously compromises hand function so reimplantation should be considered. Reimplantation of the thumb should also be considered for these reasons: The thumb constitutes 40% to 50% of the functional value of the hand because of its role in opposition and grasp, and reimplantation of the thumb has a high success rate. Reimplantation is often successful in children because they regenerate transected nerves well and readily adapt to using a reimplanted part.
Nursing process step: Evaluation

233. CORRECT ANSWER—**C.** *Rationales:* The risk for infection is high in this patient; therefore, administration of antibiotics is a priority. If other severe injuries are present and they compromise respiratory function, immediate intubation or chest tube insertion may be necessary. Insertion of a nasogastric tube is contraindicated.
Nursing process step: Intervention

234. CORRECT ANSWER—**A.** *Rationales:* A zero-base budget requires examination and justification of all expenditures each year. Cost-benefit budgeting is not a budgeting type, but a budgeting tool that shows the relation between cost and benefit to help evaluate where resources are best spent. In fixed-ceiling budgeting, the chief executive officer sets the upper limit of a budget. Flexible budgeting is a method that addresses two levels of program activity or proposed expenditure.

235. CORRECT ANSWER—**A.** *Rationales:* Intussusception occurs in an infant when the proximal bowel invaginates into the distal bowel. The condition may lead to an infarction of the bowel. Hypertrophy of the pyloric musculature causes pyloric stenosis. Volvulus occurs when a section of intestine twists on its own axis.
Nursing process step: Assessment

236. CORRECT ANSWER—**C.** *Rationales:* A sprain is the tearing of ligaments that results in inflammation and ecchymotic discoloration. An abrasion is a partial-thickness scraping away of the skin. A contusion is a closed wound in which ruptured blood vessels have hemorrhaged into the surrounding tissue and are self-contained.
Nursing process step: Assessment

237. CORRECT ANSWER—**A.** *Rationales:* The use of accessory muscles indicates worsening respiratory function. The patient also has increased pain when moving. Increased pain leads to increased blood pressure and a tendency to breath shallowly. For these reasons, it is important to provide adequate pain medication to decrease the complications of immobility.
Nursing process step: Evaluation

238. CORRECT ANSWER—**C.** *Rationales:* In a pediatric patient, one of the hallmark signs of radial head dislocation is the patient's refusal to use the affected arm. Other symptoms include limited supination and pain. No deformity may be obvious with this injury. Dislocations of the knee are associated with instability of the ligaments and do not frequently occur. Dislocations of the patella commonly present with excessive swelling. In adults, elbow dislocations present with a loss of arm length.
Nursing process step: Assessment

239. CORRECT ANSWER—**A.** *Rationales:* The antigen-antibody reaction in anaphylactic shock induces the release of histamine, which causes massive vasodilation; a reduction in arterial pressure by dilating the arterioles; and an increase in vascular permeability, creating a rapid shift of fluids into the interstitial spaces. Myocardial contractility is decreased because of inadequate venous return, resulting in decreased preload.
Nursing process step: Assessment

240. CORRECT ANSWER—**C.** *Rationales:* A fat embolism occurs after a bone fracture or surgical manipulation of bone. A fat embolus is a small fat globule that has been displaced into the blood. The origin, although largely unknown, is believed to be either from the fracture site or from altered lipid solubility brought on by the stress of the traumatic event. The fat globules can occlude blood vessels in the brain, lungs, heart, and other organs. Symptoms include a recent fracture or bone surgery, dyspnea, sudden onset of substernal chest pain, hemoptysis, cough, crackles, altered mental status, fever, and petechiae to the buccal membranes, conjunctiva, chest, neck, shoulders, or axillary folds. Because these symptoms closely mimic other syndromes, such as pulmonary embolus and myocardial infarction, careful attention must be given to the circumstances surrounding the onset of symptoms and to the patient's medical history.
Nursing process step: Analysis

241. **CORRECT ANSWER—B.** *Rationales:* The intestines should be covered with gauze moistened with sterile saline or water. Pushing them back into the abdomen may damage them further. If the intestines are allowed to dry, they may be irreversibly damaged. The abdominal portion of the pneumatic antishock garment should not be inflated if viscera are protruding.
Nursing process step: Intervention

242. **CORRECT ANSWER—C.** *Rationales:* Blood loss of 1,500 to 4,500 ml can occur with pelvic fractures. A closed femur fracture can result in 1,000 to 2,000 ml of blood loss into the surrounding tissue. Blood loss of 500 to 1,000 ml can occur with fractures of the elbow, forearm, tibia, or ankle.
Nursing process step: Assessment

243. **CORRECT ANSWER—D.** *Rationales:* Copies of all hospital records should be sent with the patient who is being transferred, if possible. Failure to send records usually requires repeating the tests at the receiving facility. Repeating tests can be painful and time-consuming and is an unnecessary expense.
Nursing process step: Planning/Intervention

244. **CORRECT ANSWER—D.** *Rationales:* The earliest indicator of a change in neurologic status is the level of consciousness. A patient who exhibits altered mental status or decreased level of consciousness should be reevaluated by nurses and doctors. A change in the reaction or shape of pupils is a late indicator of a neurologic problem. Motor response appears as a delayed sign of neurologic status changes. Capillary refill is an indicator of circulatory status.
Nursing process step: Assessment

245. **CORRECT ANSWER—A.** *Rationales:* An ongoing blood loss of 100 to 200 ml/hour from a chest tube indicates a need for surgical repair. A transfusion reaction does not cause increased chest tube output. The most common transfusion reactions include hypotension, tachycardia, chest pain, dyspnea, nausea, vomiting, chills, flushing, hives, abdominal pain, flank pain, disseminated intravascular coagulation, fever, jaundice, increased serum bilirubin levels, hemoglobinuria, and decreased serum hemoglobin levels. If the patient is thought to have a massive hemothorax, a second chest tube may be inserted to manage the blood loss.
Nursing process step: Evaluation

246. **CORRECT ANSWER—D.** *Rationales:* The definitive therapy for a patient with pneumothorax is tube thoracotomy. The first concerns are always airway, breathing, and circulation. Administering supplemental oxygen should occur while equipment is gathered to insert the chest tube. The second intervention should be insertion of two I.V. lines with large-bore needles. The patient with pneumothorax has severe chest pain, so analgesics should be administered.
Nursing process step: Intervention

247. **CORRECT ANSWER—B.** *Rationales:* A urine specific gravity of 1.050 is elevated and indicates decreased renal perfusion. It can result in dehydration. The most appropriate intervention for this patient is a bolus of crystalloid at 40 ml/kg. If urine output is less than 30 ml/hour, adequate volume replacement has not been achieved. The patient in shock may need to have an indwelling urinary catheter inserted to monitor urine output. Furosemide 40 mg I.V. is not recommended in a patient who is already volume depleted.
Nursing process step: Intervention

248. CORRECT ANSWER—**C.** *Rationales:* When patients verbalize new information within the context of integrating that information into their lifestyles, retention and utilization of the information may have been achieved. Encouraging the patient to determine how the integration of knowledge will be achieved promotes positive thinking and consideration. Pretests and posttests measure knowledge, not integration. The content of questions a patient asks can be an indication of integration but is not evidence of it. If the patient is provided with information about incorporating the information into the patient's lifestyle, the patient has less control of the situation.
Nursing process step: Evaluation

249. CORRECT ANSWER—**A.** *Rationales:* The priority intervention is to maintain airway patency. This is accomplished by suctioning. Chest tube insertion and surgical intervention are necessary after initial stabilization of the patient. If the patient is intubated, the end of the endotracheal tube must be positioned distal to the injury. The patient should be monitored for possible pneumothorax.
Nursing process step: Intervention

250. CORRECT ANSWER—**B.** *Rationales:* Hepatitis is the most likely diagnosis. A patient with hepatitis may experience low-grade fever, malaise, joint pain, headache, dark urine and pruritus. The abdominal examination reveals an enlarged, tender liver. The patient may or may not be jaundiced. A patient with Lyme disease may have flulike symptoms — headache, fatigue, joint and muscle aches — as well as a bull's-eye-shaped rash. Signs and symptoms of diphtheria include fever, which may be high or low, headache, nausea, and sore throat. On physical exam, a gray-white membrane covers the larynx and pharynx. A patient with human immunodeficiency virus may exhibit fever, diarrhea, weight loss, night sweats, fatigue, and cough. He or she may also have symptoms associated with opportunistic infections.
Nursing process step: Analysis

APPENDICES

Appendix A: Critical Laboratory Values

Critical laboratory values represent severe pathophysiologic states that are life-threatening unless immediate corrective action is taken. The chart below lists critical limits as determined by a national survey of trauma and medical centers in the United States. The chart lists low and high critical limits, as well as the low and high ranges, for tests for clinical chemistry, blood gases and pH, and hematology; it also lists important qualitative results.

Critical values in clinical chemistry

Test	Units	Low	Range	High	Range
Bilirubin	µmol/liter	N/A	N/A	257	86 to 513
	mg/dl	N/A	N/A	15	5 to 30
Calcium	mmol/liter	1.65	1.25 to 2.15	3.22	2.62 to 3.49
	mg/dl	6.6	5.0 to 8.6	12.9	10.5 to 14.0
Calcium, free	mmol/liter	0.78	0.75 to 0.88	1.58	1.50 to 1.63
	mg/dl	3.13	3.01 to 3.53	6.33	6.01 to 6.53
Chloride	mmol/liter	75	60 to 90	126	115 to 156
CO$_2$ content	mmol/liter	11	5 to 20	40	35 to 50
Creatinine	µmol/liter	N/A	N/A	654	177 to 1,326
	mg/dl	N/A	N/A	7.4	2.0 to 15.0
Glucose	mmol/liter	2.6	1.7 to 3.9	26.9	6.1 to 55.5
	mg/dl	46	30 to 70	484	110 to 1,000
Glucose, CSF	mmol/liter	2.1	1.1 to 2.8	24.3	13.9 to 38.9
	mg/dl	37	20 to 50	438	250 to 700
Lactate dehydrogenase	mmol/liter	N/A	N/A	3.4	2.3 to 5.0
	mg/dl	N/A	N/A	30.6	20.7 to 45.0
Magnesium	mmol/liter	0.41	0.21 to 0.74	2.02	1.03 to 5.02
	mg/dl	1.0	0.5 to 1.8	4.9	2.5 to 12.2
Osmolality	mmol/kg	250	230 to 280	326	295 to 375
Phosphorus	mmol/liter	0.39	0.26 to 0.65	2.87	2.26 to 3.23
	mg/dl	1.2	0.8 to 2.0	8.9	7.0 to 10.0
Potassium	mmol/liter	2.8	2.5 to 3.6	6.2 8.0 (hemolyzed)	5.0 to 8.0
Sodium	mmol/liter	120	110 to 137	158	145 to 170
Urea nitrogen	mmol/liter	N/A	N/A	37.1	14.3 to 107.1
	mg/dl	N/A	N/A	104	40 to 300
Uric acid	µmol/liter	N/A	N/A	773	595 to 892
	mg/dl	N/A	N/A	13	10 to 15

Critical values in blood gases and pH

Test	Units	Low	Range	High	Range
P_{CO_2}	mm Hg	19	9 to 25	67	50 to 80
	kPa	2.5	1.2 to 3.3	8.9	6.7 to 10.7
pH		7.21	7.00 to 7.35	7.59	7.50 to 7.65
P_{O_2}	mm Hg	43	30 to 55	N/A	N/A
	kPa	5.7	4.0 to 7.3	N/A	N/A
P_{O_2}, newborn	mm Hg	37	30 to 50	92	70 to 100
	kPa	4.9	4.0 to 6.7	12.3	9.3 to 13.3

Critical values in hematology

Test	Units	Low	Range	High	Range
Fibrinogen	g/liter	0.88	0.5 to 1	7.75	5 to 10
Hematocrit		0.18	0.12 to 0.30	0.61	0.54 to 0.80
Hemoglobin	g/liter	66	40 to 120	199	170 to 300
Partial thromboplastin time	seconds	N/A	N/A	68	32 to 150
Platelets	$\times 10^9$/liter	37	10 to 100	910	555 to 1,000
Prothrombin time	seconds	N/A	N/A	27	14 to 40
White blood cell count	$\times 10^9$/liter	2.0	1.0 to 4.0	37	10.0 to 100.0

Critical qualitative findings

Hematology	• blasts on blood smear • new diagnosis or findings of leukemia • sickle cells (or aplastic crisis)
Microbiology and parasitology	• positive culture or Gram stain from blood, CSF, or body cavity fluid • positive antigen detection for *Cryptococcus,* group b streptococci, *Haemophilus influenzae* b, or *Neisseria meningitidis* • positive acid-fast bacillus or culture • *Salmonella, Shigella,* or *Campylobacter* on stool culture • malarial parasites
Microscopy and urinalysis	• elevated white blood cell count in CSF • malignant cells, blasts, or microorganisms in CSF or body fluids • positive results for glucose or ketones in urine • pathologic crystals on urinalysis
Blood blank and immunology	• incompatible crossmatch • positive test for syphilis

Source: Kost, G.J. "Critical Limits for Urgent Clinician Notification at U.S. Medical Centers," *JAMA* 263(5):704-707, February 2, 1990.

B: Common Life-Support Drugs

Drug	Indications and precautions
adenosine	*Paroxysmal supraventricular tachycardia (PSVT) involving atrioventricular (AV) node reentry* • May cause flushing, dyspnea, chest pain, transient periods of sinus bradycardia, and ventricular ectopy. • Short half-life (less than 5 seconds). • PSVT may recur. • Theophylline decreases effectiveness. • Dipyridamole potentiates effectiveness.
aminophylline	*Acute bronchial asthma, bronchospasm associated with chronic bronchitis and emphysema* • May cause palpitations, flushing, tachycardia or other arrhythmias, nervousness, irritability, headache, and hypotension.
atropine sulfate	*Bradycardia, asystole* • Lower dose (less than 0.5 mg) may cause bradycardia. • Higher dose (more than 3 mg) may cause full vagal blockage. • Contraindicated for glaucoma patients (use isoproterenol instead).
beta adrenergic blockers (atenolol, metoprolol tartrate, propranolol hydrochloride)	*Reduce ventricular irritability in patients after myocardial infarction (MI)* • Can cause bradycardia, AV conduction delays, hypotension. • Contraindicated in bradycardia, second- and third-degree block, hypotension, or bronchospastic lung disease.
bretylium tosylate (Bretylate, Bretylol)	*Life-threatening ventricular fibrillation and ventricular tachycardia* • Generally not used to treat premature ventricular contractions unless other drugs fail. • May increase digitalis toxicity. • May lower blood pressure.
diuretics (furosemide)	*Acute pulmonary edema, cerebral edema after cardiac arrest* • Venodilator effects occur within 5 minutes; can result in hypotension. • Diuresis occurs within 60 minutes.
dobutamine hydrochloride (Dobutrex)	*Acute congestive heart failure (CHF), cardiopulmonary bypass surgery* • Don't use with beta blockers, such as propranolol. • Patients with atrial fibrillation should receive digoxin first, or they can develop rapid ventricular response. • Drug is incompatible with alkaline solutions. • Infiltration may produce severe tissue damage.
dopamine hydrochloride (Intropin)	*Shock, decreased renal function* • Don't use for treating uncorrected tachyarrhythmias or ventricular fibrillation. • May precipitate arrhythmias. • Drug is incompatible with alkaline solutions. • Infiltration may produce severe tissue damage. • Solution deteriorates after 24 hours.
epinephrine hydrochloride (Adrenalin)	*Bronchospasm, anaphylaxis, severe allergic reactions, cardiac arrest, arrhythmias* • Increases intraocular pressure. • May exacerbate CHF, arrhythmias, angina pectoris, hyperthyroidism, and emphysema. • May cause headache, tremors, or palpitations. • Monitor patients for signs of cerebral hemorrhage.
isoproterenol hydrochloride (Isuprel)	*Bronchospasm, arrhythmias, cardiac arrest* • Don't administer with epinephrine. • Don't mix with barbiturates, sodium bicarbonate, any calcium preparation, or aminophylline.

Drug	Indications and precautions
lidocaine hydrochloride (Xylocaine)	*Ventricular arrhythmias* • Don't use if bradycardia is present or if patient has high-grade sinoatrial or AV block • Don't mix with sodium bicarbonate. • May lead to central nervous system toxicity. • Light-headedness and dizziness are common.
magnesium sulfate	*Hypomagnesemia, torsades de pointes* • Serum magnesium and potassium levels should be determined. • Can precipitate hypotension.
nitroglycerin	*Angina, CHF associated with MI* • Angina not relieved with three sublingual tablets requires EMS. • May cause tachycardia, paradoxical bradycardia, headache. • Administration for more than 24 hours may produce tolerance. • Hypovolemia decreases effectiveness and worsens hypotension.
nitroprusside sodium	*Hypertension, increased systemic vascular resistance* • Continuous blood pressure monitoring is required. • Deteriorates when exposed to light; wrap in opaque container. • May cause hypotension, headache, vomiting. • Cyanide toxicity may occur after 72 hours.
procainamide hydrochloride (Pronestyl)	*Arrhythmias, malignant hyperthermia* • Can cause precipitous hypotension; don't use for treating second- or third-degree heart block unless a pacemaker has been inserted. • Can cause AV block. • Discontinue if PR interval or QRS complex widens or if arrhythmias worsen.
sodium bicarbonate	*Metabolic acidosis, cardiac arrest* • Don't mix with epinephrine; causes epinephrine degradation. • Don't mix with calcium salts; forms insoluble precipitates.
thrombolytic agents (streptokinase, urokinase, t-PA)	*Thrombolysis of clots in acute MI and pulmonary embolus* • Should be initiated within 6 hours of onset of pain. • Contraindicated with a history of recent surgery or internal bleeding.
verapamil hydrochloride (Calan, Isoptin)	*Supraventricular tachyarrhythmias, angina, hypertension* • Contraindicated in patients with aortic stenosis, hypotension, cardiogenic shock, severe CHF, second- or third-degree AV block, or sick sinus syndrome. • High doses or too-rapid administration can cause a significant drop in blood pressure. • May increase serum digoxin levels.

Appendix C: NANDA Taxonomy

The taxonomy developed by the North American Nursing Diagnosis Association (NANDA) is the currently accepted classification system for nursing diagnoses. The list of approved nursing diagnoses is grouped into nine human response patterns. The complete taxonomy is listed below.

Pattern 1: Exchanging

1.1.2.1	Altered nutrition: More than body requirements
1.1.2.2	Altered nutrition: Less than body requirements
1.1.2.3	Altered nutrition: Potential for more than body requirements
1.2.1.1	Risk for infection
1.2.2.1	Risk for altered body temperature
1.2.2.2	Hypothermia
1.2.2.3	Hyperthermia
1.2.2.4	Ineffective thermoregulation
1.2.3.1	Dysreflexia
1.3.1.1	Constipation
1.3.1.1.1	Perceived constipation
1.3.1.1.2	Colonic constipation
1.3.1.2	Diarrhea
1.3.1.3	Bowel incontinence
1.3.2	Altered urinary elimination
1.3.2.1.1	Stress incontinence
1.3.2.1.2	Reflex incontinence
1.3.2.1.3	Urge incontinence
1.3.2.1.4	Functional incontinence
1.3.2.1.5	Total incontinence
1.3.2.2	Urinary retention
1.4.1.1	Altered tissue perfusion (specify renal, cerebral, cardiopulmonary, gastrointestinal, peripheral)
1.4.1.2.1	Fluid volume excess
1.4.1.2.2.1	Fluid volume deficit
1.4.1.2.2.2	Risk for fluid volume deficit
1.4.2.1	Decreased cardiac output
1.5.1.1	Impaired gas exchange
1.5.1.2	Ineffective airway clearance
1.5.1.3	Ineffective breathing pattern
1.5.1.3.1	Inability to sustain spontaneous ventilation
1.5.1.3.2	Dysfunctional ventilatory weaning response
1.6.1	Risk for injury
1.6.1.1	Risk for suffocation
1.6.1.2	Risk for poisoning
1.6.1.3	Risk for trauma
1.6.1.4	Risk for aspiration
1.6.1.5	Risk for disuse syndrome
1.6.2	Altered protection
1.6.2.1	Impaired tissue integrity
1.6.2.1.1	Altered oral mucous membrane
1.6.2.1.2.1	Impaired skin integrity
1.6.2.1.2.2	Risk for impaired skin integrity
1.7.1	Decreased adaptive capacity: Intracranial*
1.8	Energy field disturbance*

Pattern 2: Communicating

2.1.1.1	Impaired verbal communication

Pattern 3: Relating

3.1.1	Impaired social interaction
3.1.2	Social isolation
3.1.3	Risk for loneliness*
3.2.1	Altered role performance
3.2.1.1.1	Altered parenting
3.2.1.1.2	Risk for altered parenting
3.2.1.1.2.1	Risk for altered parent/infant/child attachment*
3.2.1.2.1	Sexual dysfunction
3.2.2	Altered family processes
3.2.2.1	Caregiver role strain
3.2.2.2	Risk for caregiver role strain
3.2.2.3.1	Altered family process: Alcoholism*
3.2.3.1	Parental role conflict
3.3	Altered sexuality patterns

Pattern 4: Valuing

4.1.1	Spiritual distress (distress of the human spirit)
4.2	Potential for enhanced spiritual well-being*

Pattern 5: Choosing

5.1.1.1	Ineffective individual coping
5.1.1.1.1	Impaired adjustment
5.1.1.1.2	Defensive coping
5.1.1.1.3	Ineffective denial
5.1.2.1.1	Ineffective family coping: Disabling
5.1.2.1.2	Ineffective family coping: Compromised
5.1.2.2	Family coping: Potential for growth

*Indicates 1 of the 19 diagnoses recently approved by NANDA.

5.1.3.1	Potential for enhanced community coping*
5.1.3.2	Ineffective community coping*
5.2.1	Ineffective management of therapeutic regimen: Individual
5.2.1.1	Noncompliance (specify)
5.2.2	Ineffective management of therapeutic regimen: Families*
5.2.3	Ineffective management of therapeutic regimen: Community*
5.2.4	Effective management of therapeutic regimen: Individual*
5.3.1.1	Decisional conflict (specify)
5.4	Health-seeking behaviors (specify)

Pattern 6: Moving

6.1.1.1	Impaired physical mobility
6.1.1.1.1	Risk for peripheral neurovascular dysfunction
6.1.1.1.2	Risk for perioperative positioning injury*
6.1.1.2	Activity intolerance
6.1.1.2.1	Fatigue
6.1.1.3	Risk for activity intolerance
6.2.1	Sleep pattern disturbance
6.3.1.1	Diversional activity deficit
6.4.1.1	Impaired home maintenance management
6.4.2	Altered health maintenance
6.5.1	Feeding self-care deficit
6.5.1.1	Impaired swallowing
6.5.1.2	Ineffective breast-feeding
6.5.1.2.1	Interrupted breast-feeding
6.5.1.3	Effective breast-feeding
6.5.1.4	Ineffective infant feeding pattern
6.5.2	Bathing or hygiene self-care deficit
6.5.3	Dressing or grooming self-care deficit
6.5.4	Toileting self-care deficit
6.6	Altered growth and development
6.7	Relocation stress syndrome
6.8.1	Risk for disorganized infant behavior*
6.8.2	Disorganized infant behavior*
6.8.3	Potential for enhanced organized infant behavior*

Pattern 7: Perceiving

7.1.1	Body image disturbance
7.1.2	Self-esteem disturbance
7.1.2.1	Chronic low self-esteem
7.1.2.2	Situational low self-esteem
7.1.3	Personal identity disturbance
7.2	Sensory or perceptual alterations (specify visual, auditory, kinesthetic, gustatory, tactile, or olfactory)
7.2.1.1	Unilateral neglect
7.3.1	Hopelessness
7.3.2	Powerlessness

Pattern 8: Knowing

8.1.1	Knowledge deficit (specify)
8.2.1	Impaired environmental interpretation syndrome*
8.2.2	Acute confusion*
8.2.3	Chronic confusion*
8.3	Altered thought processes
8.3.1	Impaired memory*

Pattern 9: Feeling

9.1.1	Pain
9.1.1.1	Chronic pain
9.2.1.1	Dysfunctional grieving
9.2.1.2	Anticipatory grieving
9.2.2	Risk for violence: Self-directed or directed at others
9.2.2.1	Risk for self-mutilation
9.2.3	Posttrauma response
9.2.3.1	Rape-trauma syndrome
9.2.3.1.1	Rape-trauma syndrome: Compound reaction
9.2.3.1.2	Rape-trauma syndrome: Silent reaction
9.3.1	Anxiety
9.3.2	Fear

*Indicates 1 of the 19 diagnoses recently approved by NANDA.

Appendix D: Triage Assessment Principles

Triage involves deciding which patients should be treated before others and where the treatment should take place. Triage may also involve basic first aid and preliminary care.

Making triage decisions

To make triage decisions effectively, you must gather and interpret both subjective and objective data rapidly and accurately. Follow this rule: "When in doubt, triage up." That is, if you're uncertain as to the seriousness of a patient's condition, treat it as more, rather than less, serious. Triage activity consists of:
• obtaining a focused history of the patient's chief complaint
• performing a limited physical examination
• classifying the patient's problem for urgency
• reassuring the patient that he'll receive definitive medical care as soon as possible.

Obtain a history

Focus on the patient's chief complaint. Record it in his own words, if possible. Have him qualify his complaint as precisely as he can, using the PQRST acronym (Provocative/Palliative, Quality/Quantity, Region/Radiation, Severity scale, Timing) or a similar device.
• Also record the patient's age, current medications and time of last dose, allergies, date of last tetanus toxoid inoculation, and any other medical history, such as height, weight, and last menstrual period.

Perform a physical examination

Observe general appearance and assess vital signs and level of consciousness (LOC).
• Take oral or axillary temperature as appropriate. Rectal temperature is the most accurate; take this as indicated and if you can ensure the patient's privacy.
• Check radial or apical pulse. Note rate, rhythm, and quality. While assessing pulse, check skin temperature and capillary refill time.
• Check blood pressure as quickly and accurately as possible.

• Note rate, depth, symmetry, and quality of respirations. Also note skin color and turgor, facial expression, accessory muscle use, and any audible breath sounds.
• Assess LOC using a scale such as the Glasgow Coma Scale, or make a notation that the patient is oriented to time, place, and person.

Classifying emergency conditions

These lists help you determine which conditions to treat first.
Emergent conditions: A patient with the following conditions will probably die or lose organ function without immediate medical attention. Start lifesaving measures and call the doctor immediately if you find:
• respiratory distress or arrest
• cardiac arrest
• severe chest pain with dyspnea or cyanosis
• seizures
• severe hemorrhage
• severe head injury
• coma
• poisoning or drug overdose
• open chest or abdominal wounds
• profound shock
• multiple injuries
• hyperpyrexia (temperature over 105° F [40.5° C])
• emergency childbirth or complications of pregnancy.
Urgent conditions: Although serious, the following conditions don't immediately threaten the patient's life or organ functions. You can delay treatment for 20 minutes to 2 hours, if necessary, if you find:
• chest pain not associated with respiratory symptoms
• back injury
• persistent nausea, vomiting, or diarrhea
• severe abdominal pain
• temperature of 102° to 105° F (38.8° to 40.5° C)
• panic
• bleeding from any orifice.

Appendix E: Coma Scales

To assess a patient's LOC quickly and to uncover baseline changes, use the Glasgow Coma Scale. To assess a child's LOC, use the Emergency Nurses Association's modified Glasgow Coma Scale or the Pediatric Coma Scale. In all three scales, assign points for the best responses; the higher the score, the more alert the patient.

Glasgow Coma Scale

FINDING	SCORE	FINDING	SCORE	FINDING	SCORE
Eye-opening response		**Motor Response**		**Verbal response**	
Opens spontaneously	4	Obeys verbal command	6	Oriented and converses	5
Opens to verbal command	3	Localizes painful stimuli	5	Disoriented and converses	4
Opens to pain	2	Flexion-withdrawal	4	Inappropriate words	3
No response	1	Flexion-abnormal (decorticate rigidity)	3	Incomprehensible words	2
		Extension (decerebrate rigidity)	2	No response	1
		No response	1		

Modified Glasgow Coma Scale

FINDING	SCORE	FINDING	SCORE	FINDING	SCORE
Eye-opening response		**Motor Response**		**Verbal response**	
Spontaneous	4	Normal spontaneous movements	6	Coos, babbles	5
To speech	3	Withdraws to touch	5	Irritable, cries	4
To pain	2	Withdraws to pain	4	Cries to pain	3
None	1	Abnormal flexion	3	Moans to pain	2
		Abnormal extension	2	None	1
		None	1		

Pediatric Coma Scale

<AGE 1 YEAR	>AGE 1 YEAR	SCORE
Eye-opening response		
Spontaneously	Spontaneously	4
To shout	To verbal command	3
To pain	To pain	2
No response	No response	1

Pediatric Coma Scale *(continued)*		
<AGE 1 YEAR	**>AGE 1 YEAR**	**SCORE**
Motor response		
Spontaneous	Obeys	6
Localizes pain	Localizes pain	5
Flexion-withdrawal	Flexion-withdrawal	4
Flexion-withdrawal (decorticate rigidity)	Flexion-withdrawal (decorticate rigidity)	3
Extension (decerebrate rigidity)	Extension (decerebrate rigidity)	2
No response	No response	1

AGES 0 TO 2 YEARS	AGES 2 TO 5 YEARS	AGE 5 YEARS	SCORE
Verbal response			
Smiles; coos appropriately	Appropriate words or phrases	Oriented and converses	5
Cries; consolable	Inappropriate words	Disoriented and converses	4
Persistent inappropriate crying and screaming	Persistent cries and screams	Inappropriate words	3
Grunts; agitated; restless	Grunts	Incomprehensible sounds	2
No response	No response	No response	1

Appendix F: Laboratory Values in Toxicology

Blood or urine tests (sometimes gastric contents or lavage fluid) reveal the type and amount of substances taken in overdoses. Specific toxic levels vary with the institution and technique used. Consult standard references for therapeutic levels.

Alcohol
- (Ethanol); serum
- Toxic level: variable; if blood alcohol level is between 0.05% and 0.1% weight/volume (50 to 100 mg/dl), a person is legally intoxicated; lethal level, 350 to 500 mg/dl

Amitriptyline (and metabolite nortriptylline)
- (Elavil); serum or plasma
- Toxic level: 1,000 ng/ml

Amphetamines
- (Amphetamine); urine
- Toxic level: 30 g/ml

Barbiturates and Hypnotics
- Amobarbital (Amytal); serum
- Toxic level: 50 g/ml

Desipramine
- (Norpramin); serum or plasma
- Toxic level: 1,000 ng/ml

Dextroamphetamine
- (Dexedrine); urine
- Toxic level: 15 g/ml

Doxepin (and metabolite desmethyldoxepin)
- (Adapin, Sinequan); serum or plasma
- Toxic level: 1,000 ng/ml

Glutethimide
- (Doriden); serum
- Toxic level: 10 g/ml

Imipramine (and metabolite desipramine)
- (Tofranil); serum or plasma
- Toxic level: 1,000 ng/ml

Isopropanol
- (Isopropyl alcohol, rubbing alcohol); serum
- Toxic level: 150 mg/dl

Lithium
- (Lithobid); serum or plasma
- Toxic level: 1.5 mEq/L

Methamphetamine
- (Desoxyn); urine
- Toxic level: 40 g/ml

Methanol
- (Antifreeze); serum
- Toxic level: variable; lethal dose, 30 ml of 100% methanol

Nonnarcotic analgesics
- Acetaminophen (Tylenol, Datril); serum
- Toxic level: after 4 hours, 120 g/ml; after 8 hours, 60 g/ml

Pentobarbital
- (Nembutal); serum
- Toxic level: 10 g/ml

Phenmetrazine
- (Preludin); urine
- Toxic level: 50 g/ml

Phenobarbital
- (Luminal); serum
- Toxic level: 60 g/ml

Phenothiazines
- Chlorpromazine (Thorazine); serum
- Toxic level: 1.0 g/ml

Prochlorperazine
- (Compazine); serum
- Toxic level: 1.0 g/ml

Salicylates
- (Aspirin); serum
- Toxic level: 40 mg/100 ml

Secobarbital
- (Seconal); serum
- Toxic level: 15 g/ml

Thioridazine
- (Mellaril); serum
- Toxic level: 10 g/ml

Trifluoperazine
- (Stelazine); serum
- Toxic level: 1.0 g/ml

Hemoglobin derivatives
Carboxyhemoglobin
- Toxic level: for acute carbon monoxide toxicity, 20% to 30% of total hemoglobin

Methemoglobin
- Toxic level: for specific drug toxicity, 10% to 70% of total hemoglobin

Sulfhemoglobin
- Toxic level: for specific drug toxicity, 10 g/dl (produces cyanosis but few or no toxic symptoms)

Appendix G: Emergency Antidotes

The number of poisons for which a specific antidote is necessary or available is small. When a specific antidote can be used, it must be administered as early as possible in a monitored dose. Observe these guidelines to stop or reverse the effects of the following substances.

Acetaminophen
• Give N-acetylcysteine in an initial dose of 140 mg/kg P.O.
• Most effective within 16 hours; prevents liver damage.

Atropine
Give physostigmine in an initial dose of 0.5 to 2 mg I.V.; can be given I.M. or S.C., but slow I.V. injection is preferred; may repeat every 20 minutes until atropine poisoning is reversed or adverse physostigmine reaction occurs.

Carbon monoxide
Give oxygen.

Cyanide
• Give amyl nitrite. Have the patient inhale the contents of a crushed ampule of the drug for 30 seconds and then breathe oxygen for 30 seconds.
• Next, infuse sodium nitrite I.V. For adults, give 10 L of 3% solution (300 mg) over 3 minutes I.V. (2.5 ml/minute); for children, initially give 0.2 mL (10 mg of 3% solution)/kg.
• Then give sodium thiosulfate. For adults, give 25% solution — 50 ml I.V. over 10 minutes; for children, give 1.65 ml/kg I.V. over 10 minutes.

Iron
Give deferoxamine in an initial dose of 1 g I.V. or I.M., then 500 mg in 4 to 12 hours and a second 500-mg dose in another 4 to 12 hours, depending on clinical response.

Lead
Give edetate calcium disodium in a dose of 1.5 g/m^2 daily by deep I.M. or by continuous I.V. infusion; give with dimercaprol in a dose of 4 mg/kg I.M. In children, give dimercaptosuccinic acid (DMSA), also called succimer, in a dose of 10 mg/kg P.O. every 8 hours for 5 days.

Mercury (arsenic, gold)
• Give dimercaprol in a dose of 4 mg/kg I.M. as soon as possible
• Alternatively, give 2,3-dimercaptosuccinic acid (oral, water-soluble preparation of dimercaprol) in a dose of 10 mg/kg P.O. every 8 hours for 5 days.

Methyl alcohol (ethylene glycol)
• Give ethyl alcohol in conjunction with dialysis in a dose of 1.5 ml/kg of 50% ethyl alcohol diluted to 5% solution P.O., then 0.5 to 1 ml/kg P.O. or I.V. every 2 hours for 4 days.
• Maintain blood ethyl alcohol level of 1 to 1.5 mg/ml.

Cyanide- or drug-induced methemoglobinemia
Give methylene blue in a dose of 0.2 ml/kg of 1% solution I.V. over 5 minutes.

Opiates
Give naloxone. For adults, give 0.4 to 2 mg I.V., and repeat 3 times every 2 to 3 minutes if needed; for children, give 0.01 mg/kg I.V.

Organophosphates
• Give atropine in conjunction with pralidoxime.
• Atropine: For adults, initially give 1 to 2 mg I.V.; repeat every 5 to 60 minutes (if severe, you can give 2 to 5 mg I.V.). For children, give 0.05 mg/kg. In critical adult patients, up to 5 mg I.V. every 15 minutes may be necessary.
• Pralidoxime: For adults, initially give 1 g I.V. over 5 minutes; infusion over 15 to 30 minutes (1 g/100 ml of normal saline solution) is preferred; for children, give 20 to 40 mg/kg I.V.

Benzodiazepines
• Give flumazenil in an initial dose of 0.2 mg undiluted with I.V. running; then 0.3 mg after 1 minute if needed; then 0.5 mg repeated at 1-minute intervals.
• Each dose is given over 30 seconds. The total cumulative dose is 3 mg.

Phenothiazine
Give diphenhydramine in a dose of 1 to 2 mg/kg, slow I.V. push, undiluted.

Selected References

Baer, C., and Williams, B. *Clinical Pharmacology and Nursing*, 3rd ed. Springhouse, Pa.: Springhouse Corp., 1996.

Barkin, R., and Rosen, P. *Emergency Pediatrics: A Guide to Ambulatory Care*. Philadelphia: W.B. Saunders Co., 1994.

Bartlett, J.G. *Pocketbook of Infectious Disease Therapy*. Baltimore: Williams & Wilkins Co., 1994.

Bayley, E., and Turcke, S. *A Comprehensive Curriculum for Trauma Nursing*. Boston: Jones & Bartlett Pubs., Inc., 1992.

Budassi, S. S. *Emergency Nursing Principles and Practice*. St. Louis: Mosby–Year Book, Inc., 1992.

Cardona, V.D., et al. *Trauma Nursing from Resuscitation Through Rehabilitation*, 2nd ed. Philadelphia: W.B. Saunders Co., 1994.

Clochesy, J.M., et al. *Critical Care Nursing*, 2nd ed. Philadelphia: W.B. Saunders Co., 1996.

Critical Care and Emergency Nursing, 2nd ed. Springhouse, Pa.: Springhouse Corporation, 1994.

Critical Care Skills: A Nurse's PhotoGuide. Springhouse, Pa.: Springhouse Corporation, 1996.

Crosby, L., et al. *Emergency Care and Transportation of the Sick and Injured*. Rosemont, Ill.: American Academy of Orthopedic Surgeons, 1995.

Cummins, R.O. *Textbook of Advanced Cardiac Life Support*. American Heart Association, 1994.

Daily, E.K., and Schroeder, J.S. *Techniques in Bedside Hemodynamic Monitoring*, 5th ed. St. Louis: Mosby–Year Book, Inc., 1994.

EmergiCare Cards, 2nd ed. Springhouse, Pa.: Springhouse Corporation, 1996.

Fontaine, K.L., and Fletcher, J.S. *Essentials of Mental Health Nursing*, 3rd ed. Redwood City, Calif.: Addison-Wesley, 1995.

Hammer, J. "Challenging Diagnosis: Adult Respiratory Distress Syndrome," *Critical Care Nurse* 15(5): 46-51, 1995.

Handbook of Critical Care Nursing. Springhouse, Pa.: Springhouse Corporation, 1996.

Handysides, G. *Triage in Emergency Practice*. St. Louis: Mosby–Year Book, Inc., 1996.

Hickey, J. *The Clinical Practice of Neurological and Neurosurgical Nursing*, 3rd ed. Philadelphia: J.B. Lippincott Co., 1992.

Ho, M. *Current Emergency Diagnosis and Treatment*, 5th ed. East Norwalk, Conn.: Appleton and Lange, 1996.

Hudak, C.M., and Gallo, B.M. *Critical Care Nursing: A Holistic Approach*, 6th ed. Philadelphia: J.B. Lippincott Co., 1994.

Jacobs, D.S., et al. *Laboratory Test Handbook*, 3rd ed. Baltimore: Williams & Wilkins, 1994.

Kim, M.J., et al. *Pocket Guide to Nursing Diagnosis*, 6th ed. St. Louis: Mosby–Year Book, Inc., 1995.

Kinney, M., et al. *AACN's Clinical Reference for Critical-Care Nursing*, 3rd ed. St. Louis: Mosby–Year Book, Inc., 1993.

Klein, A.R., et al. *Emergency Nursing Core Curriculum*, 4th ed. Philadelphia: W.B. Saunders Co., 1994.

Lee, G. *Flight Nursing: Principles and Practice*. St. Louis: Mosby–Year Book, Inc., 1991.

Lynch, V.A. "Clinical Forensic Nursing: A New Perspective in the Management of Crime Victims from Trauma to Trial," *Clinics of North America* 7(3): 489-507, 1995.

Manual of Critical Care Procedures. Springhouse, Pa.: Springhouse Corporation, 1994.

Maull, K.I., et al. *Advances in Trauma*, vol. 11. St. Louis: Mosby–Year Book, Inc., 1996.

Meyer, M.U., et al. "Health Professional's Role in Disaster Planning: A Strategic Management Approach," *AAOHN Journal* 43(5): 251-62, 1995.

Neff, J.A., and Kidd, P.S. *Trauma Nursing: The Art and Science*. St. Louis: Mosby–Year Book, Inc., 1993.

Polit, D., and Hungler, B. *Nursing Research: Methods, Appraisal, and Utilization*, 5th ed. Philadelphia: J.B. Lippincott Co., 1995.

Proehl, J. *Adult Emergency Nursing Procedures*. Boston: Jones and Bartlett Pubs., Inc., 1993.

Reisdorff, E.J., et al. *Pediatric Emergency Medicine*. Philadelphia: W.B. Saunders Co., 1993.

Swearingen, P.J., and Keen, J.H. *Manual of Critical Care*, 3rd ed. St. Louis: Mosby–Year Book, Inc., 1995.

Tappen, R. *Nursing Leadership and Management: Concepts and Practice*, 3rd ed. Philadelphia: F.A. Davis, 1995.

Thelan, L.A., et al. *Critical Care Nursing: Diagnosis and Management*, 2nd ed. St. Louis: Mosby–Year Book, Inc., 1994.

Trauma Nursing Core Course Providers Manual, 4th ed. Emergency Nurses Association, 1995.

Urban, N., et al. *Guidelines for Critical Care Nursing*. St. Louis: Mosby–Year Book, Inc., 1995.

Williams, S.W. *Essentials of Nutrition and Diet Therapy*, 6th ed. St. Louis: Mosby–Year Book Inc., 1994.

Yameen, J.M. "Management Skills...EMS Management," *Emergency* 25(9): 56-57, 1993.

Index

A

Abdomen, assessing, 5, 7
Abdominal aneurysm, assessment findings in, 323
Abdominal emergencies, 2-12
Abdominal injury
  assessing, in children, 3
  signs of, 6
Abdominal pain
  assessing, 2, 5
  interventions for, 2
Abdominal trauma, interventions for, 281, 315. *See also* Blunt abdominal trauma *and* Penetrating abdominal trauma.
Abrasion, 236, 335
Abruptio placentae, 104
  symptoms of, 318
Absence seizures, 96. *See also* Seizure.
Acetaminophen overdose
  antidote for, 97, 217
  blood levels in, 225
  effects of, 222
  treatment for, 97
Acetylcysteine as antidote for acetaminophen overdose, 97, 217
Achalasia, 65
Acid burns, 44. *See also* Burn injury.
Acquired immunodeficiency syndrome, symptoms of, 59
Activated charcoal, 151
Acute respiratory distress syndrome
  laboratory findings in, 169
  nursing diagnoses for, 170
  patient positioning to improve oxygenation in, 178
  treatment goals for, 176
Acyclovir, 76, 77, 305
Addison's disease, symptoms of, 62
Adenosine, 152, 304, 331
  administration guidelines for, 156
Adolescents, developmental approach for, 155
Adrenal crisis, symptoms of, 321
Advanced directive, 315
Aerophagia in pediatric patient, 155
Affective learning, 252, 254, 315
Afterload, 24
AIDS. *See* Acquired immunodeficiency syndrome.

Air embolism
  patient positioning for, 40
  symptoms of, 332
Airway clearing as priority of care, 319
Airway management, corrosive esophagitis and, 10
Airway obstruction, epiglottitis and, 48
Alcohol intoxication, oxygen delivery in patient with, 316
Alcoholism, thiamine deficiency and, 65
Alcohol withdrawal syndrome
  nursing diagnoses for, 216
  symptoms of, 216
Alkali burns, 44. *See also* Burn injury.
Alkali poisoning
  complications of, 224
  management of, 224
  symptoms of, 224
Allen's test, 276, 308
  purpose of, 92
Allergic conjunctivitis, characteristics of, 110
Allergic reaction. *See also* Anaphylactic shock.
  interventions for, 58
  nursing diagnoses for, 209
Allergic shiners, 313
Alpha-adrenergic receptor stimulation, effects of, 192
Alzheimer's disease, characteristics of, 93
Amitriptyline, 142
Amphetamine abuse, assessment findings in, 218, 318
Amputation. *See* Traumatic amputation.
Amyotrophic lateral sclerosis, 93
Anaphylactic reaction. *See also* Anaphylactic shock.
  discharge instructions for, 238
  evaluating effectiveness of treatment for, 289, 327
  interventions for, 58, 238
  nursing diagnoses for, 209
  pharmacologic management of, 313
Anaphylactic shock, 191, 206
  initial interventions for, 206
  pharmacologic treatment of, 211
Anencephalics as organ donors, 157

Angina
  characteristics of, 28
  nursing diagnoses for, 25, 28, 330
Animal bite, pharmacologic interventions for, 228
Ankle dislocation, 124
Ankle injury
  assessment findings in, 292
  interventions for, 331
Ankle strain, nursing diagnoses for, 118
Anoxia, appearance of pupils in, 314
Anterior wall damage, ECG changes in, 20, 312
Antibiotic therapy, preoperative administration of, 312
Anticholinergic crisis, treatment for, 164
Anticholinesterase toxicity, antidote for, 91
Anticoagulant therapy, cerebrovascular accident and, 97
Antidotes, 351
Antigen-antibody reaction. *See also* Anaphylactic shock.
  histamine release and, 335
  nursing diagnoses for, 209
Antihypertensive overdose, symptoms of, 21
Antipyretics, pediatric dose recommendations for, 68
Anxiety
  acute, initial interventions for, 137
  assessment findings in, 312
Aortic aneurysm, nursing diagnosis for, 28
Aortic dissection, assessment findings in, 329
Aortic injury
  emergency intervention for, 17
  mechanisms of, 19
Aortic rupture, assessment findings in, 177, 307
Apgar score, parameters for, 108
Apical wall damage, ECG changes in, 312
Apneustic breathing, 64, 312
Apraxia, 97
Arachnoid mater, 99
Arsenic poisoning, interventions for, 220